ASSESSMENT OF TOXIC AGENTS AT THE WORKPLACE
Roles of Ambient and Biological Monitoring

National Institute for Occupational Safety and Health, Rockville, MD, USA
Occupational Safety and Health Administration, Washington, DC, USA
Commission of the European Communities, Health and Safety Directorate, Luxembourg

Assessment of Toxic Agents at the Workplace

Roles of Ambient and Biological Monitoring

edited by

A. BERLIN, R. E. YODAIKEN and **B. A. HENMAN**

1984 **MARTINUS NIJHOFF PUBLISHERS**
a member of the KLUWER ACADEMIC PUBLISHERS GROUP
BOSTON / THE HAGUE / DORDRECHT / LANCASTER
for
THE COMMISSION OF THE EUROPEAN COMMUNITIES

Distributors

for the United States and Canada: Kluwer Boston, Inc., 190 Old Derby Street, Hingham, MA 02043, USA
for all other countries: Kluwer Academic Publishers Group, Distribution Center, P.O.Box 322, 3300 AH Dordrecht, The Netherlands

Library of Congress Cataloging in Publication Data

Main entry under title:

Assessment of toxic agents at the workplace.

  Papers of an international seminar held in Luxembourg,
Dec. 8-12, 1980, and organized jointly by the Commission
of the European Communities and the United States
authorities--the Occupational Safety and Health Administration and the National Institute for Occupational
Safety and Health.
  Includes index.
  1. Industrial toxicology--Congresses. 2. Environmental
monitoring--Congresses. 3. Patient monitoring--Con-
gresses. I. Berlin, A. II. Yodaiken, R. E.

III. Henman, B. A. IV. Commission of the European Com-
munities. V. United States. Occupational Safety and
Health Administration. VI. National Institute for
Occupational Safety and Health.
RA1229.A88 1984   615.9'02   83-19423
ISBN-13:978-94-009-6764-9   e-ISBN-13:978-94-009-6762-5
DOI: 10.1007/978-94-009-6762-5

ISBN-13:978-94-009-6764-9 (this volume)
EUR 8083 EN

Book information

This volume is based on material presented at a seminar held in Luxembourg on December 8–12, 1980. The views expressed are not necessarily those of the institutions organising the seminar (Commission of the European Communities, Occupational Safety and Health Administration, USA and National Institute for Occupational Safety and Health, USA).

Publication arranged by: Commission of the European Communities, Directorate-General Information Market and Innovation, Luxembourg

Copyright/legal notice

Table of Contents

*   *   *

EDITORIAL NOTE

The papers in this report have in the main been the subject of minor editing in order to achieve consistency. The discussions required substantial editing to eliminate undue repetition; every attempt was made to adhere to the content and meaning of each contributor. Whenever possible, the English spelling and words are used. The summary report gives an overview of the proceedings.

The editors would like to acknowledge the support given by the chairmen during and after the conference.

CHAIRMEN: M.S. Baram (USA), J. Degimbe (CEC), S. Epstein (USA), F. Pocchiari (I), P. Recht (B), J.T. Wilson (USA).

RAPPORTEURS: N. Ashford (USA), C. Courtoux (F), L. De Boer (NL), J. Froines (US-NIOSH), R. Harris (USA), W. Hunter (CEC), G. Kliesch (FRG), G. Lehnert (FRG), G. Matanoski (USA), P. Recht (B), K. Robock (FRG), K.H. Schaller (FRG), A. Schuster (L), W. Sunderman (USA), A.M. Thiess (FRG), M. Weber (USA).

The editors also appreciate the invaluable assistance given by D. Logan both in the scientific planning and during the conference. Thanks are also due to A. Bonini for his technical assistance.

ASSESSMENT OF TOXIC AGENTS AT THE WORKPLACE - ROLES OF
AMBIENT AND BIOLOGICAL MONITORING

SUMMARY REPORT - A Berlin, R E Yodaiken and D C Logan

Reprinted by permission of International
Archives of Occupational and Environmental
Health. Springer-Verlag.

1. <u>INTRODUCTION</u>

1.1 Organisation and aims

This International Seminar, organised jointly by the Commission of the European Communities and the United States authorities (Occupational Safety and Health Administration and the National Institute for Occupational Safety and Health) has brought together more than 150 participants from the Member States of the European Community, from the United States, and also from Greece, Finland, Sweden and Switzerland.

The aim of the Seminar was to examine the roles of ambient and biological monitoring in protecting the health of workers exposed to toxic agents and to define a multidisciplinary approach to this monitoring.

To achieve this aim expertise from the following disciplines, directly or indirectly involved with monitoring, was called upon: medicine, industrial hygiene, nursing, biology, engineering, chemistry, epidemiology, statistics, economics and jurisprudence, and representatives from trade unions, industry and government agencies.

The difference in concepts that each of these disciplines has of monitoring and of its role in the team is fully reflected in the papers.

1.2 Current trends in occupational health and hygiene (as related to monitoring).

The primary purpose of occupational health monitoring is to help achieve a satisfactory working environment and, secondly, to demonstrate that achievement. The increased awareness of occupational health, hygiene and safety in recent years had led, both in the European Community and in the United States, to improvement in working conditions and reduction of

worker exposure to some toxic agents. However, substantial
hazards remain, the number of cases of occupational illness
due to these hazardous exposures is still high, and new cases
will continue to occur if there are no improvements. During
the past years investigations have revealed a number of
examples of unreported occupational diseases. New problems
have appeared with changes related to energy development,
biotechnology, electronics, chemicals and so forth.

There is an increasing tendency to develop essentially
ambient, but also biological limits and to develop methods of
ensuring their implementation, thereby preventing health
damage from exposure to toxic chemicals. The introduction of
both ambient and biological standards in the United States
and in the European Community, and the recognition of the
need for such standards by ILO, is an irreversible fact.
This has forced all those concerned to pay more attention to
the significance of these limits, to their application and to
the problem of achieving a common terminology at the international level.

Aspects of monitoring include providing information to help
achieve compliance with standards, validating that compliance
and accumulating information for later review of the standards.

An appreciation that setting standards requires consultation
between the social partners and must take into account socio-
economic and political factors is growing. At the same time
workers and their representatives (including health and
safety professionals) as well as management are increasingly
involved with monitoring the application of standards. More
access is being gained to ambient and biological monitoring
records and therefore it is appropriate for the social
partners to become conversant with monitoring techniques. At
present there are few provisions for epidemiological follow
up to test the adequacy of existing standards and it is
becoming clear that new strategies must place more emphasis
on toxicological and pharmacokinetic parameters.

Authorities are fully aware that an appropriate combination of ambient and biological monitoring will lead to better protection of workers' health but some uneasiness and some uncertainty still exists on how best to achieve the maximum protection.

Workers are frequently not aware of the hazards associated with substances to which they are exposed, nor of the methods for preventing exposure. Occupational safety and health programmes must therefore ensure that workers are provided with assistance and information about all known or suspected hazards. National health and safety programmes increasingly place emphasis on training and education programmes for employers and workers.

2. DEFINITIONS

The following definitions were developed within the context of the seminar:

Monitoring is a systematic continuous or repetitive health-related activity designed to lead if necessary to corrective actions. Three types of monitoring are defined: ambient, biological and health surveillance.

Ambient monitoring is the measurement and assessment of agents at the workplace and evaluates ambient exposure and health risk compared to an appropriate reference.

Biological monitoring is the measurement and assessment of workplace agents or their metabolites either in tissues, secreta, excreta, expired air or any combination of these to evaluate exposure and health risk compared to an appropriate reference.

Health surveillance is the periodic medico-physiological examinations of exposed workers with the objective of protecting health and preventing occupationally related

disease. The detection of established disease is outside the scope of this definition.

The definitions of biological monitoring and health
surveillance separate components of a continuum which can
range from the measurement of agents in the body through
measurements of metabolites, to signs of early disease. A
problem left unresolved concerns the precise place within
these definitions of certain biochemical tests such as zinc
protoporphyrin (ZPP), delta aminolaevulinic acid dehydrase
(ALA-D), delta aminolaevulnic acid (ALA) in the blood and
urine, etc... which are in fact indicators of metabolic
effects which have occurred as a consequence of exposure.

3.   ROLES OF MONITORING AND PROTECTING WORKER HEALTH

3.1 Ambient monitoring

Ambient monitoring is carried out for different reasons, for
example:

   determining ambient concentrations in relation to an
   established legal standard or consensus guideline,

   determining the relationship, if any, between the
   concentrations of agents at the workplace and the health
   of the workers,

   ensuring the effectiveness of control measures,

   evaluating the need for controls in the vicinity of
   specific emission sources,

   indicating trends in relation to an improvement or
   deterioration at the workplace,

   providing an historical record.

It was generally accepted by the participants that personal
sampling is a better measure of employee exposure than area
sampling. For example, samples of air from the breathing
zone of the worker give a more reliable estimate of the
workers's exposure. It is necessary to utilise a statistical
framework to ensure that the sampling scheme is valid; it
should also be borne in mind that the cost of individual
samples is relatively high.

Considering the many agents which should, and often have to
be, monitored, few effective personal monitoring devices are
available and it is important to recognise that personal
dosimetry is in its infancy. Recognition of potential errors
is essential both for compliance with laws and regulations,
and for quantitation of dose and dose effect in epidemiological studies.

3.2 Biological monitoring

Biological monitoring measures or evaluates exposure from all
routes. It sometimes allows a better evaluation of health
risk than ambient monitoring especially in cases where
exposure through different routes has to be considered.

Biological monitoring takes into account individual variability, the impact of factors such as personal activity, biological characteristics and life styles of the individual. When
applicable, it is a valuable adjunct to ambient monitoring,
health surveillance and other medical data. One serious
drawback at present is that is is only available for a
limited number of agents.

3.3 Examples of workplace hazards

Two inorganic toxic agents, one organic agent and a class of
organic toxic agents were selected for discussion. The criteria for selection were that the agents be of considerable
concern and provide a wide variety of problems in monitoring.

3.3.1   Carbon monoxide

Monitoring of ambient exposures is difficult due to their episodic and non-predictable nature. Ambient monitoring methods using continuous CO analysers are often inadequate; this can be improved to some extent by using currently available personal samplers or portable analysers. A better assessment of personal exposure could be obtained with the development of chemical badges.

The results from all instruments which measure CO in air are only of value if the need for making them is clearly specified. At present evaluating exposures to CO in air by measuring carboxyhaemoglobin (COHb) content of the blood is limited by the extent to which the subject has acquired CO from other sources (smoking, endogenous CO production by xenobiotic metabolism) and by the effect of physical activity on uptake or expiration of CO.

The ease with which an agent or its metabolite can be determined in a tissue, organ or biological medium depends upon several factors, such as the physico-chemical characteristics of the compound, its toxico-kinetic propeties including its half life, and the target tissue or organ. Since carbon monoxide is a gas, and a target tissue is blood, it seems evident that biological monitoring for carbon monoxide is most valuable in the alveolar air and blood.

Because it is a non-invasive method, determination of CO in alveolar gas as a measure of percent COHb has great advantages, but the method has its limitations. The most precise indicator of CO exposure and of its poten-tial medical significance is direct measurement of COHb. At present gas chromatography is the reference procedure for analysis of CO in blood. The most convenient and simple methods are spectrophotometric techniques, although they may not be highly accurate at COHb concentrations below 5%.

3.3.2   Cadmium

Preventing acute toxic effects on the lungs can only be accomplished by keeping the airborne concentration of cadmium below a certain level. Ambient monitoring techniques including the use of continuous analyses are available for this purpose. Ambient monitoring may not be sufficient to prevent undue long term absorption of cadmium. Renal dysfunction is the earliest chronic effect believed to occur when Cd concentrations exceed 200 μg/g cortical tissue.

Oral intake of cadmium, personal hygiene habits, great individual variation in the oral absorption rate and non-occupational exposure may significantly affect the cadmium body burden. For estimating the body burden of cadmium and hence the risk of health impairment, biological indicators such as cadmium in blood and in urine may be used. By combining the determination of CdU with CdB, not only recent exposure, but also the cumulative internal dose is taken into consideration. The relationship between cadmium toxicity, renal damage and hypertension clearly needs to be studied further. Atomic absorption spectrophotometry and anodic stripping voltametry are now the preferred methods for determination of Cd in biological material.

3.3.3   Benzene

Benzene is a potent haematotoxin capable of causing aplastic anaemia and acute myeloblastic leukaemia. Considerable attention was devoted to biological monitoring and health surveillance rather than ambient monitoring.

Several methods are currently being developed for the biological monitoring of benzene: benzene in expired air and blood, and urinary output of phenol. The assessment of benzene exposure through measurement in expired air must take into account the complex elimination kinetics.

Headspace chromatography provides a simple and reliable method for the determination of benzene in blood. The measurement of phenol in urine is relatively non-specific and insensitive for the individual assessment of exposure to low levels of benzene in air.

Health surveillance of workers potentially exposed to benzene is currently based on evidence of bone marrow toxicity as well as routine blood examinations.

3.3.4   Aromatic Amines

Aromatic amines includes a large number of substances with widely differing toxicological properties. For the purpose of prevention in the working environment it is appropriate either to restrict the definition of aromatic amines to a homogenous group of compounds or, from a more practical point of view, to draw up a list of specific amines on which attention should be focused.

For many of these lipotropic substances, the skin is the main intake pathway, and therefore ambient air monitoring alone is not sufficient. In view of the carcinogenic effects of many aromatic amines, very sensitive methods of detection are being developed. Indicators of body burden currently used are non-specific total urinary amino-compounds and tests for specific aromatic amines in the urine such as benzidine or its metabolites for which the bladder is a primary target organ.

Primary aromatic amines can be determined by spectrophotometry. More specific methods recently applied
employ gas-liquid chromatography, high pressure liquid
chromatography and spectrophotofluorimetry.

3.2 Quality of monitoring data

The importance of ensuring the quality of data as an integral
part of any monitoring programme was unanimously stressed.
However, it was recognised that the amount of emphasis to be
placed on standardisation, good laboratory practice and
quality control depends on the objectives of the monitoring
programme.

The concept of good monitoring practice (GMP) should be
firmly established, based on good laboratory practice guidelines currently developed at the international level for the
purpose of improving the quality of toxicological data and
achieving mutual acceptance of those data. Such GMP should
help ensure that self-generated monitoring data can be of
direct use to authorities in decision making. Introduction
of GMP should not reduce monitoring efforts, only improve the
quality.

When monitoring is used for international regulatory purposes, harmonisation (two or more methods giving the same
result) and in certain cases, standardisation (an acceptable
reference method) of sampling strategies, methods, and analytical procedures have to be achieved within the jurisdictions
covered by the specific regulation, in order to ensure
uniformity of application of the standard.

To achieve harmonisation, collaborative/cooperative studies
have been carried out and a number of quality control
programmes established. Such programmes at the international
level are particularly important for biological indicators:
considering current manpower mobility it would be highly
detrimental to workers' faith in occupational health and

safety programmes designed to protect worker health, if the numerical result for the same biological indicator varied with the place of employment or when crossing national boundaries.

The question of the accreditation of laboratories involved in monitoring was raised but not resolved.

The availability of guidelines in GMP, standard methods and quality control programmes will be of help to the worker representatives in evaluating monitoring programmes.

4.   ROLES OF THE VARIOUS DISCIPLINES IN MONITORING

4.1 Multidisciplinary approach to monitoring

The physician, the industrial hygienist, the occupational health nurse, the epidemiologist, the analytical chemist, the statistician and the engineer are all members of the occupational health team and share a goal of preventive health care in the occupational setting. Other professionals who play a role in monitoring include economists, computer scientists and lawyers or legal experts.

The engineer has an important role in the multidisciplinary team and the potential to:

-   modify processes in such a way as to reduce exposure to toxic products and eliminate or reduce toxic by-products,
-   develop and implement appropriate control technologies,
-   institute appropriate protective engineering measures for possible emergency situations.

The analytical chemist also has a critical role in the monitoring programme, being responsible for the selection of the appropriate analytical techniques, for careful and accurate measurements of samples, for assessment of new techniques, and for analytical quality control.

For ambient monitoring cost estimates, the economist in consultation with relevant members of the team must calculate capital cost of equipment, labour, maintenance and materials. Fluctuations are primarily associated with personnel and maintenance costs as well as interest rates. Labour costs tend to increase while maintenance costs may decrease with improvements in equipment reliability. For biological monitoring the worktime lost by the workers must also be taken into account. Given the goal of protecting worker health, the economist plays an essential role in workplace monitoring, by helping to achieve cost-effective methods which will add efficiency but in no way compromise worker health.

Computer experts have increasing importance in workplace record-keeping. Ambient and biological monitoring data and health surveillance information are being stored in appropriate compartments for retrieval, analysis and feedback. The computer scientist is also concerned wih assuring that confidential medical information can only be retrieved by specified and authorised personnel. Computerisation of data is important for evaluating the efficacy of such monitoring as well as providing input into research. The role of the computer scientist is also expanding as the science is applied not only to geographically separated corporate facilities but also to link up with social and health services outside industry.

The lawyer's or legal expert's role in the area of ambient and biological monitoring is in the interpretation of statutes regarding the creation, maintenance, storage and access to monitoring data by the worker, members of the occupational health team, and by the social partners. It was noted that degrees of access to monitoring information vary considerably between countries. Access of the worker to his or her individual medical record was discussed in relation to worker access to individual ambient and biological monitoring data. There was universal agreement that such access was of fundamental importance to the overall monitoring programme. Protection of the confidentiality of employee medical information was emphasised.

Some difficulties were identified in regard to the proper function of the various members of the team. It was noted that individuals often fail to utilise the skills of the others, sometimes have inadequate training in the relevant scientific fields, and may lack sufficient authority, independence, and management support to effectively fulfil their responsibilities.

Overlapping and poorly defined duties regarding the coordination of efforts, leadership of the overall monitoring programme, and implementation of appropriate steps based on monitoring results need to be identified and resolved, to ensure effective programmes. The limited number of health and safety professionals currently available for the entire international workforce is a constraint. It is important to recognise that small and medium-sized firms which make up a significant percentage of industry, will not be able to afford multidisciplinary teams of their own in the forseeable future. There are additional difficulties imposed on the implementation of biological monitoring when medical services are provided by outside physicians.

Furthermore, the rapid development of complicated monitoring techniques, both for ambient and biological monitoring, along with increasingly sophisticated analytical methodologies, will have implications and consequences for all members of the occupational health team in terms of training requirements, allocation of time and resources, and so on.

4.2 Role of the social partners and the government in relation to monitoring

Several possible roles of government labour inspectors and compliance officers were discussed during the seminar. In some circumstances, labour inspectors have direct monitoring responsibilities. Primarily through ambient monitoring but also, on occasion, through biological monitoring, these individuals help ensure compliance with standards and the adequacy of monitoring programmes. In other circumstances labour inspectors only provide an auditing function by reviewing existing programmes.

Similarly medical inspectors in some cases are able to review monitoring data and medical records either to ensure compliance with standards, or for research purposes. Medical inspectors may not, however, have access to medical records.

From the point of view of the groups who are directly involved in the problem of health protection at the workplace, viz. the workers and their representatives on one hand and the employers and their professional organisations on the other, the problem was not so much a technical one but one which focused on the policy of prevention and health protection.

One apparent disagreement between the social partners concerned the relative importance of ambient and biological monitoring in the overall monitoring programme. Everyone approved of ambient monitoring as a means of providing important information towards ensuring an acceptable workplace environment, particularly facilitating rapid intervention in the case of accidents.

Workers' representatives stressed the fundamental importance of ambient monitoring and the control of hazards at the source. They acknowledged the importance of biological monitoring in appropriate circumstances to ensure the adequacy of safety, engineering controls, other protective measures, and in epidemiological research, but expressed the fear that biological monitoring data may be misused. Industrial representatives placed more emphasis on biological monitoring in the overall safety and health programme and

encouraged active research in this area to develop additional
ways in which biological monitoring could be used to further
protect workers' health.

There was agreement that when undertaking a monitoring programme and evaluating the results the health team should do
so in consultation with representatives from both management
and workers.

4.3 Education and training

The occupational health team is diverse, and planned instruction is essential with a composite approach to training aimed
not only at understanding hazard control but also appreciat-
ing various workers' tasks and needs.

It was agreed that the worker should be educated and trained
to anticipate and avoid occupational hazards. Training of
workers may be undertaken by government, management or
labour. Some countries have compulsory training programmes
and basic training for safety organisation members. Furthermore there is specialised training for specific hazardous
jobs.

Workers should have an understanding of the hazardous
substances to which they are exposed, their effects, as well
as the limitations and capabilities of the monitoring programmes. Training can be accomplished by workshops,
conferences and pamphlets as well as through formal training
programmes.

Stress was laid on the need to provide foreign workers such
as migrants with special training in their own language.
Additionally it was agreed that both management and workers
need planned, broad-based training programmes.

It was confirmed that safety and health is not a disparate
individual responsibility for professionals concerned with

monitoring health, but everybody in the health team, as well as the social partners have responsibilities and require basic training.

In order to optimise the development of training programmes for members of the health team in relation to monitoring, the development of a matrix model was considered which would:

- identify the tasks to be carried out by the monitoring programme,
- identify the aims to be achieved by such programmes,
- indicate for each element of the matrix, where appropriate, the training profile of the person undertaking the task.

Such a model could provide an advisory function to authorities for policy development in this area and to management and labour organisations concerned with the health of the work force.

5. CONCLUSIONS AND RECOMMENDATIONS

The rapid development of monitoring techniques for both ambient and biological monitoring, along with increasingly sophisticated analytical methodologies, will have important consequences for all members of the occupational health team which should be carefully considered and evaluated.

The development of continuous personal monitoring techniques such as personal sampler chemical badges which darken when exposed to carbon monoxide should be explored since they will improve significantly the assessment of individual exposure.

As indicators of early response following exposure to non-carcinogenic aromatic amines, the measurement of methaemoglobin, blood count in special cases, and activity of liver enzymes, is recommended. To determine other specific metabolites further research is necessary to provide basic toxicological data on their metabolism and biotransformation in the human organism and to establish, if possible, a correlation between external and internal dose and between dose and effect.

Further improvements in the analytical techniques for cadmium analysis in blood and urine are required. The possible role of specific effect parameters, such as beta-2-microglobulin in urine for cadmium toxicity in biological monitoring programmes, should be determined.

The development of personal monitoring devices is needed, bearing in mind that they should not interfere with the worker's job.

Factors to be taken into account in the choice of biological monitoring tests include:

-    the test should measure or evaluate absorption of an agent,
-    it should provide reproducible results,
-    the analytical error and biological variability should be small,
-    the test should be quantitatively relatable to the relevant range of occupational exposure,
-    convenience and risk factors should be considered,
-    the concentrations of the agent measured in the various body media should be quantitatively relatable to a health effect,
-    the test should provide useful information over and above that obtained by ambient monitoring.

Regarding the quality of data the following recommendations are considered essential:

-    Good monitoring practice (GMP) should be developed internationally for epidemiological purposes and to help develop reliance on self-generated data,

- international biological quality control programmes are most urgently needed and initiatives in this area are required,
- the requirements for standardisation of methods and the need for uniform application of standards should be evaluated and specific proposals drafted.

It is recommended that although economic factors should be properly considered in determining the most effective way of achieving maximum health for workers, monitoring decisions should not be made on a cost-benefit basis.

The increasing generation of monitoring data requires adequate storage, with ease of retrieval, and this dictates that automatic record-keeping systems should be encouraged. Incentives should be provided for the extension of computer technology to allow for the collection of monitoring data, its storage for later retrieval and analysis, which should include not only workers, but their families, communities and all consumers of toxic or hazardous products.

Because of the identified problems regarding the proper functioning of the occupational health team it is recommended that each member should:

- utilise the skills of the others,
- have adequate training in the relevant scientific fields, and
- have sufficient authority, independence and management support to effectively fulfil their responsibilities.

To establish training programmes for members of the health team the development of a matrix model was recommended which would identify the tasks to be carried out and the aims to be achieved, indicating for each element of the matrix the training profile of the person undertaking the task.

INTRODUCTORY REMARKS

J DECIMDE (Director General for Social Affairs and Employment, Commission of the European Communities), in welcoming
participants from the Member States of the European Communities, the USA and other countries to the International
Seminar, spoke of the fruitful co-operation which has been
established between the Commission of the European Communities and the Occupational Safety and Health Administration
(OSHA) and the National Institute for Occupational Safety and
Health (NIOSH) since the adoption by Council on 29 July 1978
of the Action Programme on Safety and Health at Work.

M Degimbe described the Action Programme on Safety and Health
at Work as a charter on which the Commission has worked and
will continue to work, and he outlined recent developments
and projected activities. He described health and safety as
two pillars of the protection of workers and hoped that the
legislative approach, approved by the Council of Ministers,
would increase the protection of workers. He also expressed
his pleasure with the co-operation of the International
Labour Office and the World Health Organization.

M Degimbe thanked the Honourable J Santer (Minister of Labour
for the Grand Duchy of Luxembourg) for the support and help
which his Ministry has always given the Commission on all
social and health problems.

J SANTER at the outset stressed the importance of the Action
Programme on Safety and Health at Work of 29 July 1978, which
sought to promote research into occupational diseases and
accidents at work, to provide protection against dangerous
substances and machines, to ensure inspection and to improve
human behaviour at the workplace. He spoke also of the
Directive concerned with vinyl chloride monomer and the
Directive on 'The Protection of Workers from the Risks Related to Exposure to Chemical, Physical and Biological Agents
at Work' (The 'Framework Directive') of 27 November 1980.

As regards the Framework Directive, he reminded participants that it called for monitoring and inspection. One of its principles was to set limit values which could be achieved through ambient and biological monitoring. There were fundamental problems to be solved to achieve the final objective of improvement in protection of the health of workers. He hoped that the outcome of the seminar would be fruitful for the workers of the countries represented.

J LOWENSTEIN (Ambassador of the United States of America to the Grand Duchy of Luxembourg) extended the best wishes of Eula Bingham (Assistant Secretary of Labor USA) who was not able to be present. He pointed out that this International Seminar brought together experts with scientific, legal, economic and social skills, whose common purpose was to participate in the prevention of disease at work. The USA and the European Community, as full partners in achieving this end, were committed to meet the goals of worker health and industrial growth and to ensure that these two concepts remained inseparable.

With the increase in exposure to new toxic materials, monitoring was a major tool in ensuring compliance with regulations and in setting standards; ambient and biological monitoring made it possible to detect toxic materials both at the source and after absorption.

This seminar presented an opportunity to pool information and share knowledge that had been gained at various national and international levels and thus avoid duplications. He concluded by hoping that the seminar would provide a basis for future collaborations.

CURRENT TRENDS IN OCCUPATIONAL HEALTH AND HYGIENE -
GENERAL CONSIDERATIONS I

R HAYS BELL, DAVID C LOGAN AND PATRICIA STEWART (USA-OSHA)

Summary

*In the United States in 1979, close on one hundred and fifty
thousand new cases of occupational illness were experienced
by workers in the private sector. This is probably a low
estimate. The Occupational Safety and Health Administration
(OSHA) is playing a central role in reduction of these
hazards including development of standards, a consultation
service and training and education.*

*Both atmospheric monitoring and biological monitoring are
important in the measurement of worker exposure. However,
they each have distinct advantages, disadvantages and difficulties. Examples are given in this paper as are examples of
OSHA's current work in these areas.*

During 1979 workers in the private sector in the United
States experienced about 148,900 new cases of occupational illness. This estimate is probably low because occupational illnesses are often not recognized as such and therefore not reported. Uncounted thousands die from latent
occupational exposures to substances causing cancer, lung
diseases, nerve disorders and other irreversible illnesses.
Industry, labour and government have taken some crucial steps
in reducing worker exposure to serious workplace hazards such
as vinyl chloride, coke oven emissions, arsenic and acryloni-
tile. But substantial hazards remain.

The development of standards has been one of the key elements
in an effective programme for preventing health damage as the
result of exposure to toxic chemicals.

A second major element is consultation. OSHA has established
a free on-site consultation service to help employers and
employees identify and correct workplace hazards. Free consultative services are presently available in all 50 states.

A third element is that of training and education. OSHA is continuing to build a stronger education and training programme for employers and workers which can lead to voluntary abatement of workplace hazards. The OSHA "New Directions" grant programme has provided financial support to help trade associations, employee groups and educational institutions develop their institutional competence as centres for job-safety and health education. We have increased OSHA's budget for "New Directions" grants by 1000% over the past four years to help workers and employers learn about occupational hazards and ways to correct them.

Our ability to establish a sound safety and health programme depends to a large extent on our ability to measure and quan-titate toxic exposures. Quantitating the amount of a sub-stance which a worker has absorbed or is likely to absorb is the fundamental issue in establishing dose-response relationships, permissible exposure limits and ceiling levels. It is an unfortunate reality that this quantifica-tion and estimation of exposure is often so difficult. At the very basic level the analytical techniques for assaying many chemicals are frequently cumbersome or even not current-ly known. Even if the analytical methods are available, there still remains the problem of estimating worker expo-sure, either from limited atmospheric measurements of the toxic substance or from limited biological sampling where there may be difficulty in obtaining representative measure-ments. It seems clear that both atmospheric monitoring and biological monitoring are important in the effort to quanti-tate worker exposure. For specific toxic substances, either one or the other, or both may be important. They each have distinct advantages and disadvantages.

Biological monitoring can be either direct or indirect. Direct biological monitoring - for example of blood lead levels or the level of MOCA in the urine - is the direct measurement of a toxic compound or its metabolites in the body tissues. It is an indication of exposure only.

Indirect monitoring - for example of changes in cholinesterase levels in the blood following exposure to a haematoxin -
measures the effect of the compound on the body system, organ
or tissue.

Biological monitoring can supplement air monitoring in a
number of important ways. Air monitoring can only measure
the degree of exposure through inhalation. It gives no indication of possible absorption through the skin. Biological
monitoring, on the other hand, measures the exposure from all
routes of absorption.

Biological monitoring can indicate what types of controls are
needed. If biological monitoring indicates that exposures
are being controlled then the ventilation equipment is probably sufficient. However, if air monitoring reveals low
concentrations of a contaminant, but the biological monitoring continues to show high exposure, other controls (for example, work practice or personal protective equipment) may
be necessary. In addition, biological monitoring can indicate
infrequent high exposures that routine air monitoring may
miss. Also, it may reveal a body burden which, with continued low level exposure to the same compound, may cause significant risk to the employee. It may identify individuals
with unusual sensitivities due to atypical metabolic routes
or enzyme kinetics. In either of these last two cases, the
individual could be removed from the exposure and biological
monitoring could then be used to monitor improvement. It may
also allow the administration of a particular type or degree
of therapy which, without the presence of the contaminant,
could be extremely dangerous. Finally, biological monitoring
may indicate additive or synergistic effects which would not
be recognized by air monitoring alone.

There are some difficulties associated with biological
monitoring. For example, a toxin may be metabolized to a
product or several products that are not easily detected.
The timing of sample collection can influence the amount of

contaminant in the sample. The concentration of the compound may not be indicative of recent exposures due to the existence of a body burden. In some cases, there may be a time lapse before effects of the chemical are observed. The concentration may not be due to occupational exposure alone. Finally, the amount of the chemical may vary according to a number of factors unrelated to the occupational environment. These include diet, age, sex, dose and the presence of other chemicals, including drugs.

In spite of these difficulties biological monitoring is a very useful tool in assessing exposure and OSHA has been making increasing use of biological monitoring in standard setting. For example, in our standard for occupational exposure to lead, the employer is required to monitor the employee for both lead and zinc protoporphyrin. Blood levels above a stated value trigger medical examinations by a physician. They also indicate when an employee must be removed from exposure and when he/she is permitted to return. It is in this way that biological monitoring should be used: as a supplement to air monitoring which provides exposure information that air monitoring may miss.

In addition to the use of biological monitoring in standard setting activities, OSHA has been making increasing use of biological monitoring in compliance efforts.

Recently OSHA physicians and compliance personnel have been invloved in the medical investigation of several worker fatalities and serious illness at chemical plants in the USA where heavy over-exposures to pentachlorophenol (PCP) have occurred. On one investigation the company stopped production on the day before an OSHA inspection was initiated and it was therefore not possible to document excessive atmospheric levels of pentachlorophenol through air sampling. In this particular case, autopsy tissues, blood, urine, and bile were analyzed for pentachlorophenol. The levels of PCP reported enabled our physicians and medical consultants to make the determination that an excessive over-exposure had occurred. Without the biological sampling results documenting the over-exposures and establishing the aetiology for the fatality and other adverse toxicity would have been much more difficult, if not impossible.

In another case OSHA is conducting a study of workers who are potentially exposed to the chemotherapeutic agent methotrexate. This investigation was initiated on the basis of worker complaints that they were being inadequately protected. As part of this investigation, physicians from OSHA with the assistance and cooperation from the company will be taking periodic blood specimens from production workers and measuring the methotrexate content within the blood specimens.

This information will help enable us to confirm the adequate personal protective measures and engineering controls which are currently in effect. If detectable levels of methotrexate are discovered, a more careful assessment would be called for in interpreting the risk to the worker and adequacy of the current control procedures. Because of the marked sensitivity of the available methotrexate assays, non-detectable levels would provide added assurance that worker exposure is not significant.

OSHA in another case has used urinary MOCA levels as an indicator of worker exposure and has required a comprehensive medical surveillance programme for these workers on the basis of this biological indicator of exposure.

Biological monitoring is an important tool in an overall programme of protecting worker health. Efforts to explore the ways in which it can be used in the control of workplace hazards is clearly justified. In addition discussions and dialogue will undoubtedly make a useful contribution to our understanding of the potential uses, limitations and implications for research of this important form of workplace monitoring.

CURRENT TRENDS IN OCCUPATIONAL HEALTH AND HYGIENE - GENERAL
CONSIDERATIONS II

H J DUNSTER (UK)

Summary

*The aim of occupational hygiene is to achieve a satisfactory
working environment and to demonstrate that achievement. One
feature of occupational hygiene is the setting of standards
which can relate to the amount of toxic material in the
workplace environment itself, the intake by an individual or
the concentration in the body. Monitoring is concerned with
providing information to help achieve compliance with
standards. Results derived from monitoring need to be
related to the time scale of metabolic processes and of the
subsequent biological effects; to the manner in which the
measurements can be made; and to regulatory requirements. In
the context of regulatory requirements, there are practical
aspects of environmental limits and of biological limits;
these include definition of terms and method of measurement.*

*There is then a need to set quantitative limits. This poses
no particular problem for threshold effects but it is much
more difficult for non-threshold cases. Internationally,
there are difficulties arising from confusion of terminology
and from relationships between standard setting and the
introduction of new techniques of measurement.*

*There then follows a process of consultation, initially at
the professional level and then with the representatives of
the work-force. This process of consultation becomes more
difficult as the geographical scale of the discussion
increases in a limited time scale.*

Introduction

In simple terms the aim of occupational hygiene is to achieve
a satisfactory working environment and to demonstrate that
achievement. This simple aim involves not only science and
engineering but brings in wide ranging social judgements.
In particular, one feature of occupational hygiene is the
setting of standards which define a satisfactory working
environment and this is rarely, if ever, merely a matter of
science and engineering.

Monitoring is then concerned with providing information to help achieve compliance with these standards and in testing that compliance. It is also concerned with accumulating information for later review of the validity of standards.

Standards for toxic materials in the workplace may be environmental and are then usually expressed in terms of the concentration of the toxic material in air. Other standards relate to individuals and are expressed either as the concentration breathed or as the intake per unit time. Finally, they may be biological, such as the concentration or amount of toxic materials or their metabolites in body fluids and organs.

The physical quantities to which all these standards relate vary in place and time and decisions have to be taken about the way in which results are averaged before being related to the standard. These decisions depend on the time scale of the metabolic processes and of the subsequent biological effects. There are also practical considerations imposed by practical restrictions on the way the measurements can be made and by the regulatory need to test for compliance with the standards.

Monitoring capability

It is not always recognised that the selection of a standard and its quantification depends in part on monitoring capability. In the context of this seminar this is particularly important because of the complex relationships between environmental measurements, biological measurements and the consequences for individual workers.

Environmental monitoring is a form of sampling in space and time. The intake by the workers is another sample taken at different times, in a different way, and at different locations. It is far from obvious that the monitoring sample is representative of the workers' sample. Problems such as the sensitivity and complexity of detection methods influence the duration and number of samples that can reasonably be taken.

In the same way, biological monitoring will have practical limitations because of the difficulty of obtaining representative measurements, even for materials retained for long periods in the body. If the relevant metabolic processes are rapid the results may be critically dependent on the time at which the sample is taken or the measurement made.

These practical features have a substantial effect not only on the design of the monitoring programme but also on the way in which results are related to standards and on the form in which those standards are expressed.

Regulatory implications

Although the basic aim is to protect individuals the regulatory aim is more specific and may be expressed in terms of the exposure of individuals or the intake by them of toxic materials, or it may be expressed in terms of the working environment.

The older view, derived from conventional industrial safety, was to make the working environment safe. This is still valid for substances with clear thresholds of effect. The working environment will never be completely free from contamination by the materials in process, and if it cannot be assumed that these have a threshold of biological effect, a more sophisticated approach is required. Controls can then extend beyond the concentrations in the environment and will include systems of work and the selective use of personal protection. These will all be aimed at limiting the exposure of individuals because of the existence of residual risks from exposures even below the limit values set in standards.

There are obvious regulatory difficulties in defining individual exposure, and this accounts for the continuing emphasis
on environmental rather than individual monitoring. Biological monitoring poses even greater problems. However, the
possible use of biological monitoring results to reinforce,
or relax, controls applied to the working environment is now
a subject of much discussion. The additional information
from biological monitoring can be used to indicate whether
the use of good or bad working practices is causing the
practical situation to differ significantly from the model
postulated in setting environmental standards. Biological
monitoring is particularly important if inhalation is not the
only significant route of intake of the toxic material into
the individual.

Practical aspects of environmental limits

There is a need to relate a regulatory environmental limit to
a precise definition of the quantity to be measured and limited. Thus if a concentration is to be defined, it is essential to state the period over which the concentration can be
averaged. Words like "instantaneous" are meaningless since
any measurement must provide some form of time-weighted
average, albeit over a very short time. Words like "ceiling"
must be carefully defined to be scientifically defendable.
In practice, all concentration limits are time-weighted
averages and should be stated as such. The period of averag-
ing ranges from the order of a second or so up to perhaps as
much as a year.

For the protection of workers, it may be necessary to use
several limits to control the different effects of one substance. A long term limit will be appropriate for protecting against the effect of continued chronic exposure, while a
higher short term limit may also be required to prevent acute
effects when the exposures are very non-uniform in time.
Short term figures are sometimes used for plant control
purposes but these should not be regarded as limits. They are
action levels for operational purposes.

The specification of a limit must also include information about the method of measurement. Points to be considered are fixed sampling, individual sampling, continuous sampling, intermittent and spot sampling. There is great merit in the use of statistical techniques to relate non-continuous measurements to long term averages, or averages over one length of time to averages over another.

Practical aspects of biological limits

Except in relation to radioactive materials, there has been considerable reluctance to introduce limits applicable to the results of biological monitoring. There seems no fundamental reason why limits should not be set but the practical difficulties are usually formidable. It has been more common to set action levels so that results in excess of the action level call for various forms of investigation leading to improved conditions, or possibly to action involving the individual. Such action may be removal from further exposure for a period, or it may require some form of therapy.

In the longer term it should be possible to relate the likelihood or severity of future biological consequences more closely to the results of biological monitoring than to the results of environmental monitoring. If the practical problems of the biological monitoring programme are not too severe, the results can be used as the primary basis for demonstrating compliance with the fundamental objectives of occupational hygiene, while the environmental monitoring programme can be more practically oriented to give early warning of departures from satisfactory operating conditions in the workplace. The two programmes interact in that consistently satisfactory environmental monitoring results imply little or no need to carry out biological monitoring except as an occasional confirmatory check. In the other direction, if biological monitoring either as part of a regular programme or as a confirmatory check indicates unsatisfactory conditions, the design and intensity of the environmental monitoring programme will need reconsideration.

Standard setting

Once the basic objectives have been defined there is a need
to set quantitative limits. This poses no particular problem
in principle for threshold effects, although it may be difficult to establish the toxicological data. It is much more
difficult for non-threshold cases, e.g. some, or perhaps
most, carcinogens. For these substances as a matter of principle, and for others as a matter of prudence, the use of a
limit alone is insufficient. There must also be some reflection of the general principle of good industrial hygiene to
keep all exposures as low as can reasonably be achieved. The
UK approach is to put a general duty on employers to remove
hazards so far as is reasonably practicable. This means that
if a limit is established and there is some residual risk
from exposures at or below this limit then there is a continuing duty to do all that is reasonable to reduce exposures
still further. This procedure compares closely with that
which has been a part of radiological protection for the last
few decades.

Internationally, there is considerable confusion of terminology. "So far as is reasonably practicable" and "as low as
reasonably achievable" have much the same meaning. Phrases
like "best engineering practice", "all feasible methods", or
"technology based limits" appear, at least on the surface, to
be very different. The problem is posed by the fact that
engineering practice and modern technology can achieve almost
anything, given the necessary application of resources.
Standards based on limits of detection can vary dramatically
with the introduction of new techniques. Although the use of
standards derived in these ways is at best intellectually
sterile and at worst intellectually dishonest, they have in
practice proved useful in the hands of regulators and enforcement agencies who are prepared to inject a reasonable
degree of flexibility into their application. It seems,
however, more appropriate that the regulatory development
should be in the direction of recognising a proper balance

between the risks to society and society's commitment of resources to reducing these risks. In this way a somewhat more consistent component of social judgement could be introduced into the process of standard setting and subsequent application and enforcement.

Consultation

Once the technical policy has been clarified, the process for quantitative setting of a standard should involve a process of consultation, initially at the professional level and then with the representatives of the workforce.

This process is difficult and time-consuming and properly means that the final choice of standard is based on a very wide range of factors, not all of which are concerned with toxicology and health. Nevertheless, toxicological studies are essential and if they can unequivocally define thresholds of significant effects then they make the process of standard setting very much easier for those materials that have such thresholds. In general, however, the concept of health-based standards or limits is intrinsically unsatisfactory.

The process of consultation gets more difficult as the geographical scale of the discussion increases. It is not always easy to get agreement across several industries within one country. It is correspondingly more difficult to get agreement across a number of countries. Although there are tripartite discussions between the two sides of industry and officials on occupational hygiene and industrial safety problems in the Community, it can be argued that these are not sufficiently representative to justify the inclusion of occupational hygiene standards, and in the form of binding limits, in Directives. Certainly, if binding limits are required, the preparation of such Directives has got to involve a good deal more scope for discussions and consultation at the national level than can be achieved in the timescale which the Commission of the European Communities usually wishes to impose.

Conclusions

The concept of a control limit, whether environmental or biological, is now much more complicated than was thought to be
the case some years ago. It is important that the logical
basis, the terminology and the policy for the application of
these limits should all be clarified. Much of the international and Community confusion about limits stems from the
present lack of clarity.

Monitoring is a necessary part of occupational hygiene.
Control limits are a useful adjunct to that monitoring.
Occupational hygiene is very much more than the combination
of monitoring and control limits and the current emphasis on
limits to the detriment of the development of strategies for
improving working environments is to be deprecated.

CURRENT TRENDS IN OCCUPATIONAL HEALTH AND HYGIENE - GENERAL
CONSIDERATIONS III

A ROBBINS (USA-NIOSH)

Summary

*In 1970 the Congress of the United States adopted the
Ocupational Safety and Health Act which provided for the
creation of the Occupational Safety and Health Administration
(OSHA) and the National Institute for Occupational Safety and
Health (NIOSH). These two bodies have contributed to the
growth in occupational safety and health since that time.*

*This paper is aimed at a look forward to new industries, new
workers and new research. Some of these new industries will
produce new jobs with new hazards, together with more of the
old hazards; new research can expand opportunities for
preventing occupational disease.*

*A new OSHA standard gives a worker access to his medical
records and exposure records; medical screening is a common
practice in industry and is generally required as part of
OSHA health standards or recommended in NIOSH criteria
documents and hazard assessments. NIOSH is engaged in an
extensive evaluation of medical screening and has been
comparing screening in industry with screening in the general
population; it will then analyse requirements in OSHA health
standards and its own recommendations for screening in
criteria documents in order to determine the efficacy of
those recommendations.*

In 1970 the Congress of the United States adopted the Occupational Safety and Health Act (OSH Act) which provided for the
creation of the Occupational Safety and Health Administration
(OSHA) and of the National Institute for Occupational Safety
and Health (NIOSH). During the past 10 years, the implementation of the OSH Act has dominated the practice of occupational health in the United States. Today, the United States is
at a watershed with respect to occupational safety and
health. What direction the country will take in this vital
area is now an open debate, the resolution of which will
occur during this second decade, following the passage of the
OSH Act. Since the passage of this legislation, there have
been significant strides in protecting workers' health. For
example, OSHA promulgated standards for exposure to asbestos,
coke ovens, vinyl chloride, cotton, lead, arsenic, dibromo-

chloropropane (DBCP), acrylonitrile plus 14 others. A very
important standard was implemented giving workers and their
representatives access to their medical and monitoring records. OSHA established a cancer policy which defined the
agency's policy toward the definition of carcinogens and established toxicology as the basis for that definition. Within
this period, thousands of workplaces have been cleaned up to
provide for more safe and more healthy work environments.

There is no question that there has been a significant growth
of interest in occupational safety and health in this country
in the past 20 years. OSHA has impacted significantly on the
consciousness of labour, of management and of the general
public.

There has been a clear change in union involvement in safety
and health in the United States. A few years ago there were
half a dozen professionals in labour who were involved in
safety and health on a full-time basis. Today, the number is
greater than 100. The efforts at education and training with
respect to workers have increased remarkably. Three years
ago, OSHA spent approximately $700,000 on training and educa-
tion. OSHA provides $14 million a year in grants to labour,
the private sector, universities and others to facilitate
worker education in occupational health and safety.

NIOSH has established 12 educational resource centres to
facilitate manpower training in the field of occupational
safety and health. Occupational medicine, industrial hygiene, safety and nursing represent the primary curricula
in the centres.

NIOSH criteria documents and our field research have clearly
led to an expanded knowledge of the safety and health problems in the workplace. Public concern and awareness have
grown remarkably. Occupational health has become a new
issue. The science has become public. The courts have
upheld OSHA in, for example, cases involving asbestos, vinyl
chloride, lead and cotton.

Turning to our research into occupational disease, as with infectious disease in the beginning of its studies, the big picture of occupational disease, its dimension, and causation is not yet well-developed. We have of necessity been preoccupied with small pieces of a large puzzle. Our reporting and surveillance mechanisms, though complex and sophisticated, are not yet adequate to state with certainty the relevance or incidence of various occupational health problems, nor to evaluate long-term trends of the problems.

Moreover, we are still plagued by the difficulty in determining aetiology or diagnosing accurately.

But despite our imperfect knowledge and uncertainty which we must acknowledge, we must act conservatively because our research is showing that when you look for disease in the workplace you find it. No matter how you describe it, occupational disease is an ever present reality to thousands of American workers. And unfortunately, unlike many public health problems, for most occupational diseases there is little or no therapeutic relief, no immunisation, and we have virtually no examples of eradicating disease once its aetiological agent in the workplace has been discovered.

For example, recent NIOSH studies continue to document and describe disease associated with well-known substances, lead, cotton dust, and silica, and physical agents such as vibration. The old problems have not disappeared and new issues keep surfacing as our investigations have demonstrated. These have included investigations into brain tumours in the petrochemical industry, the teratogenesis associated with exposure to cellosolves, the peripheral neuropathies associated with exposure to 2,5 substituted hexanes and stress related disorders in machine paced work.

What our research has shown, therefore, is that the magnitude of the occupational disease problem is much greater than we or even the framers of the Act in the 1960s ever expected. The question is .... Where do we proceed with such information at this time?

A look beyond the frontier in occupational medicine forecasts new industries, new workers, and new research. Most important, it will reveal new approaches to prevention of occupational disease. If these predictions are correct, we will increase our ability to protect workers; but the ways that our society responds to workplace hazards also will be critical to our effectiveness. Some of the rapidly growing sectors of the economy will produce new jobs with new hazards, as well as more of the old hazards. New research can expand opportunities for preventing occupational disease.

New industries

Although gross shifts in employment do not characterise all of the new hazards, some generalisations are possible. Service industries now provide more than half of the jobs in the United States. Since 1969 there has been no increase in the number of jobs in the manufacturing sector. At the same time, the service sector -wholesale, retail, and government - has grown from 33% of the workforce in 1950 to 53% in 1978. Non-toxic problems of the work environment will become increasingly common or apparent. Already, ergonomics issues are more common. Today, millions of workers, find themselves seated all day in front of video display terminals where they experience stress and discomfort that are not related to any chemical or radiation exposure. The shift to service employment involves new enterprises, new technology, and new capitalisation. There is a chance to address ourselves to these non-toxic aspects of the work environment from the start. There is a chance to use design to prevent problems, rather than training to alter the habits of the worker, or ad hoc engineering to modify the machines, as problems appear.

Energy

The country's determination to maximise use of energy sources other than oil will restructure the entire energy industry. Greater numbers of workers will be employed in coal, solar,

and synthetic fuel production. Mining of coal, particularly
underground, is still extremely hazardous. Directly related
to an increase in coal output will be increases in disease,
injury, and death among miners. Although the nature of
mining hazards are known to occupational medicine, efficient
and effective methods for their prevention have yet to be
fully explored and implemented. Further information on
mining hazards should play a fundamental role in decisions on
energy-production. Increased emphasis on alternative energy
sources will also create new safety and health hazards to
workers. The manufacture of photovoltaic cells used to
transform sunlight to electricity exposes workers to arsenic
and cadmium. Although the data on exposure are inconclusive
at this writing, a recently completed industrial hygiene
survey of the solar energy industry has documented potential
exposures to toxic substances.

Experience with synthetic fuel production dates back to World
War II. A coal gasification/liquefaction plant has been in
continuous operation in South Africa since 1954. The United
States plans to produce petroleum by these techniques, as
well as from oil shale commercial plants by 1987. It is
estimated that there will be as many as 24,000 workers
involved in synfuel production by the year 1992. Many of the
process materials used in, and products and byproducts of,
the synthetic fuel industry are known carcinogens. Moreover,
reliability of new equipment under high pressures and high
temperatures with erosive/corrosive slurries has not been
assured. Maintenance work in the industry will involve exposures to poisons, carcinogens, and high temperatures. Much
is known today and occupational safety and health ought to be
considered in today's decisions, not after epidemiological
results describe death and disease 20 years from now.

Biotechnology

Recombinant DNA technology is only one of many new biological
approaches to industrial production. Energy, chemical,

agricultural, and pharmaceutical industries are all exploring
new production based on genetically modified micro-organisms.
The current proliferation of recombinant DNA technology has
produced a boom of new companies and new capital. Risks
associated with exposure to modified micro-organisms, their
biological products and by-products, and to possible inadver-
tent expressions of novel genetic information have not been
fully assessed. Experience from laboratories, drug companies
and other production facilities using biotechnologies are
relevant starting points for a full review of occupational
biohazards. The companies involved with the new technology
all acknowledge the need for control technology, medical
surveillance, environmental surveillance, and worker
education. Yet there is no consensus on how to proceed.

Electronics

The electronics industry has emerged as one of the basic
elements of the global economic system. Its technological
development has proceeded at a pace exceeded by few, if any,
other major industrial sectors. Semiconductor technology has
allowed rapid growth and development in computer and
information-processing systems. The latest technologically
advanced circuit is the microcomputer or "chip". The
industry employs the conventional materials of precision
engineering, such as steel, copper, aluminium, glass, and
plastics, but special materials such as germanium, silicon,
for semiconductors.

Only now are we becoming aware of previously overlooked
health hazards of the work environment in electronic-
component manufacturing and recycling plants. These workplaces appear to be clean as compared with many in heavy
manufacturing. However, neurological, respiratory, cardiovascular, and bone illnesses in workers have been causally
linked with the absence of effective ventilation systems, and
workers have been found to develop dermatitis in work where
the skin comes in contact with the metals and solvents used
in making the chips.

In the rapid expansion and competition among several large
corporations, occupational health concerns seem to have been
overlooked. The potential size and stability of this market
should be an incentive to invest in hazard-preventing
engineering controls. Will occupational medicine address
these issues from the desired perspective of prevention, or
will it respond only to already identified hazards in the
electronics industry?

New research

There is increased interest in reproductive hazards and
neurobehavioural toxicology. The range of reproductive
hazards was not recognised in the past: simple teratology,
where maternal exposures during pregnancy affected physical
characteristics of the child, attracted all the attention.

The findings that exposures to lead, and to DBCP cause reduced fertility or infertility, brought new attention to the
range of reproductive hazards. New findings that reproductive hazards can manifest themselves as behaviour or cancer
lead ineluctably to the conclusion that women, men and future
generations may be impaired. The costs of reproductive
damage may be as large as from occupationally caused cancer.
Toxicologists are also exploring the subclinical neurological
impairments which result from a variety of materials -
including low-level exposures to lead and carbon disulphide.
(Preventive ageing is the kind of charge that previously went
undetected.) The challenge here is more and progressive than
isolating causes and effects, but making the almost impercep-
tible dysfunctions a target of preventive medicine.

Finally, in light of the rapidly escalating rate at which
chemicals are entering commerce, we must develop and validate
tests which predict human toxicity cheaper and faster than
full-scale bioassays. To address the effects of those chemicals already in commerce, we must develop screening methods
for use in the field which predict toxic effects in man.

Prevention strategies

To become effective, knowledge of occupational hazards and their effects must be shared with the general medical profession, and not viewed as a narrow specialism. Occupational medicine must complement a retrospective, body-counting orientation with one of anticipation and prevention. This public health approach focuses on eliminating dangerous processes and substances, and spreading knowledge of these dangers.

Predictive tests - and predictions from tests

New uses of laboratory toxicology strengthen decision making for prevention. It is now possible to predict the likelihood of particular substances causing cancer in humans. For those suspected carcinogens, the OSHA has issued standards for evaluation of scientific evidence and development of protective policies. The Toxic Substances Control Act goes further, requiring the testing of new chemicals to be completed before their introduction into the market.

The use of laboratory science by administrative agencies to make public health policy has brought the courts forward to deal with challenge by the regulated industries.

Although costs are involved, the original decisions are debated largely by scientists. The public is not expected to comprehend or participate in the tally. Industry seems willing to accept the process that uses experts and the courts and keeps the public at a distance.

One problem of using laboratory results to develop public health policy is the way that statistics are used in the laboratory. Traditionally, very stringent requirements must be met in order to call results positive. Public health, on the other hand, always demands protective approaches to decision making and action. How stringent a standard of proof is appropriate if the potential harm is great or if the cost of avoiding the hazard is low? In such a situation, even the slightest hint from the laboratory might appropriately trigger public health action. It is often wrong to wait for laboratory certainty; instead we must minimise false negatives to achieve moderate public health management.

Control technology and substitution

Predictive tests, epidemiological studies, and experimental research contribute to much more than new standards for preventing health hazards. All point toward the same solutions: control technology and substitution of safe materials and processes for those that are hazardous.

Costs generate interest in control technology. The effects of the workplace hazards show up both in health insurance rates and in workers' compensation premiums. Workers' compensation is more expensive partly because of rapidly rising costs in medical care and partly because it is now possible to obtain compensation for occupational disease - not just injuries. The high cost of modifying engineering controls has also produced new interest in designing control technology for new plants. When occupational health is considered during the design of production processes the ultimate cost of compliance is far less. The textile industry is experimenting with washed cotton to prevent dust-related byssinosis, and the aluminium industry is examining reduction processes with closed pot rooms to minimise toxic exposures. Cotton processing free of disease-causing dust and aluminium reduction without carcinogen exposure reflect the preventive orientation of control technology to occupational health hazards. Furthermore, applied control technologies can have an energy-saving effect. Recycling of unused materials, recovery of by-products, and recirculation of wastes are examples of methods used to reduce health hazard exposures and energy consumption.

Substitution of safer materials for those found to be hazardous like control technology, must be considered every time
an occupational health problem is identified. This is the
case with asbestos and benzidine-based dyes which must be
replaced by safe substitutes. Undoubtedly, the list will
continue to expand. Occupational medicine must insist on the
safer alternatives.

Informing workers

The acid test of an occupational health programme is whether
workers are provided with assistance and information about
known or suspected hazards. Studies about occupational
hazard exposure information repeatedly show that workers are
not aware of the hazards of substances to which they are
exposed, the dangers involved, or the methods for preventing
exposures to them.

Programmes that improve workers' knowledge will increase
demands on occupational medicine. Occupational health professionals will be asked to serve this informed constituency.
A new OSHA standard has given a worker access to his medical
records and to exposure records. Workers must also be told
about the exposure and health of the whole plant (without
individual identifiers). The employer is asked to recognise
the physician's responsibility to his patients.

Medical screening is a common practice in industry, and is
generally required as part of OSHA health standards or
recommended in NIOSH criteria documents and hazard assessments. While there exists considerable literature evaluating
screening in the general population, relatively little has
been written about the special aspects of screening in the
workplace. As a first attempt to analyse the benefits and
problems involved in occupational screening, NIOSH is engaged
in an extensive evaluation of medical screening. NIOSH
intends to pursue a multistep approach to the evaluation.
First, NIOSH has been comparing screening in industry with

screening in the general population. We have reviewed the concepts pertaining to screening in the general population, including objectives, suitable diseases, suitable tests, frequency of testing, appropriate groups for testing, evaluation of screening programmes, and ethical issues in screening. We have discussed these aspects as they apply to screening in the workplace. Preplacement and pretermination physicals have been analysed as special cases of occupational screening.

Following this initial evaluation NIOSH will proceed to analyse the requirements in OSHA health standards and our recommendations for screening in criteria documents in order to determine the efficacy of those recommendations. For example, we believe even the most advanced OSHA standard with respect to biological monitoring of lead, merely sets a norm. There are no provisions for epidemiological follow-up of biological and environmental monitoring to determine the adequacy of the standard. NIOSH will attempt to develop additional recommendations for screening based on the conclusions derived from the previous evaluations. The preliminary conclusions upon which our subsequent activities will be based are set out below:

Conclusions

1. Screening is a medical procedure of limited usefulness that can advance the time of diagnosis for certain diseases.

2. All screening programmes have physical and psychological adverse effects. For this reason, all programmes should be scrutinised and evaluated for their medical and ethical merit.

3. Evaluation of a screening programme is best done by an experimental random clinical trial. Only this method can eliminate three important biases of screening

programmes - self-selection, lead-time bias, and length bias. Due to economic, ethical, and practical draw-backs, however, it may not be possible to do a random clinical trial of screening. In these cases, non-experimental methods of evaluation must be used.

4.   Screening is never a substitute for primary prevention. From a health standpoint, instituting primary prevention to <u>avoid</u> disease, is always preferable to screening for early detection of disease. While primary prevention is often initially more costly in the general population, it appears that public policies will be better directed to encouraging health-producing personal behaviours than to the promotion of further screening and other medical preventive measures. In the workplace, screening must be part of a larger effort to make the workplace as safe and healthful as possible.

5.   In the workplace, screening is always used in conjunction with other methods of disease prevention and hazard detection. Compared to its use in the general population, screening has an expanded role in the workplace. It may be used for untreatable as well as treatable diseases, for epidemiological surveillance, for monitoring the entire preventive standard, and for fixing liability for occupational disease.

6.   Due to possible conflicts of interest, occupational screening must be conducted with safeguards to ensure objectivity, fairness, and proper reporting and use of the results of screening tests.

7.   Screening in the workplace is generally more cost-effective than general population screening for three reasons:

      i)   in the workplace, screening may be used for multiple purposes.

ii)   in the workplace, the prevalence of disease
       tends to be higher, leading to a lower cost
       per case detected; and,

iii) the added cost of screening is often lower
       in the workplace because screening can be
       incorporated   with other in-plant health
       activities.

8.   Preplacement physicals are required by OSHA to establish
     a baseline health appraisal for workers, to detect con-
     ditions   that would place workers at increased risk of
     exposure, and to detect conditions that would confuse or
     render difficult the identification of work-related
     signs and symptoms of disease.

9.   Hypersusceptibility screening is a growing and contro-
     versial type of screening, that can benefit workers, but
     can   also be abused.   Hypersusceptibility screening
     should be subject to the same criteria of medical and
     ethical evaluation as any other screening programme.

CURRENT TRENDS IN OCCUPATIONAL HEALTH AND HYGIENE - GENERAL
CONSIDERATIONS IV

D HENSCHLER (FEDERAL REPUBLIC OF GERMANY)

Summary

Traditionally, efforts towards the protection of workers in areas with exposure to chemicals have been oriented to set standards for airborne gases, vapours and particulate matter in terms of concentration and time of exposure. These efforts turned on the view that there was a threshold below which no harm would result from exposure to a chemical. In keeping with this view, tolerance levels have been set in many countries; classically the concept of safe levels of airborne contaminants in the workplace is based by air monitoring on the eight hour time-weighted average value. However, many chemicals in a great variety of technical processes occur in widely varying concentrations. In order to deal with this problem two different approaches have, in the past, been proposed - the fixing of excursion factors and the fixing of 'ceiling' values. Recently, in the Federal Republic of Germany, a new concept has been proposed which subdivides all occupational chemicals into five main categories, designated according to effect, and characterized by constant analytical criteria.

In contrast there are, as yet, no official standards in European countries for biological monitoring; these may be introduced by 1982 and there are promising developments in testing for carcinogenic effect. Within this paper there is a review of some of these developments.

Introduction

Traditionally, efforts towards the protection of workers in
areas with exposure to chemicals have been oriented to set
standards for airborne gases, vapours and particulate matter
in terms of concentration and time of exposure. The first
standards were published by K. B. Lehmann, based on medical
examinations of populations at exposure in connection with
chemical analyses of the air in the workplaces, and on some
animal experimentation. This early work, starting in 1887
(1), and the conclusions drawn from it were based on some
vague arguments like the famous statement of Paracelsus that
it is the dose which makes a thing (a chemical) not a poison
(2); hence, threshold doses must exist below which no harm
will result.

The first experimental demonstration of a no-effect level of
an airborne chemical and the mathematical substantiation were
provided by Flury and Heubner with hydrogen cyanide (3): a
definite concentration exists below which no fatal poisoning
occurs for unlimited periods of exposure, due to a constant
elimination (detoxification) rate (4). This knowledge encouraged the establishment of some 100 tolerance levels in
Germany (4) and Switzerland (5) in the twenties and thirties.
Since the early forties, the Threshold Limit Values (TLV)
list of the American Conference of Governmental Industrial
Hygienists (ACGIH) in the United States has been published
and, with annual revisions, enlarged to the current list of
approximately 650 compounds(6). It is used, in part by preparing reprints without changes, by some Western European
countries. Other countries prepare their own lists, e.g. the
FRG since 1966, with Switzerland and Austria as satellites.
More recently, Holland and Sweden have provided their own
lists, with some differences not only in the threshold
values, but also in the basic philosophies and argumenta-
tions. There is one feature in common for the independent
European lists as compared with the American TLV list: a more
detailed documentation of the arguments and backgrounds for
decisions for the establishment of values. However, legislative backgrounds and executive compliance differ widely in
these countries and therefore one should be cautious in
trying to use the threshold limit values in these lists for
comparison of health protection standards.

New strategies in air monitoring

The classical concept of safe levels of airborne contaminants
in the workplace is based on the 8 hour time-weighted average
value. Several factors may be responsible for that: (a) experimental exposures, in human as well as in animal studies,
were almost exclusively performed with constant concentrations of the test chemical in the air, the results therefore
being regarded as valid only for this pattern of exposure;
(b) epidemiological studies have only been retrospective in

most instances, the exposure values being based merely on rough calculations from single analytical determinations, or on speculations only in terms of long-term averages; (c) the analytical methods available previously were rather insensitive, and only rarely suitable for following the divergencies of actual concentrations, mostly irregular in type, in the course of a work shift.

The necessity for having acceptable concentrations for short-term peak exposure had been realised from the very beginning (1, 4). Early monographs of occupational exposure standards often quoted short-term tolerable concentrations (4, 7). These, and other recommendations for introducing short-term emergency levels (8) have not been successful, and have never enjoyed general acceptance. Nevertheless, the need for such types of exposure limits continues to be propagated.

In order to deal with the problem that many chemicals in a great variety of technical processes occur in widely varying concentrations, the U.S. -TLV list has proposed, several years ago, two different approaches towards a solution. One is the fixing of excursion factors from the average value for peak exposure limits, the factors increasing with decreasing orders of magnitude of the TLVs. The other one fixes, for some types of compounds, the TLV as a "ceiling" value which should never be exceeded. Both concepts are unsatisfactory from a scientific point of view: the first one does not take into consideration well established rules of the dose-response relationship in pharmacology and toxicology; the second one lacks substantiated toxicological criteria and does not comply with the basic requirements of chemical-analytical air monitoring.

A new concept has recently been proposed in the FRG (9). It combines both toxicological and analytical requirements, and by compromise subdivides all occupational chemicals into five main categories. These categories (table 1) are designated according to toxicological and/or pharmacokinetic parameters which have priority over analytical criteria or requirements. Each category is further characterised by constant analytical criteria: a factor of maximum deviation from the 8 hour time-weighted average, a maximum deviation period, and a limit of the frequency of deviations per 8 hour shift. The combination of toxicological criteria (local/systemic activity, reversibility, half-life of compound(s) or metabolites, slope of dose-response curves, type and strength of subjective impairments, etc.) and limitations posed by analytical short-comings (sensitivity of methods, type of available methods of determination, statistical tolerance) can only be achieved on a pragmatic basis. A first tentative evaluation of some 400 chemicals in the MAK-list (Maximum Concentrations at the Workplace) revealed that more than three-quarters may be categorised according to the presently available data in the literature. The practicability of the new concept is now being tested with some model compounds. It is intended to include, in the case of positive experience, the categories, together with deviation factors, periods and frequencies in the MAK-list.

Table 1. Limits for peak exposures (9)

Category	Type of Effect	Deviation Factor	Deviation Period	Frequency per 8 h
I	Local Irritants	2	5 min	8
II	Systemic Activity Latency for effects < 2 h			
	Half-Life 1/2 - 2 h	2	30 min	4
	Half-Life 2 - 5 h	5	30 min	2
III	Systemic Acitivity			
	Half-life > 5 h	10	30 min	1
	(highly cumulative)			
IV	Very low toxic potential (MAK $\gtreqless$ 500 PPM)	2	60 min	3
V	Strong Odorants			
	Smell not persistent	5	5 min	4
	Smell persistent	2	5 min	2

Biological monitoring: standards and methods

The system of air monitoring has constituted a useful means
for health protection for almost a century. Some of its
shortcomings have been long recognised: it only determines
exposure conditions of groups of people but cannot measure
the uptake, or body burden, of an individual. Biological
monitoring which is always based on analytical determinations
with individual persons has been suggested and practised for
a limited number of compounds for many years. However, there
have been no official standards introduced in European
countries up to now. At present, groups of scientists in
several countries are preparing for the introduction of
standards for biological monitoring, to my knowledge at least
in Holland, Sweden, Finland and West Germany. In the FRG, a
very active group has already formalised the framework of
possibilities, uses and limitations of biological monitoring,
and it is intended to include this as an official part of the
list of recommended standards (MAK-list) in 1981 or 1982.

The classic biological media for monitoring of individual
exposure, urine, faeces, blood and breath, and the determination of occupational chemicals and/or their metabolites are
no longer the only means in this field. Recent developments
are broadening the scale of monitors, and we are experiencing
a fascinating and rapid development of methods which no
longer focus on the chemical itself but measure the type and
amount of reaction products with biological materials, thus
representing toxic reactions and damage immediately, rather
than the possibility of their occurrence. This kind of monitoring, now being applied mostly for genotoxic actions, has
had some precursors, as in the field of cholinesterase inhibition by some pesticides and related compounds, the significance however being restricted to a very few compounds and
occupational places only.

Biological monitoring of occupational carcinogens:
future developments

Occupational hygiene and toxicology have dramatically shifted
their main interests from conventional acute and chronic
effects to carcinogenesis and mutagenesis. The lists of
proven or suspected occupational carcinogens are lengthening,
year by year, with an exponential tendency. The main reasons
for this development may be seen in the following facts: (a)
as a result of chemical development and production, new
compounds, some with increased biological reactivity, are
being added at ever increasing rates to work areas; (b)
spectacular events in the detection of carcinogenicity in
humans caused by certain chemicals long in use have stimulated the vigilance of occupational hygienists and the medical
profession to seek further examples; vinyl chloride,
bis(chloromethyl)ether, and asbestos may be cited as out-
standing instances; (c) since the early fifties, molecular
biology has uncovered the mechanism of damage to genetic
material, which lead to mutations as a trigger-event for
cancer, by using reactive chemicals such as alkylating
agents, thus providing a means for identifying chemicals
capable of creating genetic damage; (d) on the basis of this,
geneticists have developed simple methods for screening
chemicals in microbial or cell culture systems for genotoxic
activities; the lists of suspected carcinogens according to
the Ames Test or similar techniques are already legion.

One of the first methods used in biological monitoring was
the determination of mercapturic acids in urine, as an
indicator of the formation of electrophilic metabolites which
react with the most important soluble nucleophile in the
cell: glutathione. This procedure proved of some value if, as
in the case of vinyl chloride (10), a given indirect carcinogen was taken up and metabolised in considerable amounts by a
well defined population. There are, however, some important
limitations: interference with non-carcinogens (non-specificity), short half-lives of mercapturic acids, and inaccuracy

(insensitivity) in the range of very low exposures, which are
the rule under the modern protective procedures used in the
workplace.

Mutagenicity testing of urine voided by occupational populations is another approach. The problems with this method
are, besides non-specificity, the extreme sensitivity and
lack of quantification of exposure. Nevertheless, it might
be useful as a crude identification of work areas with a
potentially carcinogenic or mutagenic exposure for initiating
further and more specific and accurate work for confirmation
or exclusion of a suspected risk (11).

Most promising in this field are those methods which identify
and quantify the reaction products of electrophilic chemicals
or the metabolites of occupational toxicants with nucleo-
philic macromolecules in situ. The best approach up to now
seems to be the determination of chemically altered haemoglobin. Alkylating species react, in an electrophilic substitution reaction, with the N3 of histidine, which can be
identified by sophisticated mass spectrometric methods (12)
after hydrolysis of haemoglobin and chromatographic separation. Since these reaction products are stable and the biological turnover of haemoglobin is well known, one can extrapolate for the body burden of alkylating activity for more
than one day, possibly for several weeks. This approach seems
to work well with vinyl chloride, ethylene oxide and possibly
ethylene, which is metabolically activated to ethylene oxide
(13). This type of biological monitoring comes much closer
than other methods to the genotoxic damage itself. It has
been shown that the covalent binding of carcinogenic metabolites is independent of dose over a wide range of five orders
of magnitude (14), following strictly first order kinetics,
that the proportion which reacted with haemoglobin is representative for the binding in fixed tissues, too, and that the
factors for the distribution of alkylating activity in
several tissues, perhaps potential target tissues for carcinogenesis, can be determined by suitable animal experiments.

It is expected that improved derivatisation and separation
methods will allow monitoring of alkylated haemoglobin down
to realistic exposure levels for a variety of carcinogens.
Occupational hygiene and toxicology will benefit here from
the fascinating advances of molecular biology and
pharmacokinetics.

The last methodological approach to be mentioned related to
biological monitoring of carcinogenic substances is the
search for biological endpoints in human tissues, i.e. for
mutations in cells available for repeated analysis. Chromosomal aberrations in lymphocytes constitute a sensitive but
obviously, unfortunately, rather non-specific monitor. More
recent methods aim at demonstrating changes in the fine
structure of DNA on the physical level. Another possibility
is to look for changes in the protein patterns of such cells
due to point mutations. Bone-marrow cells and spermatocytes
may also be used for that purpose. None of these procedures
has, however, arrived at a stage where practicability for
field application can be predicted.

In general, the classic chemical techniques for biological
monitoring will be substituted, step by step, by more
sophisticated and more representative methods for determining
minute biochemical and biological changes, and these will
provide better information on the toxic risk at the
individual level.

References

1. K.B. Lehmann: Arch. Hyg. (Berl.) 7, 231 (1887)

2. Paracelsus, B. Th. v. Hohenheim: 3. Karntner Defension
    (15)

3. Flury, F., Heubner, W.: Biochem. Zschr. 95, 249 (1919)

4. Flury, F., Zernik, F.: Schadliche Gase. Springer, Berlin
    1931

5. Hess, W.: Med. Inauguraldiss., Zurich 1911

6. Threshold Limit Values. Amer. Conf. Gov. Ind. Hyg., Cincinnati 1953-80

7. Hendersson, Y., Haggard, H.W.: Noxious Gases. Reinhold Publ. Corpn., New York 1943

8. Threshold Limit Values, Appendix D. Amer. Conf. Gov. Ind. Hyg., Cincinnati 1979

9. Henschler, D., zur Muhlen, Th., Drope, W.: Arbeitsmed., Sozialmed. $\underline{14}$, 191 (1979)

10. Heger, M., Muller, G., Norpoth, K.: Annual Meeting Dtsch. Gesellsch. f. Arbeitsmed., Innsbruck 1980, in press.

11. Rosenkrantz, H.S., Poirier, L.A.: J. Ntl. Cancer Inst. $\underline{62}$, 873 (1979)

12. Osterman-Golkar, S., Hultmark, D., Segerbak, D., Calleman, C.J., Gothe, R., Ehrenberg, L., Wachtmeister, C.A.: Biocem. Biophys, Res. Commun. $\underline{76}$, 256 (1977)

13. Ehrenberg, L., Osterman-Golkar, S., Segerbak, D., Calleman, C.J.: Mutat. Res. $\underline{45}$, 175 (1977)

14. Neumann, H.-G.: Arch. Toxicol., Suppl. $\underline{3}$, 69 (1980)

CURRENT TRENDS IN OCCUPATIONAL HEALTH AND HYGIENE - GENERAL
CONSIDERATIONS V

L PARMEGGIANI (ILO)

Summary

*One of the constitutional objectives of the International
Labour Organization (ILO) is the protection of workers,
throughout the world, against occupational hazards. This
objective is pursued on a tripartite basis.*

*In 1953, the ILO set formal international standards for pro-
tection of workers against chemical hazards with special
reference to air monitoring. Some twenty years later, the
ILO brought forward provisions including the carrying out of
biological or other tests or investigations which may be
necessary to control the degree of worker exposure.*

*In 1978, the ILO launched the International Occupational
Safety and Health Hazard Alert System and currently is join-
ing the World Health Organization and the United Nations
Environment Programme in the International Programme on
Chemical Safety.*

The protection of workers against occupational hazards
throughout the world, and in particular in its 144 member
States, is one of the constitutional objectives of the
International Labour Organization (ILO). This objective is
pursued by means of a tripartite endeavour aiming at a
balance between social and economic development. For six
long decades the ILO has been accumulating experience in this
field, accumulating achievements and overcoming difficulties,
thus enabling the Organisation to see some of these problems
in deep perspective.

The priority areas of the ILO activities in the field of
occupational safety and health include the most severe
hazards to workers' life and health. In the '50s, ionising
radiations seemed to be the most severe occupational hazard.
Later on, and because of a number of unexpected events at the
operational level, and progress in the scientific field,
there has been a gradual focusing on the hidden hazards of

chemicals both as consequences of long term relatively low exposure and as major accidents. In the '70o, the general feeling was that chemicals must remain our priority target among the most widely-diffused occupational and environmental hazards with a high degree of severity.

For many years, protection against chemical hazards was limited to administrative measures. Later, a scientific and professional approach became gradually possible, due to the advance in knowledge of the mechanisms of toxicity and dose-response relationship.

The first international standard of the ILO introducing this type of professional approach dates back as far as 1953. ILO Recommendation No. 97 concerning the protection of the health of workers in places of employment lays the ground for modern industrial hygiene practice with special reference to technical measures for the control of occupational hazards, and environmental monitoring.

Paragraph 5 stipulates:

(1) "The atmosphere of workrooms in which dangerous or obnoxious substances are manufactured, handled or used should be tested periodically at sufficiently frequent intervals to ensure that toxic or irritating dusts, fumes, gases, fibres, mists or vapours are not present in quantities liable to injure health. The competent authorities should publish from time to time, for the guidance of all concerned, the available information regarding maximum allowable concentrations of harmful substances.

(2) The authority concerned with the protection of the health of workers in places of employment should be empowered to specify the circumstances in which it is necessary to test the atmosphere of such workrooms and the manner in which the tests are to be carried out. Such tests should be conducted or supervised by qualified personnel and, where appropriate, by qualified medical personnel who possess experience in occupational health."

Of course, one could not expect that biological monitoring could have been recommended in 1953, because of lack of knowledge and analytical facilities. After the adoption of this recommendation, truly of a pioneering nature, almost 20 years had to elapse before the matter was taken up again by the International Labour Conference. Convention No. 136, which stipulates a ceiling value in the workroom air for benzene, is the first instrument enforceable after ratification which introduces an exposure limit in the international standards. In Convention No. 139 on the prevention of occupational cancer, adopted in 1974, a further step was made, with the provisions of article 5 referring to biological tests or other investigations to be carried out on workers exposed to carcinogenic substances or agents. Finally, Convention No. 148 and Recommendation No. 156, adopted in 1977, concern directly the working environment. This Convention urges the competent authority to establish criteria for determining the hazards of exposure to air pollution in the working environment and specify exposure limits on the basis of these criteria. In the elaboration of the criteria and the determination of the exposure limits, the competent authority is required to take into account the opinion of technically competent persons designated by the most representative organisations of employers and workers concerned.

May I draw your attention to the difference that exists between the exposure limits established according to such a procedure and the health-based permissible limits which are being investigated by WHO study groups since 1979? The latter represents, in the opinion of the study groups, the levels in workroom air at which there is no significant risk of adverse health effects and which do not take into account technological and economic considerations.

The Convention stipulates that the criteria and exposure limits shall be established, supplemented and revised regularly in the light of current national and international knowledge and data, taking into account, as far as possible, any increase in occupational hazards resulting from simultaneous exposure to several harmful factors at the workplace. Each member State is required to provide appropriate inspection services for the purpose of supervising the application of the provisions of this Convention or satisfy itself that the appropriate inspection is carried out. Recommendation No. 156, supplementing the Convention, adds further provisions including the carrying out of biological or other tests or investigations which may be necessary to control the degree of worker exposure, keeping of biological and medical records and environmental data for epidemiological and other research, and the reference to the most recent codes of practice or guides established by the ILO in prescribing measures for the prevention and control of air pollution.

So far, the Benzene Convention (No. 136) has been ratified by 23 member States, the Occupational Cancer Convention (No. 139) by 17 member States, and the Work Environment Convention (No. 148) by five member States. These are Ecuador, Finland, Norway, Sweden and the United Kingdom. We do hope that the example among the countries represented here of the United Kingdom and that of the United States Public Law 91-596, the Occupational Safety and Health Act, may lead all the member States of the European Community to law and practice conditions enabling them to ratify the Convention, as it appears that the general trend in the Community is towards a greater legal value of the exposure limits in use at the operational level. The endeavours of the Commission of the European Communities towards the harmonisation of criteria among its member States are very promising in this context. For similar reasons, the Governing Body of the ILO has this year approved a Code of Practice on Occupational Exposure to Airborne Substances Harmful to Health. Codes of practice and technical standards may be more suitable in this field than legal requirements for many countries, because of greater flexibility in the adoption and amending procedures.

The world-wide coverage of the ILO involves very large differences in the work environment and in the socio-economic
development of the member States. Environmental and particularly biological monitoring are most valuable methods where
and when sampling, analytical measurement, and interpretation
of results are fully reliable, technically competent inspection services are available and traditional safety and health
measures exist. The validity of exposure limits for prevention is also linked to employer awareness, and worker participation in occupational health and safety.

The ILO is preparing a global instrument on occupational
safety and health and the working environment which has
passed the first discussion at the 66th Session of the
International Labour Conference a few months ago. The
revision of Recommendation No. 112 on Occupational Health
Services is under consideration. To strengthen technical
cooperation activities in this field, a special International
Programme in the Improvement of Working conditions and
Environment has been in operation since 1976. The ILO is
joining WHO and UNEP in the International Programme on
Chemical Safety which is becoming operational. At the
suggestion of the United States Federal Government and with
its support, the ILO launched, two years ago, the
International Occupational Safety and Health Hazard Alert
System which is a new international tool to draw attention to
newly discovered and/or poorly known occupational hazards.

Thus the ILO employs a variety of means of action in this
area to increase the benefits of international cooperation in
long dated activities for the promotion of occupational
safety and health.

RECENT AND POTENTIAL ADVANCES APPLICABLE TO THE PROTECTION OF
WORKERS' HEALTH - AMBIENT MONITORING I

A SCHUETZ AND W COENEN (FEDERAL REPUBLIC OF GERMANY)

Summary

*In order to carry out ambient monitoring to good effect, it
is particularly important to select the measuring point, the
time and duration of measurement and the method to be used.
Each of these aspects is examined within the paper and procedures are set out. Examples are given of the pattern of
vinyl chloride concentration at a workplace over a variety
of periods and its relevance to the EC Directive on vinyl
chloride.*

Dangerous agents may take the form of dusts, gases or vapours
in the air at the workplace and these can be inhaled by
workers in the area. There are substances which can also be
taken up through the skin. There is a health risk if the
toxic substances or their metabolites are found in the body
or in the body fluids in quantities which exceed specific
values (biological monitoring) and/or measurements taken at
the workplace or in the working area show that concentrations
of toxic substances in the air exceed given limit values
(e/g/ MPCs) (ambient monitoring). While the results of
biological monitoring always relate to individuals and show
at a later date the effects which substances have produced
earlier, the results of ambient monitoring relate usually to
the workplace and describe the concentrations of toxic agents
present at the time of actual measurement.

Figure 1 shows how a direct comparison of the results of
ambient and biological monitoring is very often
unsatisfactory. For decisions about technical protection
measures, including the use of personal respiratory
protective equipment, ambient monitoring is therefore always
preferable. Biological parameters are, however, more useful
for decisions about individual exposure - e.g. for
occupational medical examinations.

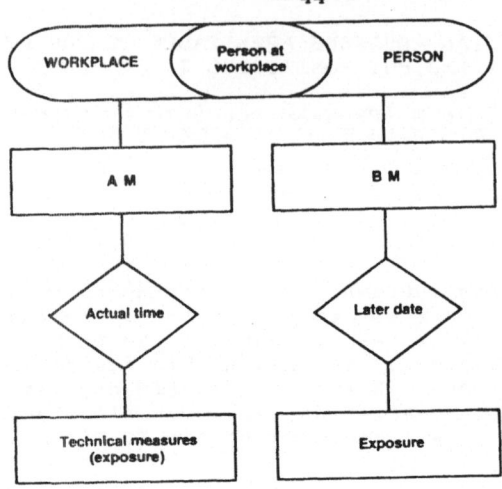

Figure 1.   Ambient (AM) and Biological (BM) Monitoring

Figure 2 sets out the purpose of measurements of concentrations of toxic agents at work. The usual procedure is to
establish the levels in the works or plant and compare these
with the limit values for the substance in question in order
to find out whether the workplaces represent a health hazard
and if so to take the necessary steps.

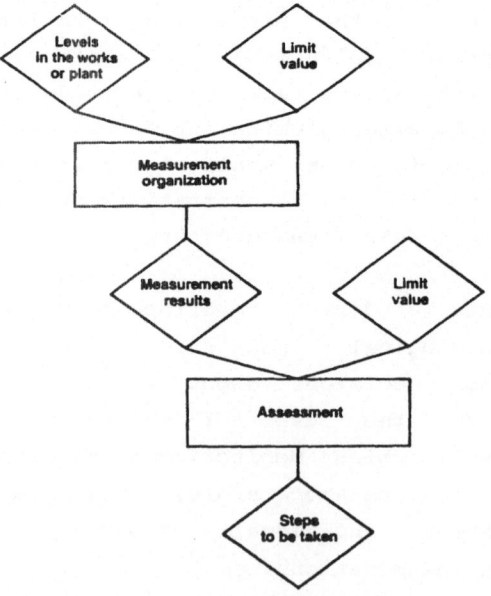

Figure 2.   Ambient Monitoring

The organisation of the measurements is particularly important and involves selecting the measuring point:
- the time and duration of measurement (personal measurement, stationary measurement, recording throughout a shift, mean value over a shift, representative for the shift, repeat measurements)
- measurement method (sampling - analysis, specificity correctness, accuracy - detection limit)

The measuring point should be chosen so that toxic agents in the working area and the exposure of those working there can be assessed on the basis of the results obtained.

It can be achieved by monitoring the individual using samplers worn by him (personal sampling), the advantage being that it provides an immediate reading for the exposure of the wearer; this method is recommended particularly for people whose workplace changes (e.g. drivers). The disadvantages are that it does not really provide direct information about concentrations of toxic substances and analysis is expensive because of the small number of samples and/or the large number of appliances used.

Also it can be achieved by monitoring the environment using fixed appliances (stationary measurements). The advantage here, particularly with gases and vapours, is that it is possible to analyse and record at the same time. Furthermore, with a measuring-cum-recording installation incorporating a switching system, samples from a variety of working areas can be taken. The disadvantage is that attributing the concentrations measured by a stationary apparatus to the people working in the area can give rise to certain errors.

The decision about which of the two methods to use in individual cases depends on the toxic agent, the nature and efficiency of the measurement method and, particularly, on the working process.

In choosing the time and duration of measurement particular attention must be given to the fact that concentrations of toxic agents at the workplace vary in time. Another point is that with so-called continuous work processes the distributions of concentrations can usually be represented lognormally. It is possible with continuous and recorded measurements to indicate the course taken by the concentration at the measuring point and to establish the required mean. In many cases, however, this is either impossible, or not justified because of the high cost, or not really necessary. It is only advisable with particularly critical, highly toxic substances or to monitor areas where leakage may cause high peak concentrations and an alarm signal is required. In the vast majority of cases, it is sufficient to take random samples according to specific rules. Statistical analysis gives a sufficiently accurate picture of whether the limit values have been exceeded. When the effects are constant spot checks should be made on random days and at random times during the working period. When the effects last for only a short time, the samples must of course be taken within this period.

The concentration thus measured (and this is essential for measurement organisation and assessment) depends on the duration of measurement - that is, the 'mean' period (see Figure 3).

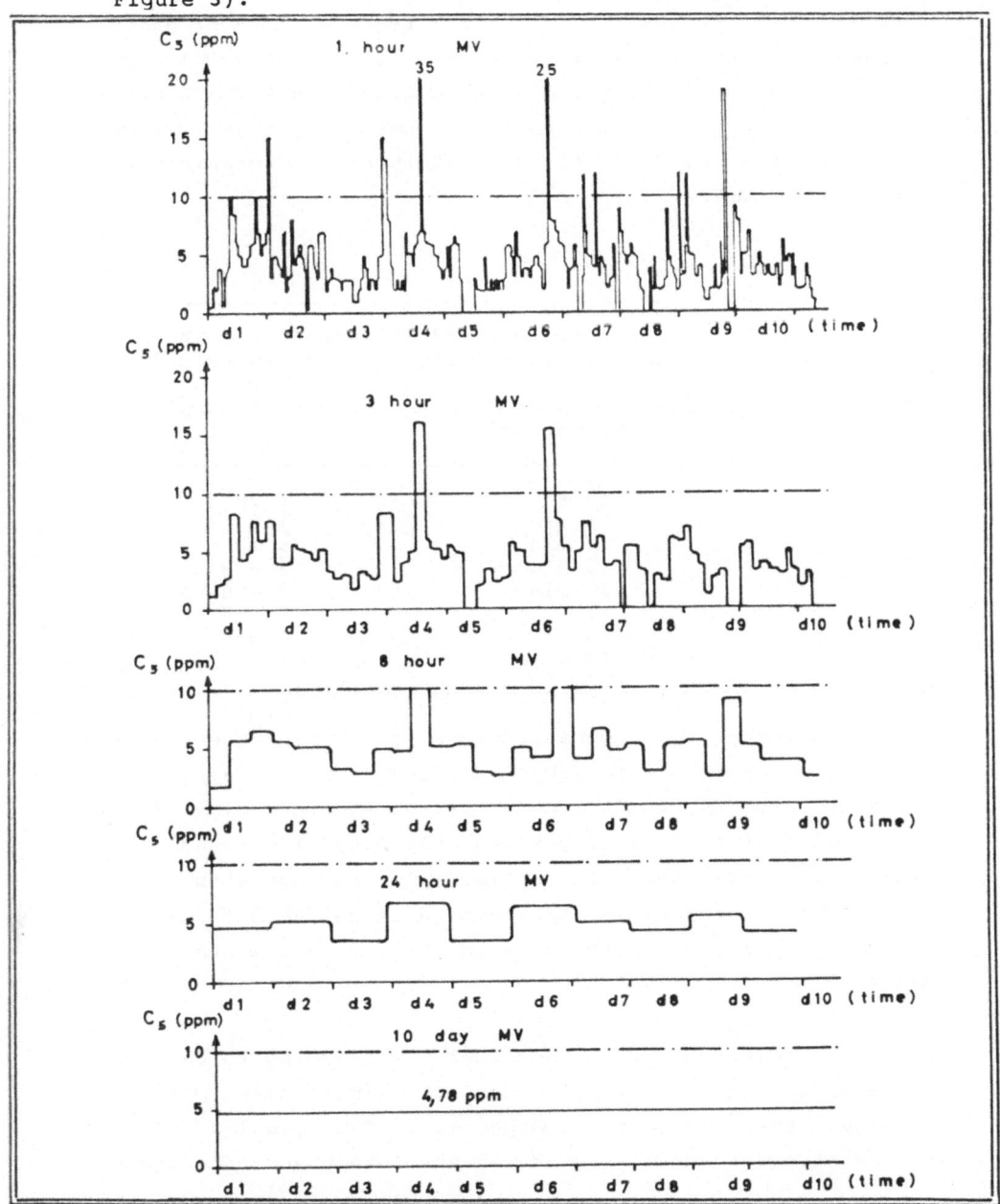

Figure 3 Vinyl chloride concentration at a workplace; mean values (mv) for a series of periods
d = day

The shorter the measurement or sampling period the more samples or spot measurements are required in order to obtain, for example mean value for the shift. Table 1 shows this relationship. Measurement methods using short sampling periods (of seconds or minutes) require 10 - 30 samples because of variations in concentration; these samples must also be taken at intervals throughout the working shift. Sampling periods of 1 to 2 hours are better as they provide a representative picture of the safety of the workplace with only 1 - 3 samples.

Table 1. Number of samples required in relation to the sampling period (mean duration of measurement)

Sampling period ('mean' period)	Number of samples per shift
10 s	$\geq$ 30
1 min	$\geq$ 20
5 min	$\geq$ 12
15 min	4 - 8
30 min	3 - 6
1 h	2 - 4
2 h	1 - 2
>4 h	1

The measurement of concentrations of toxic agents at the workplace consists of sampling and analysis. Sampling and analysis can be conducted either at the same time (from a technical point of view, particularly easy with gases) or at different times and places (usually the case with dusts). Measurement methods may be regarded as suitable for ambient monitoring if they comply with the requirements set out below.

i) The measurement method must be adapted to the toxic agent under investigation, the limit value applicable and the working atmosphere. The results of the measurement must provide an absolutely accurate account

of the concentration of the constitutent to be
measured. The measurement values must be expressed in
the terms used for the limit values (mg/m^3) or in an
easily convertible form. The measurement value should
not be distorted by more than $^+$ 10% by the effects of
.. temperature, humidity or sensitivity to other agents in
the working atmosphere.

ii) The correctness of the measurement method must be
checked by control tests, e.g. with standardised
methods, or mixing tests, e.g. using test gases.

iii) The detection limit, sensitivity and accuracy of the
method must be adapted to the limit value concerned.
It must be possible to measure concentrations of the
toxic substances in question at levels of at least 1/5
to 3 times the limit value.

iv) The measurement method must have been tried out in
practice and should not be too expensive for routine
workplace monitoring. (Methods which work in a laboratory are not necessarily sufficiently resistant and
interference-free for practical use).

From a layman's point of view, the choice of methods for the
technical monitoring of the working atmosphere has become
almost infinite as a result of the rapid development of
sampling and analysis techniques in the past ten years.
Personal measurements, stationary measurements at a
particular place, continuous or discontinuous measurements,
separate sampling and analysis, or immediate concentration
recording techniques are all possible and can be combined in
a number of ways.

Very often the only reason for going no further is that the
expenditure is not justified or the techniques are too
complicated for routine use in the works or plant. Despite
the apparently vast number of possibilities, it is often

difficult in practice to find a suitable method which fulfils
all the organisational requirements described here.

The assessment of concentrations at the workplace by means of
ambient monitoring is a task which requires a standardised
method following specific rules as highlighted in Figure 4.
The results possible are that:

- the limit value has definitely been exceeded and
  protection measures are required;
- the limit value has definitely not been exceeded and no
  measures are required;
- a clear assessment is not possible (with the result
  laying in a 'grey area') and further measurements will
  have to be made before a decision can be reached.

"Assessment" means comparison of the measuring results
against the limit values for the toxic agents concerned.

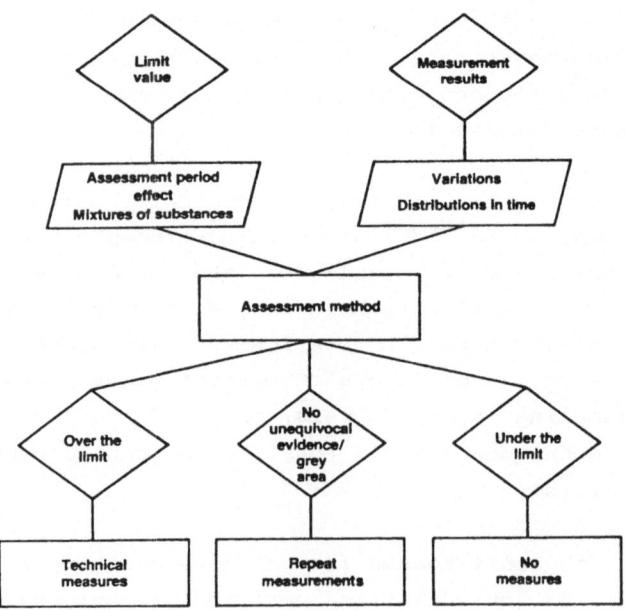

Figure 4.   Ambient Monitoring - assessment

For the assessment method to work the limit values must fulfil a number of requirements. From a technical point of view the assessment period- the period for which the limit value represents a mean value - must be clearly laid down (e.g. hour, day, year).

It would also be logical for the assessment period of the limit value to be adapted to the effects of the agent. Limit values for mixtures are also required.

Because concentrations at the workplace are known to vary considerably in time and each measurement value represents a mean value for the concentration over the measurement period, statistical procedures must be used to assess whether results are over or under the limit values.

Figure 3 gives examples of the pattern of vinyl chloride concentrations at a workplace over a variety of periods. The top diagram shows the 1 - hour mean values over a period of 10 days with three shifts a day. The highest values on the concentration curve are above 20 ppm. The diagram below this shows the 3 -hours mean values at the same workplace over the same period. The highest levels are about 15 ppm. If the mean for the shift is taken, the highest levels for the same period at the same workplace are only 10 ppm. The 10-day mean value (bottom diagram)is under 5 ppm.

For consistent assessment of the content of measurement values:

- the distribution of the measurements in time must be fixed or
- the limit values must be graduated according to the distribution of the measurement values in time.

In the first case the choice of measurement and monitoring methods is restricted for technical and practical reasons. Thus when the EC Directive on vinyl chloride was drawn up, preference was given to the idea of graduating the limit values according to the distribution of the measurement values in time. This procedure suggested itself if only because of the need to take the differing measurement and monitoring rules of the Member States into account, without allowing differences in workplace assessment to result.

The graduation of limit values according to the EC Directive is set out in Figure 5 where the limit value set for the long-term mean concentration of a toxic agent may not be exceeded and where the annual mean for this is 1.0. The limit is being respected as long as the 1 - hour mean values (or 95% of these values) remain under a limit value of 2.5.

The mean limit values for a shift, a week and a month are similarly graduated. The figures on the limit value curve are to be regarded as factors. Thus, if the annual limit value is x, the limit values for shorter periods are calculated from the factors in Figure 6 by multiplying by the value x.

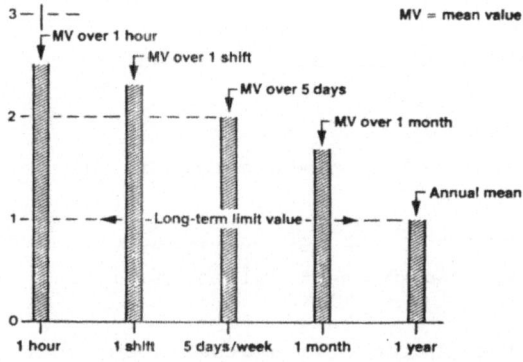

Figure 5. Graduation of Limit Values - vinyl chloride Directive

The problems of the distribution of concentration measurements in time and its effect on assessment was discussed in
detail when the Directive on vinyl chloride was being drawn
up. They apply in principle to all airborne pollutants
encountered at the workplace. There is therefore no point in
discussing these basic statistical questions every time a
Directive is being drawn up on a particular substance. For
cases where the EC Directive on Vinyl chloride is not an
appropriate example a standard definition for the statistical
analysis of measurement results using limit values is
urgently required for further Directives on toxic substances.

RECENT AND POTENTIAL ADVANCES APPLICABLE TO THE PROTECTION OF
WORKERS' HEALTH - AMBIENT MONITORING II

M. CORN (USA)

Summary

Major advances in the conceptualisation of environmental sur-
veillance for determining employee exposure are discussed,
including the strategy of sampling and the evaluation of
total and respirable dust. The acceptance of personal
samplers worn by individual workers and their role, as well
as that of area samples, is now well understood. The
availability of personal samplers specific to chemical agents
is limited and requires vigorous development. Record-keeping
has advanced to include computerised data retrieval systems
for environmental and medical surveillance data. A plea is
made for international exchange of surveillance data in order
to judge efficacy of control methods and to broaden the
population base for epidemiological studies.

Introduction

It is not possible to address recent and potential advances
in ambient monitoring without first indicating the large
number of purposes which drive those who undertake ambient
monitoring in the workplace.

The first and most important purpose of monitoring is to
determine adherence to an established legal standard or
consensus guideline for the quality of the air breathed by
the employee. At the present time, in the United States, all
such standards and guidelines are for individual chemical
species, with the exception of the entities referred to
as total suspended particulate matter ("nuisance dust"), coke
oven emissions and acid mist (expressed as hydrochloric
acid). These each contain many chemical species, but the
legal standards are for the entire weights of material
collected on the sampling filter. Because the effects of air
contaminants in the workplace on the human body vary from
acute to chronic manifestations of disease, the strategy of
sampling for agents having an acute effect or chronic effect
differ. The theory of the relationship between sampling

periods to estimate the dosage of ambient agent to the employee and biological action of the agent was investigated by Roach (1). In general, if the purpose of ambient monitoring is to determine adherence to legal standards, for practical reasons we have proceeded with short-term sampling for both acute and chronic agents. The first purpose of ambient monitoring is to determine if the sample obtained adheres to a standard for agent concentration that was promulgated by a regulatory agency or adopted by an expert consensus group.

Within the framework of sampling to determine adherence to an established standard or accepted guideline, there is the issue of whether to place the sampler on the employee or at a location in the environment. These two types of samples and the associated procedures are referred to as personal and area sampling. In general, it is widely accepted in the USA that personal sampling yields a better measure of employee exposure than does area sampling. In fact, one of the major advances of the industrial hygiene profession in recent years has been the coming to terms with personal sampling, developing satisfactory techniques, and substituting it, wherever possible, when adherence to legal standards and guidelines for personal exposure is to be evaluated.

Another very important purpose of sampling is to indicate trends in improvement or deterioration of the work environment with respect to the contaminant of interest. Such a determination can be carried out utilising either personal or area samples, depending on the context in which the data will be used for decision making.

Ambient monitoring can be carried out at many plant locations. In this case, procedures serve the purpose of a "watchdog" for ensuring the effectiveness of control measures. By placing an ambient monitor in close proximity to the source of chemical contamination, one can determine if leakage increases or decreases and can key the monitor to audible or visual alarms which trigger corrective measures.

Ambient monitoring can be undertaken to provide a historical record of the condition of the workplace. The strategy of sampling for a historical record may be different from the strategy of sampling for the purpose of measuring personal exposure or for determining overall trends.

Ambient monitoring may be undertaken for the purpose of evaluating the need for controls in the vicinity of specific emission sources in the workplace environment.

Ambient monitoring may be undertaken to determine if there is any relationship between parameters of environmental quality and complaints or symptoms of employees. This purpose differs from that of measuring exposure in that employees already have a perception of the inferior quality of the environment. The monitoring is undertaken to support or refute this perception and a suitable sampling strategy is required.

The above assembly is incomplete; there may be other purposes for programmes of ambient monitoring. One of the major advances of recent years is that we have come to recognise the different purposes of ambient monitoring and that different strategies are necessary prior to undertaking each programme of ambient monitoring.

This paper reviews some of the advances in sampling philosophy, strategy and methods that have characterised recent efforts to further the science and the art of determining the quality of the airborne environment in the workplace.

Concepts of ambient monitoring

A major advance in legal and professional thinking in the
United States has been the recognition that the employee has
a right to be informed of the potential hazards of the job in
which he or she is employed. The potential chemical contamination of work-place air is considered such a hazard.
Therefore, in all promulgated standards of the Occupational
Safety and Health Administration in the United States, the
employer is obliged to give the employee a determination of
the quality of the workplace air. The initial determination
of employee breathing zone air quality is usually required
within 30 days of initiation of employment. It is unfortunate that there are still very few such OSHA standards, but
the seminal advance which cannot be ignored is that we have
viewed the satisfactory nature of air quality in the workplace as a right of the employee; the pace of promulgation of
standards will change with economic, political, and professional manpower conditions, but the trend will always be
to produce additional standards. It should be noted that in
promulgated standards in the United States, the employee's
right extends to his own measurement of his air environment,
i.e., a personal sample. The employer may, by analogy to an
identical job classification, indicate to the employee the
character of his/her workplace air environment, but for
different job classifications and different activities the
employee receives his own measurement. Thus, this parameter
of work is viewed in an analogous manner to measurements of
an employee's biological parameter such as blood components
or pulmonary function. After the initial determination, if
the chemical hazard remains in the environment, periodic
assessments of air quality are required. The frequency with
which such assessments are made under the law are related to
whether the standard is met or exceeded. If the standard is
exceeded, measurements must be made more frequently until it
is demonstrated that the standard is being met. The philosophy extends to respirable dust in the mining environment,
which is covered by the Mining Health and Safety Act of 1977.

In my own efforts to counsel managers in the private sector
with regard to their obligations under the General Duty
Clause (2) of the Occupational Safety and Health Act of 1970,
I have indicated that if a material in the workplace has been
associated with known toxicological properties but is not yet
covered by a standard promulgated by law, it still behoves
the employer to fulfill his obligations for an intitial
determination of the potential hazard to which an employee is
exposed. The General Duty Clause is that section of the Act
which requires an employer to provide a safe and healthful
environment for every employee.

A second major advance in the philosophy of sampling ambient
air has been the concept of the personal sampler. The
original evidence for the inadequacy of area sampling was
from the radiation industry, where so-called "hot particles"
were inhaled by individual employees when fixed area monitors
indicated the satisfactory nature of airborne radioactivity
in the area. Subsequent comparison of samplers worn by
individuals and those at fixed locations demonstrated the
discrepancy between results not only in the workplace, but in
outdoor ambient air. It is now widely accepted that by
carrying a sampler which samples air from the breathing zone
of the worker a more reliable estimate of his or her daily
exposure is obtained. There is currently some concern about
variations in results obtained with samplers within and in
close proximity to the breathing zone of sampling, e.g., what
is the breathing zone? Samplers mounted on the same
individual, but at slightly different locations of the upper
body show significant differences in results. However, the
thrust of current effort is to place samplers on the
individual, rather than samplers in the working environment
at a fixed location; personal sampling is and will continue
to be a trend with steady progress at sorting out associated
problems. I shall later discuss the current state of
technology for matching practical sampling procedures in the
field with the philosophical intent of switching to personal
samplers for all determinations of exposures to toxic agents

in the occupational environment. Suffice it to say that our
desires currently exceed our capabilities to perform
measurements for most airborne contaminants.

The third area of major philosophical change with respect to
ambient monitoring in the United States involves the
retention of sampling records. A major goal of the
Occupational Safety and Health Act of 1970 was to lay the
groundwork for understanding the relationship of occupational
environmental factors and disease. The law is explicit in
its intent to develop a body of knowledge so that future
generations will not be exposed to the same potentially toxic
agents which current generations are exposed to, either alone
or in combination. Therefore, our law treats environmental
and medical surveillance records in the same manner. In
general, the sampling records must be kept for a period of
time consistent with the incubation period of the disease in
man with which the agent is associated. Retention times vary
from 40 years for carcinogenic agents such as asbestos, to 5
and 10 years for irritant materials. Table 1 summarises
retention periods for environmental and medical surveillance
records for selected air contaminants.

Table 1. Retention periods for environmental surveillance
under OSHA standards.*

Agent	Retention Time, Years
Asbestos	40 years or employment + 20 years
DBCP	40 years or employment + 20 years
Coke Oven Emissions	40 years or employment + 20 years
Carcinogens	
Formaldehyde	5 years
Phenol	1 year
Nickel (NIOSH Proposed)	40 years after last exposure

*See individual OSHA standard or NIOSH Criteria Document.

A fourth change in the philosophy of ambient monitoring in the workplace has been the movement towards certification of both the individuals who perform monitoring and the laboratories which analyse the samples collected. The underlying reason for this requirement has been the necessity to compare values for concentrations of airborne agents at all locations in the United States. Thus, a government agency (OSHA) is charged on a nationwide basis with sampling and issuing civil and possibly criminal citations for violation of the accepted standard. It has been necessary to establish very detailed procedures for sampling and to gain some assurance that the individuals performing the sampling are fully qualified and capable of performing the technical tasks. The American Industrial Hygiene Association certifies hygienists, and it is viewed as desirable that certified hygienists or safety professionals (the latter certified by the Certified Safety Professionals, a counterpart of the American Industrial Hygiene Association) do perform the sampling. After the sample is collected, laboratories certified by the American Industrial Hygiene Association usually perform the analyses. A list of certified laboratories is published several times a year in the American Industrial Hygiene Association Journal In cases which reach the courts for resolution, one is in a much stronger position if a certified laboratory has analysed the sample. Qualifications for laboratory certification involves satisfactory performance of the laboratory in round-robin testing with standard samples. Other requirements for certification include the supervision of the laboratory by a competent industrial hygiene chemist. The certification of ambient sampling in the United States has both advantages and disadvantages(3). The trend towards certification in the USA continues.

The National Institute for Occupational Safety and Health has issued a large number of recommended procedures for sampling and analysis. Adherence to these procedures is optional: adherence to procedures specified in a standard promulgated by OSHA is required.

Technical aspects of ambient air monitoring

Major recent advances in the technical aspects of sampling
and analysis for airborne contaminants are in the realms of
strategy of sampling and of personal monitoring.

The strategy of sampling is directed at obtaining the minimum
number of valid samples to either (a) ensure compliance with
an existing legal standard for an airborne agent, or (b) to
determine the average exposure of a large number of employees
who are similarly exposed to airborne agents. In the first
case, it is not possible to sample each employee every day,
or even every week. The cost of individual samples is high:
in the case of fibre counts for asbestos or man-made vitreous
fibre, the total cost of an individual sample, including pump
calibration, filter preparation, final counting, and the cost
of sending individual technicians or hygienists to the field,
was approximately $225.00 (4,5). Therefore, it is necessary
to utilise a statistical framework to ensure that the
sampling scheme is valid.

Leidel, Busch and Lynch (6) have offered sampling strategies
to ensure adherence to an existing legal standard. The
strategies are based on assumption of a logarithmic normal
frequency distribution for the agent concentrations in air,
and a lognormal frequency distribution of the sample results
obtained. Within a given confidence interval, it is possible
to estimate the average value of exposure based on a given
number of samples. The standard geometric deviation of the
pollutant concentration in the work environment is not known;
it can be either assumed or based on previous sampling
experience; a limited number of samples can also be obtained
to generate an estimator of the standard geometric
deviation.

In the case of support of epidemiological investigations,
where given work zones (7) are utilised as representing the
environment of designated workers, a statistical framework

based on the assumption of a logarithmic normal distribution of pollutant concentrations has been assumed and shown to be valid (8). With this approach, the value of a strategy of sampling manifests itself in several ways. First, the work zones with the highest exposures are immediately apparent. Second, the contributing values of individual employees (personal sampling) which do not fall within the range of values for the zone are noteworthy because they indicate those employees are receiving exposures not typical of employees in the work zone. The gradation of exposures among work zones can then be related to the findings of medical surveillance of employees in the workplace. Table 2 illustrates data obtained by zoning a man-made vitreous fibre plant (9). Approximately 25% of the employees in the plant could be sampled using an exposure zone concept to obtain approximately the same information that would have been obtained if each employee was sampled. This conclusion was arrived at by literally sampling every employee in the plant and then randomly selecting from the total population of exposure values different numbers of employees for hypothetical sampling. The efficiency of sampling rapidly decreased with worker zone assignments after approximately 20% of employees were sampled. Table 3 indicates results of sampling if random sampling rather than zoning was used. The richness of Table 2 insights into plant problem areas is apparent.

The conscious sampling strategy approach to environmental surveillance has been one of the major advances in ambient monitoring in recent years. Much remains to be done to further improve existing strategies. In the absence of continuous monitoring, it is essential that a strategy of sampling be adopted.

Table 2. Manmade vitreous fibre plan - Results of sampling using zoning and 40, 40 samples

Case 1 - Zoning with 40 samples

Zone	Population at Risk	Sample Size	Range of Agent Concentration				Sample Parameters				Number of Employees Expected to Exceed Standard	
			Entire Zone		Sample						Sample	Entire Zone
			low	high	low	high	median	mean	og	∅ (calculated)	observed	(calculated)
Production A	30	8	1.80	75.47	2.30	75.47	12.56	31.30	3.86	-0.94	7	25
Production B	18	4	1.02	36.2	1.29	15.74	3.97	9.15	3.64	-0.10	2	10
Production C	24	6	1.30	103.7	1.47	8.12	3.49	4.08	1.74	0.01	3	12
Moulding	20	5	1.04	2.33	1.11	2.21	1.64	1.70	1.30	2.89	0	< 0.1
Curing	10	3	1.19	2.94	1.46	1.81	1.62	1.63	1.11	7.38	0	< 0.1
Shipping	8	2	0.92	2.29	1.94	2.00	1.96	1.97	1.02	29.3	0	< 0.1
Quality Control	8	2	0.69	3.06	1.76	2.84	2.23	2.36	1.40	1.33	0	0.7
Maintenance	14	4	0.52	2.34	0.60	2.34	1.27	1.51	1.79	1.74	0	0.6
Forming	14	4	0.70	2.90	0.97	2.59	1.60	1.80	1.64	1.58	0	0.8
Isolated	8	2	0.32	0.94	0.32	0.79	0.50	0.61	1.89	3.05	0	< 0.1

Case 2 - Zoning with 70 samples

Zone	Population at Risk	Sample Size	Entire Zone low	high	Sample low	high	median	mean	og	∅ (calculated)	observed	(calculated)
Production A	30	14	1.80	75.47	1.97	75.47	8.77	19.14	3.49	-0.73	9	23
Production B	18	9	1.02	36.2	1.02	8.24	2.79	4.00	2.33	-0.27	3	7
Production C	24	11	1.30	103.7	1.47	94.0	6.06	14.20	3.69	-0.42	5	16
Moulding	20	10	1.04	2.33	1.04	2.21	1.63	1.67	1.27	3.20	0	< 0.1
Curing	10	5	1.19	2.94	1.64	2.94	2.06	2.11	1.26	2.29	0	< 0.1
Shipping	8	3	0.92	2.29	0.97	2.29	1.61	1.82	1.64	1.57	0	0.5
Quality Control	8	3	0.69	3.06	0.83	2.87	1.61	1.96	1.87	1.24	0	0.9
Maintenance	14	6	0.52	2.34	0.52	2.24	1.05	.24	1.77	2.11	0	0.2
Forming	14	6	0.70	2.90	0.79	2.90	1.58	.83	1.71	1.48	0	1
Isolated	8	3	0.32	0.94	0.38	0.61	0.48	0.49	1.27	8.31	0	< 0.1

Note: In the ∅ (calculated) column, values shown as "< 0.5" indicate less than 0.5; in the Entire Zone (calculated) column, values shown as "< 0.1" indicate less than 0.1.

Table 3. Results of sampling 40, 50, 70 employees using random selection and sampling entire employees in manmade vitreous fibre plant

| Type | Sample Size | Concentration | | | | Sample Parameters | | Number of Samples Expected to Exceed Standards | | Calculated Number of Employees Expected to Exceed Standard in Entire Plant |
		low	high	median	mean	og	θ	calculated	observed	
Entire Plant	154	0.32	103.7	2.52	4.38	2.86	0.31	58	43	58
Random	40	0.37	36.2	2.10	2.94	2.28	0.62	11	5	41
Random	50	0.37	103.7	2.66	5.22	3.19	0.24	20	12	62
Random	70	0.38	94.0	2.40	4.48	3.05	0.34	26	16	56

Table 4. Ambient airborne chemical agents or physical agents which can be assessed with personal monitors

Agent	Device(s)	Comment	Reference
Suspended Particulate Matter Respirable Total	Various electrostatic precipitation	1) Preselector used for respirable dust evaluation 2) Sample content analyzed by a variety of methods	9
Solvent Vapours	Charcoal tube	Absorbed material extracted and analyzed by a variety of methods	10
TDI Phosgene	Sensitized tape	Colour density of tape determined	11
Mercury	Passive diffusion tube with chemically treated surface		12
NO_2	Passive diffusion tube with chemically treated surface		13
Noise	Electronic device	Automatically integrates and computes time weighted average exposure by frequency band, if desired	14
Ionizing Radiation	Film Badge Ionization Chamber	These were the earliest possible dosimeters	

Monitoring

There are few effective personal monitoring devices for specific pollutants, when one considers the broad range of pollutants which should be and often have to be monitored. Table 4 is a summary of the state-of-the-art of commercially available personal monitoring devices for evaluation of employee exposure to potentially hazardous agents during an eight hour workshift. The table also has a column with subjective comments on the ease of use, reliability, and accuracy of these devices. Improved devices for measuring individual employee exposures to toxic agents are desperately needed. The devices that we now have are rudimentary by any standard. Often they are subject to interferences; their sampling efficiency is less than 100%. In the case of charcoal tubes, each compound must be evaluated for collection efficiency. The influence of several simultaneously present compounds has not been assessed. They are also, in many cases, uncomfortable for the wearer. Employees have, in my experience, refused to wear these devices because they interfere with their work tasks. The latter has occurred most frequently with the personal sampling pumps when equipped with cyclones required for sampling respirable dust.

There are relatively sophisticated personal samplers in the area of noise measurement. The personal sampler stores the entire spectrum of sound intensity received in the vicinity of the employee's hearing zone. The sampler is collected at the end of the working day, and by attachment to a device which, in a relatively brief time (seconds), reads the stored signal; an output of average decibel exposure for the time period the device was worn is indicated. The average exposure is based on either A or C scale weighting. Certainly, it is easier to perform this type of signal operation with a sound intensity meter than it is with a chemical monitoring device. However, the goal of personal dosimetry for chemical agents is similar to the current capability for measurement of sound intensity exposure.

The dosimeter for ionizing radiation, i.e., film badge, is
another example, albeit less sophisticated, of our capability
to place upon the employee a relatively simple device and to
obtain by a relatively straightforward evaluation method the
average exposure for the work shift. There have been
experiments in recent years with treated chemical tapes which
receive a stream of air impinging on them or drawn through
them. The tape moves at a slow rate of speed and thus, has a
memory for the amount of agent that caused discoloration
while air was drawn through the tape. After removal from the
wearer, the tape is played back in a sensing device which
detects discoloration and, the tape having been previously
calibrated for discoloration, it is possible to calculate the
average concentration of pollutant in the airstream drawn
through the tape. This is a relatively primitive approach to
the personal monitoring of the chemical agent, but it is a
beginning and indicates the direction we must move.

Because personal dosimetry is in its infancy, there are
numerous errors associated with each measurement. Explicit
recognition of these errors is essential for both regulatory
compliance procedures and estimation of dose for
epidemiological studies. In the USA, OSHA lists Standard
Analytical and Sampling Errors (SAEs) for airborne
contaminants in its Field Operations Manual. Table 5
indicates SAEs for single samples as listed by OSHA. The SAE
is added to or subtracted from the ratio of the measured
contaminant concentration to the Permissible Exposure Level
(PEL) to obtain the lower (LCL) and upper (UCL) values of the
95% confidence limit for the result. Thus, if a Coke Oven
Emissions result (benzene soluble fraction) is $200 \mu g/m^3$,
the PEL is $150 \mu g/m^3$ and the SAE is 0.21, the SAE is used
as follows:

$$\text{Ratio} = \frac{\text{(Measured Concentration)}}{\text{PEL}} = Y = \frac{200 \mu g/m^3}{150 \mu g/m^3} = 1.33 \quad \ldots\ldots(1)$$

$$LCL = Y - SAE = 1.33 - 0.21 = 1.12$$

$$\ldots\ldots(2)$$

$$UCL = Y + SAE = 1.33 + 0.21 = 1.54$$

Table 5   Sampling and analytical error (SAE) for single full
          shift sampling of selected contaminants (15)

Contaminent and type of sample	Collection method	Analytical method	SAE
Coke oven emissions (personal)	Silver membrane filter	Extraction-gravimetric	0.21
Lead and its inorganic compounds (personal)	Mixed cellulose Ester filter	Atomic absorption spectroscopy	0.12
TDI (area)	10 ml nitro reagent	High pressure liquid chromatography	0.10
Vinyl chloride (personal)	Activated charcoal (2 tubes in series)	Gas liquid chromatography	0.15
Asbestos (personal)	Mixed cellulose Ester filter	Phase contrast microscopy	0.25
Sulphuric acid (personal)	Mixed cellulose Ester filter	Ion chromatography	0.14

In this case, the hygienist presumably knows with 95%
confidence that the true result was between 168 and 231
$\mu g/m^3$. For regulatory purposes, the sample was a clear
violation of the PEL. The explicit recognition of uncertainty
in a result due to errors of methodology is a major step
forward in ambient monitoring.

Record-keeping

The Occupational Safety and Health Act of 1970 has stimulated
the development of large amounts of medical and environmental
surveillance data. In moderate to large size organisations,
the data rapidly become unmanageable unless they are stored
on tape. Thus, automatic record-keeping systems have become
common (16). They offer the advantage of permitting data to
be retrieved rapidly and to be analysed for trends and
associations. In some organisations, an entire year of
ambient monitoring can, at the touch of a keyboard, be
printed out at approximately 540 words per minute, by plant

location, employee, work zone, agent measured, etc.
Certainly, the movement to maintain medical and environmental
surveillance records as sales and shipping records are
maintained has been a major advance; methodology continues to
be improved.

Future needs in ambient monitoring

We are in the early stages of transition whereby the art of
ambient monitoring to determine personnel exposures becomes a
science. Each of the areas described above as representative
of major recent advances now requires additional extensive
development. It should be possible to develop personal
samplers that transmit a signal to a central location when
the wearer exceeds a predetermined exposure dosage (concentration x time). The strategies of sampling heretofore
presented require verification in the field. It may be
possible to further improve the efficiency and effectiveness
of these strategies. Finally, there is a need to share
environmental and medical surveillance data nationally and
internationally for the purposes of judging efficacy of
control methods and for broadening the base of populations
studied by epidemiological methods. The precedent has been
set in the pollution field where global watch efforts are in
progress; the purposes differ, but the desire to achieve
together what cannot be accomplished alone is the same motive
which should prompt organised efforts to share occupational
surveillance data on an international basis.

In summary, I have focused on major trends in ambient monitoring, rather than on details of methodological progress.
Improvements in the conceptual and technical bases of monitoring are clearly distinguishable. The task before us is to
increase the pace of development and to establish mechanisms
for international exchange of the data captured by the technical and scientific advances in methodology. The advanced
state-of-the-art of record-keeping will enable this exchange
to occur; the organisational steps must be initiated.

Finally, I would be remiss not to indicate the growing awareness and acceptance of the need for monitoring of individuals for total exposure. It is necessary, but not sufficient to evaluate ·occupational exposure alone. Exposures indoors ("indoor air pollution") and outdoors, as well as the superimposed burden of personal pollution contribute the total dosage to the target organ (18,19). Surveillance of individual exposures in this sense has hardly begun.

References

1. Roach, S: A more rational basis for air sampling programs American Ind. Hyg. Assoc. J.: 1966: 27, 1-8.

2. US Congress, Occupational Safety and Health Act of 1970.

3. Corn, M.: Influence of legal standards on the practice of industrial hygiene. Am. Ind. Hyg. Assoc. J. 1976: 37, 353-356.

4. Corn, M., Y. Y. Hammad, D. Whittier and N. Kotsko: Employee Exposure to airborne fiber and total particulate matter in two mineral wool facilities. Environ. Res. 1976: 12, 59-74

5. Esmen, N. A.., M. Corn, Y. Hammad, D. Whittier and N. Kotsko: Summary of measurements of employee exposure to airborne dust and fiber in sixteen facilities producing man-made mineral fibers. Am. Ind. Hyg. Assoc. J. 1979: 40, 108-117.

6. Leidel, N. A., K. A. Busch, and J. R. Lynch: Occupational Exposure Sampling Strategy Manual, U. S. Dept. of Health, Education and Welfare, NIOSH Pub. No. 77-173, Jan. 1977.

7. Woitowitz, H. J., G. Schacke and R. Woitowitz: Ranking Estimation of the dust exposure and industrial-medical epidemiology, Staub Reinhalt Luft, 1970: 30, 15 (Eng. translation).

8. Corn, M. and Esmen, N. A.: Workplace exposure zones for classification of employee exposures to physical and chemical agents, Am. Ind. Hyg. Assoc. J. 1979: 40: 47-57.

9. Lippman, M.: "Respirable Dust Sampling" in Air Sampling
    Instruments, 5TH Ed. 1978 Amer. Conf. Govt. Ind.
    Hygienists, P. O. Box 1937, Cincinnati, Ohio 45201, G-1
    to G-23.

10. NIOSH Manual of Analytical Methods, 5 Vols., Dept.
    Health, Education and Welfare Publications.

11. MDA Scientific, Inc. 808 Busse Highway, Parkidge, Ill.
    60069.

12. Marketed by the 3M Company, Minneapolis, Minnesota.

13. Palmes, E. D., A. F. Gunnison, J. DiMattio and C.
    Tomczyk: Personal sampler for nitrogen dioxide. Am. Ind.
    Hyg. Assoc. J. 1976: 37 570-577.

14. Several US manufacturers market these units.

15. US Department of Labor, Occupational Safety and Health
    Administration, Industrial Hygiene Field Operations
    Manual, Vol. VI, OSHA 3058, Section IX. 1980.

16 For example, see Lichtenberg, F. W. and G. E. Devett:
    The Medical Data Base System of Owens-Corning Fiberglass
    Corporation. Am. Ind. Hyg. Assoc. J. 1980: 41, 103-112.

17 Budiansky, S.: Indoor air pollution. Environ. Sci.
    Tech. 1980:

18. US Environmental Protection Agency, Contract No. 68-
    02-2294: The Status of Indoor Air Pollution Research,
    1976.   Final Report by Goemet, Inc., 15 Firstfield Road,
    Gaithersburg, Md. 20760, Oct. 1976.

RECENT AND POTENTIAL ADVANCES APPLICABLE TO THE PROTECTION OF
WORKERS' HEALTH - BIOLOGICAL MONITORING I

P. HUGHES (USA)

Summary

Monitoring consists first of making and recording measure-
ments on health and environmental indices and second of
collating and interpreting data arising with a view to
detecting changes in the health status of populations and
their environment; the first requires planning and standard-
isation and the second analysis and evaluation.

The purpose of monitoring overall is to assess recognised
occupational health risks and to evaluate their control;
of environmental monitoring to measure the dose of the
hazardous agent absorbed by the worker at his place of
work; and of biological monitoring among other things to
provide base-line data and to identify persons likely to
be vulnerable to certain exposures. Environmental and
biological monitoring should be viewed as being complementary
and not as alternative procedures. However, there are
circumstances that do not permit joint monitoring and it then
becomes necessary to give greater emphasis to one or the
other and in this paper the relative appropriateness of each
is considered together with criteria for the selection of
tests. Examples are given of medical surveillance of
workers exposed to chemical hazards on the job.

Introduction

The accepted objectives of an occupational health programme
are met in large part by identifying and bringing under
control at the workplace all chemical, physical, mechanical,
biological and psychosocial agents that are known to be or
suspected of being hazardous.

The techniques used for measuring the characteristics of the
work environment and for determining the biological response
characteristics of man constitute the basis of the modern
practice of occupational medicine and hygiene. Such practice
includes the routine assessment of control measures to ensure
that exposure levels are kept within prescribed limits for
continued health maintenance or to provide early warning of
impending ill health, this indicating the need for additional

preventive action. The experience gained so far demonstrates the need for the continuing monitoring of health and
the environment in workplaces.

In the preparation of the introductory portion of these
remarks, I have drawn upon two reports from the World Health
Organisation, one documenting the contributions of an expert
committee called to examine issues in environmental and
health monitoring, (1) and the other conveying the views of a
study group convened to consider some broader aspects of the
medical surveillance of workers exposed to chemical and
physical hazards on the job.(2)

The value of monitoring

Monitoring has two distinct functions: first, the making of
routine measurements on health and environmental indices and
the recording and transmission of these data and, second, the
collation and interpretation of such data with a view to
detecting changes in the health status of populations and
their environment. The distinction is important because
these functions involve different types of skill. The first
requires careful planning and the use of standardised techniques and methods of data collection. The second requires
analysis and evaluation, which lead to recommendations for
preventive action. It will be possible to broaden the
coverage of health surveillance of working populations by
making fuller use of technicians and, where available,
automated procedures for monitoring. One of the most
important aims in current practice is to raise the efficiency
of monitoring and to ensure comparability of data from
different groups of research workers (and within the same
group over a period of time) by standardisation of
techniques.

Monitoring is carried out in order to assess recognised
occupational health risks and evaluate their control by
(i) providing the necessary data to ensure that environmental

protective action is initially taken against health risks and to ensure that workers arc placed in jobs suiting their capacities; (ii) providing continuing evaluation to ensure that adequate protection is maintained; (iii) obtaining an accumulating body of data for epidemiological use to show the comparative effectiveness of the engineering and medical aspects of preventive programmes and, where appropriate, to permit the redefinition of permissible levels of exposure.

Environmental monitoring

Environmental monitoring (or occupational hygiene monitoring, as it is often known) makes use of an extensive battery of instruments to assess a variety of physical and chemical exposures at work.

The purpose of the procedures used for environmental assessment is to measure the dose of the hazardous agent absorbed by the worker at his place of work. This means that the assessment of the environment is not just an exercise in physical or chemical analysis but has its base in the biological characteristics of man, and the relevance of the results depends on the adequacy of the "biological calibration" of the analytical procedures.

Biological monitoring

Preplacement medical examinations serve the purpose of proper job placement according to the physical and mental capabilities of the worker, but also make it possible to identify persons likely to be vulnerable to certain exposures; for example, those with chronic obstructive pulmonary disease can be identified and excluded from work in dusty occupations. Another function is to provide baseline data that make it possible to measure early adverse effects of exposure in persons at risk.

Periodic medical examinations serve several purposes: to detect early impairment of health; to evaluate the effectiveness of preventive measures; to detect workers showing undue susceptibility to a particular environmental exposure; and to reveal trends in the health status of groups of workers.

Such examinations utilise the particular diagnostic procedures and the additional physiological, biochemical, and other tests that are required to demonstrate the presence of health impairment, if any, and its extent and severity. Their specificity and sensitivity depend on the depth and detail of knowledge of the cause-and-effect relationship in question and on the extent to which various monitoring systems have been evaluated, discarding the less reliable for the more reliable techniques. In the monitoring of lead workers, use is made of clinical signs and symptoms of lead absorption such as levels of porphyrins, delta-aminolaevulinic acid and aminolaevulinate dehydratase. In hearing conservation, temporary threshhold shift of hearing acuity is used as an early indicator of permanent threshhold shift.

Complementary roles of environmental and biological monitoring

The two approaches - measurements of environmental exposures and health assessment of exposed workers - should not be regarded as alternative procedures. They are, in fact, complementary and should be carried on in parallel to ensure the proper management of the occupational health maintenance programme. This is especially true when dealing with newly reognised hazards for which the dose/response relationships are not fully known.

There may be circumstances that do not permit joint environmental/biological monitoring, and it then becomes necessary to give greater emphasis to one or the other.

There is no complete agreement on the relative importance of environmental and medical monitoring. Some would rely entirely on environmental exposure limits, arguing that the workers should not be used as sampling devices. Others believe that the only meaningful index of hazard is "absorption" and that it makes little difference what the stress levels are in the work environment as long as workers are protected through periodic health examinations. Both these views are extreme, and not generally held.

The environmental monitoring of physical and chemical agents may be emphasised when the hazard is a specific one for which a permissible exposure limit is known and when occupational hygiene personnel are available. Biological monitoring, on the other hand, should be emphasised as the main tool for evaluating environmental control measures and is the only means for detecting total health effects. When occupational hygienists are not available, complete dependence must be placed on medical monitoring, which may, however, be expanded to include consideration of environmental factors.

Other factors should be considered when choosing between environmental or health monitoring: the level of risk, the number of subjects exposed, the latent period between exposure and onset of ill effects, variations in individual responses, exposure by routes additional to inhalation, and the range of fluctuations in exposure. Continuous environmental monitoring is necessary if the effects of exposure are serious or acute, if there is a danger of sudden high exposure, if the population at risk is large, and if the permissible limit is a ceiling value.

Using man as a biological monitor may or may not give a better estimate of magnitude of exposure than direct measurement of environmental concentration, depending on how well the measured internal concentration reflects the magnitude of the effective dose in critical organs or sites within the body. (1)

Changes in biochemical parameters as measured in various biological fluids may often be among the more sensitive indicators of early changes in health due to hazardous agents in the work environment. Such changes represent a reaction to the exposure to the hazardous agent and may, in some cases, indicate an actual effect on health. In other cases, they may only indicate homoeostatic and compensatory mechanisms, which are reversible. In still other cases they may indicate minor cellular damage for which regenerative processes are sufficient to preclude health inpairment. Thus, quantitative evaluation of biochemical parameters and the establishment of dose-effect/response relationships are essential.

Advances in analytical technology have made it possible to identify and quantify numerous biochemical parameters that were previously unrecognised. Many of these parameters are still only of value in research studies - some because they require complex instrumentation, others because the significance of the observed changes has not been established. Thus, in the choice of specific biochemical parameters their predictive validity as regards exposure and impending or actual health impairment is an important criterion. Only a few have a well-established predictive validity; some only have value when used in adequately designed epidemiological studies. Automatic analysis with microtechniques has not only promoted the measurement of multiple components but has also helped to provide a profile that may be important in health evaluation.

Since cells and tissues generally respond in a limited number of ways to a wide variety of different stresses, the changes observed are often not specific. At times the quantitative nature of the change provides somewhat greater specificity, but in most cases an independent means of establishing exposure to a particular agent will be a prerequisite for confirming a cause-effect relationship. In a specific work environment with an established exposure to

one or more hazardous agents, certain biochemical parameters
may be considered as specific for practical purposes. This
is particularly true when the pre-exposure values for the
biochemical parameters have been determined. Non-specific
tests may have particular utility in that they show the
integrative effect of exposures to combinations of hazardous
agents and stresses. (2)

Criteria for selection of tests

The choice of tests for examining groups of workers may be
limited for certain practical reasons:

- the test should not carry a risk to health and
  should not be too inconvenient to the subjects
  examined;
- the test data should be in the relevant range of
  occupational exposure, at a dosage range below or
  around permissible limits;
- levels of the contaminant measured in exhaled
  air, blood, or urine must be quantitatively relatable to an adverse health effect;
- measurements of metabolites or biochemical
  changes resulting from the inhalation of contaminants, must also be quantitatively relatable to
  an adverse health effect;
- biological tests must yield information on potential health risks equal or superior to the information obtained by air sampling;
- facilities for accurate biological measurements
  must be readily available.

In addition, the following criteria should be adhered to if
possible:

- high validity (sensitivity, specificity) i.e.,
  the test data should reflect the true situation
  under investigation;
- with increasing exposure (intensity and/or
  duration) the deviation from normal of the test
  data should increase quickly i.e., there should

be a steep dose-effect/response curve;
- the analytical error and biological variability should be small in comparison with the changes in data to be expected.

The test may often be conducted in several stages, advancing from simple procedures with less predictive validity as a screening mechanism, to more elaborate tests with better predictive validity, limited to a selected population.

It should be stressed that the test methods should be clearly specified and standardised; evaluation requires rigid adherence to such standardised methods, otherwise the data will not be comparable. At present there is a great lack of data on comparability of methods applied in various occupational health studies. The use of reference substances is desirable in order to provide a basis for comparison of the predictive validity and reliability of multiple methods, especially in cases where a new biological testing technique is being introduced and where its suitability and sensitivity for testing a certain type of action is to be checked. (2)

Among the biochemical tests proposed for use in biological monitoring are those designed to measure changes in enzymatic activity caused by damage to specific organs such as liver, kidney or bone marrow; in non-enzymatic proteins as detected by electrophoretic and immunochemical methods; or in neuro-humoral responses. The development of analytical techniques continues as further research elucidates significant metabolic pathways.

Clinical considerations in biological monitoring in the field

The clinical evaluation of several types of chemical intoxication may include the determination of the concentration of the suspected toxin in blood, urine, or breath, its metabolite in urine, or an affected enzyme in serum. The biological monitoring of exposed workers on a periodic basis is also

of value in maintaining surveillance of the health of those
exposed to certain metals such as lead, mercury, cadmium,
arsenic, selenium, tellurium, thallium, zinc and manganese,
as well as to fluoride. Useful tests in emergencies include:
carboxyhaemoglobin with suspected carbon monoxide exposure,
methaemoglobin with aniline and a few other chemicals, phenol
in urine with benzene exposure, trichloroacetic acid in urine
with trichloroethylene, and cholinesterase in serum with
organophosphates. The detection of arsenic in hair and
fingernails might also be mentioned in the evaluation of a
suspected chronic exposure.

These are among the simpler, longer established procedures.
We could now add to the list changes in the pattern of serum
proteins, chromosome aberrations, the presence of circulating
antibodies and perhaps sputum cytology. Considering biological tests in general, many score high in sensitivity, but
unfortunately, rather low in specificity. The results are
then difficult to interpret.

But in fact, only a few of the more basic tests are now used
widely in occupational health practice, such as fluoride in
urine, and lead in blood and urine. These are well validated
procedures, with which there has been a good bit of clinical
experience. The absorption, distribution, and excretion both
of fluoride, and of lead, has been studied carefully over the
past forty years or more. The literature provides a sound
basis for the interpretation of findings, and in turn, a
reliable measure of the level of exposure of the individual
to the substance.

There are, in fact, only a quite limited number of biological
procedures that have proven to be this useful, although many
others have been proposed. Even the long established practice of determining mercury in urine has not been entirely
satisfactory; while it is of some value in estimating absorption, there is no generally accepted critical level of
mercury in urine above which intoxication can be expected.

The same limitation applies to the interpretation of manganese levels in the urine.

More recently, a number of tests have been introduced based upon the effect of the toxic agent on metabolic processes. Returning to lead, the inhibition of delta-aminolaevulinic acid dehydrase (ALA-D), an enzyme involved in porphyrin synthesis, leads to an increase in levels of delta-aminolaevulinic acid (ALA) in blood and urine. The blood and urine levels of coproporphyrin III, and free erythrocyte protoporphyrins (FEP), are also usually elevated. FEP combines with zinc in the blood to form zinc protoporphyrin (ZPP), which is the half assayed. While ALA-D, ALA, coproporphyrin III assays, and blood examinations for haemoglobin, reticulocytes, and stippled red cells may be useful in the assessment of the health of the exposed worker, no one of these measurements alone is an accepted specific index of lead absorption in the same manner that the determination of the lead level in blood in useful.(3)

So while the search goes on for chemical tests relatively simple to perform, yet of a high degree of specificity, the results of which may be interpreted with reasonable confidence, there are not very many such tests at hand today.

That is not to say that we don't have useful methods for monitoring the health of individuals exposed to chemical and physical hazards at work. There are a number of tests and procedures which, used in combination, carefully performed, and interpreted intelligently, permit judgments as to the relative hazard of a job, especially when employed along with environmental monitoring.

A multitest approach is often utilised, preferably as part of a physical examination. This practice, when related to chemical or physical hazards of the job, constitutes medical surveillance.

In our practice in one aluminium and chemical company, we
first identified by industrial hygiene means all of the
chemical and physical exposures encountered in our work
processes, setting these down on a chart, and listing for
each, among other things, any biological monitoring that
should be employed, as well as other techniques of medical
surveillance.

We selected our procedures from three sources: from an OSHA
health standard if one has been promulgated for that chemical
or physical stress, from a NIOSH criteria document if one has
been compiled, and from the experience we gained as contrac-
tors to NIOSH in drafting medical surveillance requirements
for substances covered by the NIOSH/OSHA Standards Completion
Project of 1974-76.

We produced a large chart covering all the hazards to which
any of our employees are exposed, the jobs on which exposures
occur, the health effects of overexposure, and medical
surveillance requirements including techniques of biological
monitoring. From the chart, we constructed the scope of
examination to which each employee is entitled, based upon
job assignment.(4)

For example, a potroom worker in an aluminium smelter is
exposed to fluoride and to particulate polycyclic organic
matter, (PPOM), both released from the large electrolytic
cells (pots) in which aluminium oxide is reduced to metallic
aluminium. Since the electrolytic bath operates near
$1000^{O}C$, there is exposure to heat, as well as to noise.

Overexposure to fluoride causes irritation of the eyes and
respiratory tract. Absorption of excessive amounts over a
long period of time may cause increased radiographic density
of bone; i.e., osteosclerosis due to deposition of fluoride,
detectable by pelvic X-Ray, which we utilise.

Since the main avenue of excretion of fluoride is through the kidneys, a screening urinalysis for sugar, protein, and blood is required to determine if kidney function is adequate. We also determine the pre-exposure urinary fluoride concentration for a baseline - step one in biological monitoring.

Because of the risk of respiratory irritation, chest X-Ray and pulmonary function tests are desirable.

As regards the other exposures of the potroom worker: PPOM is suspect of producing an increased risk of lung cancer and perhaps of leukaemia, based upon recent mortality studies, so we are interested in early methods of detection, such as sputum cytology for lung cancer, and a complete blood count for leukaemia.

Adding together the medical surveillance requirements for fluoride, PPOM, heat and noise, the preplacement and periodic examination of the potroom worker includes, in addition to medical history and physical examination these monitoring procedures: complete blood count and determination of haemo-globin, routine urinalysis plus urinary fluoride level, sputum cytology, pulmonary function, X-Ray of the chest and the pelvis (the latter at only six year intervals), electro-cardiogram and audiogram.

We utilise the preplacement examination to establish a baseline, and we repeat the procedures yearly - more frequently if indicated by the findings.

This is a flexible system. As we encounter new chemicals, or as epidemiological investigation suggests previously unrecog-nised hazards, or as new biological monitoring procedures are introduced and validated, the examination procedure can be modified quite readily.

Conclusions

Certain conclusions may be drawn from this brief overview of
the medical surveillance of workers exposed to chemical
hazards on the job.

    i) Many changes detected by biological monitoring
       are non-specific if observed in an individual
       worker. However, the specificity may increase
       when a group of workers is examined and compared
       with a control group.

   ii) Many changes are not sensitive if no baseline
       values are known. The sensitivity can be increa-
       sed by measuring pre-exposure levels, or by
       comparison with control groups.

  iii) The sensitivity and specificity of changes may
       increase if several parameters are examined at
       the same time.

   iv) The specificity of changes will also increase if
       the hazardous work factor is taken into account,
       particularly if the exposure is measured quanti-
       tatively (degree and duration of exposure); i.e.,
       if health evaluation is combined with environ-
       mental monitoring. Only then can dose-response
       relationships be established.

References

1. World Health Organisation. Environmental and health
    monitoring in occupational health. Geneva: World Health
    Organisation, 1973. (Technical report series No. 535)
    5-8; 11-15; 20.

2. World Health Organisation. Early detection of health
    impairment in occupational exposure to health hazards.
    Geneva: World Health Organisation, 1975. (Technical
    report series No. 571) 27-28; 38-39; 71.

3. Proctor, N.H., Hughes, J.P. Chemical hazards of the
    workplace. Philadelphia: Lippincott, 1978, 307-309.

4. Proctor, N.H., Hughes, J.P. Chemical hazards of the
    workplace. Philadelphia: Lippincott, 1978, 12-21.

RECENT AND POTENTIAL ADVANCES APPLICABLE TO THE PROTECTION OF
WORKERS' HEALTH - BIOLOGICAL MONITORING II

R L ZIELHUIS (NETHERLANDS)

Summary

*In the recent past there has been confusion as to the defini-
tions of ambient monitoring (AM), biological monitoring (BM),
and health surveillance (HS). This paper presents new
definitions of AM and BM which should more clearly define
the various concepts and help to distinguish them from HS.
It also presents a short review of the attitude of national
authorities of the countries of the European Community to
biological monitoring and discusses points of ethics concerning the introduction of BM in occupational health practice.*

Definitions

In 1977 the Commission of the European Communities, the World
Health Organisation and the Environmental Protection Agency
(CEC-WHO-EPA) organised an international Seminar on the Use
of Biological Specimens for the Assessment of Human Exposure
to Environmental Pollutants (Berlin et al, 1979). Ambient
(or as it is often called: "environmental") Monitoring (AM)
was defined as "systematic collection of environmental
samples for analysis of pollutant concentrations" and
Biological Monitoring (BM) as: "systematic collection of
biological specimens for which analysis of pollutants is for
immediate application". This year (4-9 Aug.1980) an
International Course on Biological Monitoring was organised
in Helsinki (Aitio (Ed) 1981). During this course the terms
AM (EM), BM and Health Surveillance (HS) were repeatedly
discussed, because apparently confusion existed. Taking into
account the discussions during the Course I proposed new
definitions of BM and of AM, which are not contradictory to
the 1977-definitions, but which - in my opinion - more
clearly define the various concepts (Zielhuis 1981a).

I will maintain the specific limited definition of BM as
agreed upon by CEC-WHO-EPA in 1977, and in various meetings
of WHO and of CEC. Too many experts still apply a much

broader definition which comprises both periodic assessment
of exposure and health risk and .periodic assessment of health
status (effects). They combine the limited definition of BM
and the term Health Surveillance (HS) (or Health Effect
Monitoring). Quite different approaches are taken together
and, moreover, in an erratic way. This conference should once
again decide upon a specific definition of BM, in order to
prevent further confusion.

At first we have to consider the term "Monitoring".
According to various dictionaries "monitoring" implies:
testing, watching, observing; a continuous or repetitive
activity; a specified objective; a comparison of the
data observed with a reference level. Moreover, if there
exists a discrepancy between the observed data and the
reference level, corrective action has to be undertaken, -
depending on the sign of the difference - in negative or
positive direction. These aspects should be retained in the
definitions of AM and of BM. So, I came to the following
definition of BM: "systematic continuous or repetitive
activity for collection of biological samples for analysis of
concentrations of pollutants, metabolites or specific non-
adverse biochemical effect-parameters for immediate application, with the objective to assess exposure and health risk
to exposed subjects, comparing the data observed with a
reference level, and - if necessary - leading to corrective
action". This definition of BM contains the essential
elements of the term monitoring and also those of the
definition agreed upon in 1977. It has to be operationalised
for BM in occupational health, in environmental health, in
clinical practice, and also in ecotoxicological studies. The
specific objective, referring to specified agents and to
groups exposed, has to be precisely defined. In contradic-
tion to monitoring in general, there is only one direction of
corrective action (except in clinical practice): decrease of
exposure levels, because in the case of xenobiotic agents the
reference level, which is a maximal individual ceiling or
group average level, is never a goal to be aimed at, but a

level not to be exceeded. In addition to the pollutants or
their metabolites, a few rather specific, non-adverse and
reversible effect-parameters can be included, e.g. inhibition
of ALA-D-levels or increase of ZPP-levels in erythrocytes in
the case of exposure to inorganic lead, inhibition of ChE-
levels in erythrocytes in the case of exposure to organo-
phosphate-insecticides.

HS as such should clearly be distinguished from BM, because
HS aims at measuring health effects, adverse and/or non-
adverse, reversible and/or non-reversible, specific and/or
non-specific effects, and - per definition - is not a
preventive action as such. However, in practice both BM
and HS often are combined, particularly when the BM levels
approach the reference level. Ultimately, AM, BM and HS
serve the same objective: prevention of health risk and
health impairment.

Two Objectives

Both AM and BM assess exposure and health risk, whereas HS
assesses the health status. This dual purpose of BM and AM
needs further clarification, because it proved to be a point
of confusion in Helsinki. Moreover, this will give me the
opportunity to clarify the difference in information to be
derived from AM and from BM.

If one speaks of exposure, one should distinguish three
concepts:
1. Exposure in the general sense
    One measures concentrations (C) in e.g. air, food,
    beverages. C is expressed in mg/m^3 (air), mg/kg
    (food), mg/l (beverages), mg/m^3 or mg/l (skin).
In addition the frequency, duration and variability in time
(T) has to be considered.

2. Intake (I)

    One measures the amount offered to various routes
    of entry:
    - inhalation: C x respiratory volume (m^3)
    - ingestion : C x weight (kg) or volume (l)
    - skin   : C x exposed (cm^2) x thickness of
                  layer (for liquids: cm)

Consequently, I is expressed in e.g. μg, mg, g, kg. This
corresponds to the dose administered in clinical therapy. I
also takes into account physical activity. Because usually
in AM measurement of C only allows to approximate the
dose, one hesitates to apply the term dose-effect/response-
relationships, but one prefers to speak of exposure-effect/
response-relationships.

3. Uptake (U)

    U is the amount absorbed, i.e. I multiplied with
    the various functional absorption factors for e.g.
    lung, gastrointestinal tract, skin.

The kinetics of agent A_i in subject B_i is determined by
both the physico-chemical properties of A_i and the biological characteristics (e.g. liver-, kidney function, clearance
in respiratory tract, pregnancy, fatty mass, age, sex) of
subjects B_i. Together they determine the internal dose and
the concentration at the effector sites (C_{eff}). If C_{eff}
exceeds the critical concentration, adverse health effects
may occur (not: do occur).

Taking into account T, there exists a relation between C and
I, as measured or approximated in AM, and with U and C_{eff}
as measured or approximated in BM. It is evident that in AM,
even when the concentration in all environmental media (air,
food, beverages, or skin) are measured, many factors are not
taken into account, which determine the relation between C
(and T) and U and C_{eff}. If I is measured, and not only C,
the predictability of U and of C_{eff} will be improved. When
concentrations in biological specimens or amounts excreted
are measured, U and C_{eff} will be better approximated than
in AM, not in the least because also the biological characteristics of the subjects exposed are taken into account.

In <u>routine</u>-AM and BM the following triangle is assumed to be known:

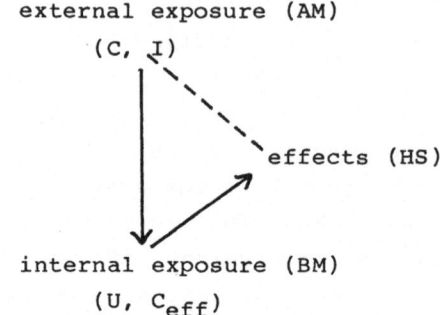

The broken arrow is only hypothetical. AM too easily relies on this <u>hypothetical</u> relationship, whereas BM takes into account the <u>actual</u> relationship. Only in the case of agents which exert a local effect, the broken arrow signifies the actual relationship; in that case BM is not feasible.

It is evident that AM first of all measures or approximates external exposure, and indirectly the health risk (C_{eff}). BM measures or approximates internal exposure and indirectly external exposure by means of parameters which allow a better estimation of health risk than in the case of AM.

<u>AM and/or BM?</u>

Whether one applies AM or BM in occupational health depends upon the specific objective, the state of the art, the available expertise and equipment. It is not a matter of principal preference for one approach. In the design of technical preventive measures AM will be preferred, but in the case of assessment of exposure and of health risk, both approaches may have their place, either subsequently or in combination, either primary or secondary. BM has one great drawback: at this moment routine BM can only be applied for a limited, although widely used number of agents. However, if available knowledge exists, BM has great advantages over AM: assessment

of total exposure; the impact of activity and of dermal
absorption is taken into consideration; it may require less
time and expenditure of manpower. From the health point of
view, BM has much to be preferred: it takes into account the
biological characteristics, and so allows to elucidate the
inter- and intra-individual variability in internal exposure
and in health risk. BM is a medico-biological approach,
which may serve to assess the actual exposure and health risk
more adequately than AM alone.

In this Seminar practical, legislative and ethical aspects
will be discussed. I will not do this at this moment. Up to
now various reviews have already been published on the
advantages and limitations of B.M., e.g. Zielhuis (1978,
1979, 1981b, 1981c), Lauwerys (1981).

BM in the European Community

The Director of the Health and Safety Directorate of CEC
asked me to present in this introductory paper a short review
of the attitude of national authorities (Labour Inspectorate,
Ministry of Labour and Social Affairs, Ministry of Employment, Health and Safety Executive) of the nine CEC-countries.
I have put the following three questions which could be
answered by "yes" or "no" to the nine representatives of
these national authorities.

1. Does your Department consider biological monitoring
   as a method to be promoted as an important measure
   in the prevention of health impairment?

2. Does your Department consider to introduce in the
   future biological "standards" for some agents,
   which will have in your country about the same
   significance as standards for concentration in air
   (e.g. MAC, TLV)?

3. Does your Department take initiatives to promote
   and finance research activities for development of
   biological monitoring methods, in order to broaden
   the application in practice?

I have received answers from 7 governments. Some representatives presented a lengthy sentence to express their view from which I had to extract a "yes" - or "no" - answer. I take the responsibility for my interpretation, without binding the governments to my "black-white" answers. Nevertheless, I am convinced that "yes" corresponds to a very positive attitude of various governmental authorities.

	Question 1 (BM as such)	2 (BM-standard)	3 (promotion and financing BM-research)
Denmark	yes	yes	yes
Belgium	yes	yes (part of medical examination, and submitted to administrative regulations)	no (very limited budget)
Federal Republic of Germany	yes	yes (also by means of regulations of occupational health insurance)	yes
United Kingdom	yes	yes	yes
Ireland	yes	yes	no (not yet)
Italy	yes	yes	yes
The Netherlands	yes	yes	yes

The CEC itself also promotes the BM-approach viz the publication of small monographs on BM-methods, and, moreover, by imposing a lead in blood standard (CEC, Directive December 1979).

At this moment a biological standard for lead in blood (Pb-B) is already in force or is expected to come into force in the near future in all countries mentioned. If this step is taken, then the road is open for more biological standards, e.g. for COHb in non-smokers ZPP in blood, trichloroacetic acid (TCA) in urine or blood, mandelic acid (MA) in urine, cholinesterase inhibition (ChE) in blood.

Ethical Aspects

Finally I will discuss shortly three points of ethics, concerning the introduction of BM in occupational health practice, which I discussed more at length previously (Zielhuis 1978, 1979, 1981b), and which will be discussed more fully in this seminar.

One of the respondents wrote to me that "BM should be carried out where the tests are simple, specific, economic, acceptable to the worker, etc.". I do not agree fully with this statement. Too easily one wants to rely on simple tests, which are assumed to present a valid estimate of exposure and of health risk. Of course, one should apply simple and economic tests, if available. But first of all one should apply valid tests. The Pb-B test is by no means a simple test, because it requires very experienced personnel and expensive equipment. Fortunately, the simple ZPP-test very probably can predict whether Pb-B will exceed 600 g/l, and so can be added as a simple prescreening test. TCA in urine may allow an estimate of group average exposure to trichloroethylene, but TCA in blood at the end of the workweek probably will present a much more reliable indicator of exposure and of health risk. Although blood analysis will be more inconvenient to the worker, he will agree to it, if he can be convinced that such an analysis offers better assessment of his individual health risk. No manager will use simple tests to check the risk of bad performance of his machinery, if more costly tests allow him a more valid answer, and in the end will save money. Sophisticated tests will then be economical. There certainly is no reason to take another attitude to the workers, who are valuable as human beings, the value of whom, however, cannot be expressed in money.

BM is a biomedical approach, and, therefore, it should be in the hands of the occupational health department. Evaluation of the ambient environment requires the expertise of the industrial hygienist; evaluation of biological data requires

the expertise of a well educated physician, because the biological levels are determined both by exposure and by individual biological characteristics. Moreover, in the view of
the worker, it is a part of his/her medical examination.
This requires specific training of the occupational health
physician in e.g. the toxicokinetics and toxicodynamics of
various agents. Moreover, I fully agree with one of the
respondents who wrote: "Biological results are the property
of the individual and cannot be released in any identifiable
form to the company or any other. Biological results cannot
be hidden from the individual worker". BM-data should be
evaluated, often together with data on the health status by
the occupational physician, and communicated and discussed as
personal data within the client-physician relationship. Only
grouped data, not identifiable to individual workers, can be
presented to management, workers' councils, and the
Inspectorate of Labour.

Finally, some antagonists of BM sometimes refer to BM as
experimentation, in which workers are treated as
"experimental rabbits": expose the rabbits and look whether
"effects" occur. They tend to emphasise ambient monitoring,
because this portrays external exposure, which may lead to
technical measures to decrease exposure. However, they
neglect the fact that the actual health risk is determined
by internal exposure, which also depends upon biological
characteristics of the workers. If a worker is exposed
externally he will also be exposed internally. Internal
exposure levels are not to be considered "effects", but they
indicate the probability of effects ad hoc or in the future.
BM allows a better prevention of group and individual health
risk than AM alone, at least if occupational health physician,
management and Labour Inspectorate actually use the BM data
as a preventive tool. The reference level not to be exceeded
should be a topic of ongoing study. The responsible
authorities should never try to regard this reference level as
an optimum to be achieved; moreover, management should clearly
show its willingness to decrease exposure if indicated, by

technical measures and by e.g. making facilities available for frequent washing of hands, clothes, etc.

Because BM is a medico-biological approach, the ethical aspects of prevention in occupational health perforce become more easily in the open than by relying on AM alone, because BM is a more personal approach, which cannot be carried out without active cooperation of the workers themselves.

I am convinced that further development of BM-methods, and - subsequently - wide application in practice, will serve the prevention of health impairment in workers. However, if we want to achieve this, we at first must have a clear and consistent idea what BM is.

Conclusion

A modified definition of biological monitoring (BM) is presented: "systematic continuous or repetitive activity for collection of biological samples for analysis of concentrations of pollutants, metabolites or non-adverse biochemical effects for immediate application, with the objective to assess exposure and health risk to exposed subjects, comparing the data observed with a reference level, and - if necessary - leading to corrective action". BM more validly estimates the concentration in effector organs and the health risk than ambient monitoring. Within CEC there is a very positive attitude to promote BM and to set biological standards. Sophisticated tests may have to be applied for sake of optimal prevention of health risk. Because BM is a bio-medical approach, the data should be treated as personal data, not to be identified as such to others.

References

1. Aitio, A. (Ed.). Proceedings Course on Biological
    Monitoring. Helsinki, Aug. 1980; in the press 1981.

2. Berlin, A., A.H. Wolff, Y. Hasegawa. The use of
    biological specimens for the assessment of human
    exposure to environmental pollutants. The Hague,
    Nijhof, 1979.

3.. Council European Economic Community (CEC). Proposal
    for a Directive, December 1979.

4. Lauwerys, R. General aspects of biological monitor-
    ing. In: Aitio (Ed.), 1981.

5. Zielhuis, R.L. Biological monitoring. Scand. J.
    Work Environment. Health 4 (1978) 1-18.

6. Zielhuis, R.L. General aspects of biological monitor-
    ing. In: Berlin et al (1979), p. 341-359.

7. Zielhuis, R.L. Concepts of biological and environmen-
    tal monitoring, and of health surveillance (1981a).
    In: Aitio (Ed).) 1981.

8. Zielhuis, R.L. Theoretical and practical considera-
    tions in biological monitoring (1981b). In: Aitio
    (Ed.) 1981.

9. Zielhuis, R.L. Approaches in the development of bio-
    logical monitoring methods: Laboratory and field
    studies (1981c). In: Aitio (Ed.) 1981.

CURRENT USE OF AMBIENT AND BIOLOGICAL MONITORING: REFERENCE
WORKPLACE HAZARDS. INORGANIC TOXIC AGENTS - CARBON MONOXIDE I

E. P. RADFORD (USA)

Summary

With modern methods of measuring carbon monoxide in air, or in workers themselves, now widely available and well tested, it should be mandatory that these techniques be applied wherever carbon monoxide exposure is likely to be frequent in the work place. The relative merits of area, personal, and individual biological monitoring of exposure are discussed. While continuously recording area monitors and portable or personal samplers are useful, supplementation of these techniques by alveolar gas or blood measurements is often necessary.

Introduction

Medical effects of exposure to carbon monoxide (CO) have been known for nearly 100 years, and the mechanisms by which CO affects oxygen delivery to optical organs have been extensively studied. As a result, we are able to predict the effects expected from exposure for varying times to different concentrations of this colourless, odourless gas (1). We are concerned not only with acute exposures to CO that can be rapidly life-threatening, when the fraction of haemoglobin found to the CO in the blood reaches 50% or more, but also with repeated exposures to lower concentrations, which may be associated with chronic effects on the nervous system or predispose to myocardial ischaemia, even if no acute symptoms are experienced (1).

In view of the extensive physiological and medical knowledge concerning the risks of exposure to CO, it is incomprehensible that workers in industries where the presence of CO is likely to occur usually do not have adequate assessment of their exposures, necessary to assure that preventive measures are, in fact, effective. In small operations, such as in automobile repair shops, extensive monitoring equipment is usually not practical, and education and appropriate exhaust removal are the principal methods that have to be invoked to prevent over-exposure. But even in these cases, routine monitoring of CO by simple colorimetric methods (see below) carried out by regulatory personnel on an occasional basis can detect shops in which infractions of good practices may lead to potentially serious exposures.

In large industrial operations involving furnaces, roasting procedures or other situations where incomplete combustion occurs routinely, or when CO is used as a fuel, as in the steel industry, there is no excuse for the occurrence of over-exposure to CO. Repeated episodes when workers are overcome means negligence on the part of medical and supervisory personnel.

The most common control method employed in these kinds of operations is to install continuous CO analysers as area monitors. These commercially available devices can be set to sound an alarm when the concentration exceeds a preset level. In my experience, however, this approach is often inadequate, for several reasons. First, area monitors may be placed too far from potential sources, especially accidental leaks; substantial concentration gradients can exist within even a well-ventilated building when the CO at the source is at high concentration. Thus serious exposures can occur even though the monitor may indicate low concentrations. Second, because clinical symptoms of CO poisoning are slow in onset and are relatively non-specific in nature, excessive exposure can often occur even if none of the workers complain of symptoms. In this case, warning alarms may come to be ignored because supervisors assume that nothing is wrong and it is the analyser that is in error, or that the hazard is negligible even if the alarm is sounding. Third, even if the alarms are heeded, the usual advice to workers is to go outside for a short period until the hazardous condition has been corrected, at which time they are returned to work. Such brief removal from exposure does not mean that the concentrations of blood carboxyhaemoglobin will be reduced, because the time for elimination of CO is on the order of hours when the worker is breathing CO-free air at standard conditions.

Monitoring of exposure conditions can be improved both by personal samplers or by simple portable analysers. Portable analysers include variants of the monitoring devices, cited above including the Ecolyser, a relatively inexpensive commercially available portable device that depends on electrochemical oxidation of CO to produce the output signal. In my experience, however, colorimetric tubes through which a standard volume of air is drawn (such as e.g., Draeger tubes) are sufficiently accurate if used properly that they are adequate local monitors even for low concentrations, and they have the advantage of low cost and long shelf-life.

The problem with portable air samplers is that CO exposures in the workplace may be episodic and not predictable, and thus intermittent grab samples may not be very informative. Similar problems exist for personal samplers, such as pump-operated air samplers. The exposure may have occurred long before the results are obtained from chemical analysis of the sample. One eminently practical solution is to use, as personal samplers, chemical badges exposed directly to the air and which darken when exposed to CO. These devices, which usually involve reaction of palladium salts with CO, would have to be tested for cross reactions with other air-borne constituents of the particular work environment. More-over, their sensitivity under conditions of concern remains to be determined.

It is evident from the above discussion that continuous, spot sampling or personal monitoring of CO in air is not fully satisfactory in assessing potentially hazardous occupational exposures to this gas, especially acute exposures. In some applications these methods may be satisfactory, but I believe that in general the best monitoring device is to evaluate the men themselves. Under any condition where exposure is suspected, there should be available an area where a personal biological sample can be obtained. Either alveolar gas or blood can be used to assess cumulative exposure.

Alveolar gas sampling

Because it is a non-invasive method, determination of CO in alveolar gas as a measure of percent carboxyhaemoglobin in blood has great advantage, but the method has its limitations. Sampling has to be done in an area free of CO, and there should be time taken to allow the alveolar gas to equilibrate with CO-free inspired air. Also, this method cannot be used with persons who have chronic lung disease, in whom the alveolar gas composition tends to be extremely variable. Moreover, the subject's cooperation is essential. Despite these difficulties, skilled personnel can achieve reliable results.

The theory of measuring carboxyhaemoglobin by measuring alveolar gas is based on the idea that under certain conditions the gas in the lungs will equilibrate with the blood. Measurements of the gas phase can then be applied to determine carboxyhaemoglobin by use of the Haldane relationship:

$$HbCO = M \frac{pCO}{pO_2} HbO_2$$

The oxygen partial pressure in the arterial blood, pO_2, can be assumed; pCO, the carbon monoxide partial pressure, is the measured quantity, $\underline{M}$ is the Haldane constant (equal to 220 with very little individual variation at physiological pH); and oxyhaemoglobin concentration is assumed to be appoximately 1 -carboxyhaemoglobin concentration.

The problem in using this method is to approximate equilibrium conditions when the gas composition is actually changing at all times. Two manoeuvres have been tried to achieve equilibrium conditions, rebreathing and breath holding. With rebreathing, the subject breathes in and out into a bag. A gas sample is taken after a specified number of breaths. Since oxygen is being continuously removed and carbon monoxide concentrations are a function of both the oxyhaemoglobin present as well as the total volume of the lungs and bag, this is a complex system with equilibrium difficult to achieve. For this reason the rebreathing method has been replaced by the breath-holding method (2).

Jones et al. (2) have shown that when a subject holds his breath, alveolar carbon monoxide concentration increases initially as carbon monoxide leaves the blood to equilibrate. As the alveolar oxygen falls, however, carbon monoxide is reabsorbed into the blood due to the fall of oxyhaemoglobin and the Haldane relationship. Thus alveolar pCO will go through a maximum depending on the duration of breath holding. Jones et al. (2) concluded that 20 seconds was the optimum period of time for both practical and theoretical reasons and this technique is now standard.

The subject expires to residual volume, inspires maximally, holds his breath for 20 seconds, and then breathes out as far as possible. With the aid of a three-way valve, the first 500 ml of expirate is discarded, and the remaining gas is collected by turning the valve to an air-tight bag. The gas in the bag is then analysed with standard gas analysers. For field use the Ecolyser has proved to be a rugged and reliable instrument.

Theoretically, based on the Coburn-Forster-Kane equation (3), the slope of the graph relating the percent concentration of carboxyhaemoglobin to alveolar pCO in ppm should be about 0.155 at sea level for carboxyhaemoglobin value equivalent to between 0 to 50 ppm, and progressively lower for higher concentrations. Various researchers have reported discrepancies in the results. Forbes et al. found a ratio of 0.14 (4), Sjostrand found 0.16 (5), and Ringold et al. found 0.20 (6). Smith (unpublished observations) showed that the slope

was about 0.18 and did not decrease at higher carboxyhaemoglobin percent concentrations, as would be expected, because
equilibrium was reached less effectively. A calibration
curve relating measured CO in alveolar gas to carboxyhaemoglobin concentration should be established by each group
using the method.

Spectrophotometric measurement of carboxyhaemoglobin in blood

The most precise indicator of CO exposure and of its potential medical significance is direct measurement of carboxyhaemoglobin. The most convenient and simple methods are spectrophotometric techniques. Although they may not be highly
accurate at carboxyhaemoglobin concentrations below 5%, they
are capable of detecting higher concentrations with sufficient reliability. The spectrophotometric determination of
carboxyhaemoglobin is dependent on the difference between the
carboxyhaemoglobin absorption curve and the absorption curve
for other forms of haemoglobin that are present at certain
wavelengths of electromagnetic radiation.

A number of spectrophotometric procedures have been developed
that vary in sophistication and accuracy. Klendshoj et al.
(7) diluted blood 1:100 with dilute ammonia, added solid
hydro-sulphite, and measured the absorbance at 555 and 480
nm. The addition of the hydrosulphite prevents presence of
any other but the two pigments, carboxyhaemoglobin and
reduced haemoglobin.

Both of these have the same absorbance at 555 nm but different absorbances at 480 nm. The ratio of absorbance, 555/480,
decreases with increasing carboxyhaemoglobin. It is evaluated using a standard curve prepared by analysing known
standards. This method is simple, rapid, and sufficiently
accurate to determine a 2-5% change in carboxyhaemoglobin
concentration.

Small et al. (8) used blood diluted about 1.70 in dilute ammonia and made absorbance measurements in the Soret Region (410-435 nm) at four wavelengths with a 1-nm light path. A series of simultaneous equations are used to estimate the percent carboxy-haemoglobin, the percent methaemoglobin, and by difference the percent oxyhaemoglobin. The accuracy of this method is $\pm$ 0.6% at low carboxyhaemoglobin concentrations and $\pm$ 2% methaemoglobin at concentrations below 20%.

The most convenient spectrophotometric procedure is automated differential spectrophotometry carried out with a carbon monoxide oximeter (manufactured by the Instrumentation Laboratory Co.) described by Malenfant et al. (9). In this method measurements of the three-component system containing reduced haemoglobin, oxyhaemoglobin, and carboxyhaemoglobin are made at three appropriate wavelengths: 548, 568 and 578 nm. The instrument carries out three simultaneous absorbance measurements at the three wavelengths on an automatically diluted, haemolysed blood sample. The signals are then processed by an analogue computer and displayed in digital form as total haemoglobin and the percent concentration of oxy- and carboxyhaemoglobin. This instrument is commercially available and widely used and accurate measurements at carboxyhaemoglobin concentrations above 5% can be carried out readily.

Conclusions

Carbon monoxide is a gas commonly associated with combustion processes in industry. Its pathologic physiology and potentially lethal effects have been well known for decades, thus there is no reason why adequate protection of workers from it cannot be achieved. Because very significant exposures can occur with minimal symptoms, an important element of protection is in knowing the degree of exposure by use of one of the methods described above.

References

1. Carbon Monoxide. Committee of Medical and Biological Effects of Environmental Pollutants. Nat'l. Acad. Sciences, Washington, D.C., 1977.

2. Jones, R.H., M.F. Ellicott, J.B. Cadigan and E.A. Gaensler. The relationship between alveolar and blood carbon monoxide concentrations during breathholding. Simple estimation of COHb saturation. J. Lab. Clin. Med. 51:553-564, 1958.

3. Coburn, R.F., R.E. Forster and P.B. Kane. Considerations of the physiological variables that determine the blood carboxyhaemoglobin concentration in man. J. Clin. Invest. 44:1899-1910, 1965.

4. Forbes, W.H., F. Sargent and F.J.W. Roughton. The rate of carbon monoxide uptake by normal men. Amer. J. Physiol. 143:594-608, 1945.

5. Sjostrand, T. A method for the determination of carboxy-haemoglobin concentrations by analysis of the alveolar air. Acta. Physiol. Scand. 16:201-210, 1948.

6. Ringold, A., J.R. Goldsmith, H.L. Helwig, Finn, R., and F. Schuette. Estimating recent carbon monoxide exposures. A rapid method. Arch. Environ. Health 5:308-318, 1962.

7. Klendshoj, N.C., M. Feldstein and A.L. Sprague. The spectrophotometric determination of carbon monoxide. J. Biol. Chem. 183:297-303, 1950.

8. Small, K.A., E.P. Radford, J.M. Frazier, F.L. Rodkey and H.A. Collison. A rapid method for simultaneous measurement of carboxy- and methaemoglobin in blood. J. Appl. Physiol. 31:154-160, 1971.

9. Malenfant, A.L., S.R. Gambino, A.J. Waraksa and E.I. Roe. Spectrophotometric determination of haemoglobin concentration and per cent oxyhaemoglobin and carboxyhaemoglobin saturation. Clin. Chem. 14:789, 1968.

CURRENT USE OF AMBIENT AND BIOLOGICAL MONITORING REFERENCE
WORKPLACE HAZARDS. INORGANIC TOXIC AGENTS - CARBON MONOXIDE
II

P.J. LAWTHER (UK)

Summary

*The different advantages of monitoring the ambient air and of
biological monitoring for carbon monoxide are demonstrated.
Techniques are reviewed ranging from the detector tube,
through the canary, to blood carbon monoxide analyses.*

The purpose of this short essay is to demonstrate, by
reference to a common and dangerous toxic gas, the different
advantages of monitoring the ambient air and of 'biological'
monitoring by which is meant the measurement of some index of
the body burden of a pollutant. For many reasons which will
be discussed, it would be difficult to select a pollutant
better suited than carbon monoxide to illustrate the
differences in techniques.

Though the title of the session implies that attention be
confined to hazards in work places, the relevance of the
selection of carbon monoxide as a model pollutant for the
illustration of the points mentioned above is enhanced by the
fact that there are many adventitious sources of this gas
which may alter the extent to which the working environment might be blamed for the body burden attained. The Chief
Employment Medical Adviser's Notes of Guidance (published by
the Employment Medical Advisory Service of the Health and
Safety Executive in the UK) begins its note on this gas:

"Of all the gases which have poisonous effects on man and
animals, carbon monoxide, CO, is the most widely met. Over
half of all reported industrial gassing fatalities are caused
by carbon monoxide."

It is well known that its hazardous nature is enhanced by the
fact that it is colourless, odourless and non-irritant. It is
produced wherever carbon-containing substances are burned in
an inadequate supply of air. Such processes include many

industrial activities, but include domestic heating and cooking, the burning of petrol in motor cars, and the smoking of tobacco. There are other processes, such as inert gas-shielded welding and the manufacture of certain synthetic compounds using CO as a raw material, which may be hazardous. Clearly, the value of monitoring of the air in the workplace will have limitations in the light of the non-industrial sources to which the worker may often be exposed.

The methods used for monitoring the concentration of CO in ambient air of workplace, home or street (remembering that the home or the street is the workplace of many people) will depend on the use to which the results will be put. They may be needed to make 'spot' measurements in a confined space to determine whether or not the atmosphere is safe enough for a workman to enter it for a short time; there may be a need to monitor carbon monoxide in a vehicular tunnel so that an alarm might sound if the CO concentration reached a selected value; a common need is to monitor the air in work places so that the Threshold Limit Value (commonly 50 ppm) is not exceeded. A comprehensive account of the methods available (though not necessarily all are recommended nor are they in common use) is given by Commins in the useful publication of the proceedings of a European Colloquium 'Health Effects of Carbon Monoxide Environmental Pollution' held in Luxembourg in December 1973, under the auspices of the Commission of the European Communities (EUR 5242 defin). No attempt will be made here to cover the same ground; reference may be made to that paper or to standard text-books on the measurement of air pollutants. A few of the commonly used methods will be mentioned.

For spot checks the detector tube has many advantages. Air is drawn by means of a calibrated hand pump through tubes packed with an absorbent impregnated with chemical reagents which change colour when exposed to CO. The length of the stain or the colour shade is used to indicate the concentra-

tion of the gas. They necessarily lack precision but are
easy to use and accurate enough to be used to test atmospheres for safety for short exposures. The use of non-
dispersive infra-red analysers enables continuous monitoring
to be carried out and is useful for the analysis of spot
samples collected in bags. Electro-chemical reactions have
been exploited in instruments which give a rapid response
time; the measurement of the heat of reaction when CO is
oxidised by catalysts such as hopcalite gives satisfactory
results. 'Wet' chemical methods are more suited to individual research projects which do not merit the acquisition of
analysers. Mass spectometry, dual isotope fluorimetry, gas
chromatography have their special advantages and advocates
for use in continuous monitoring. The results from all
instruments which measure the concentration of CO in air are
of value only if the need for making them is clearly
specified. Their value in predicting the COHb content of the
blood of those exposed to contaminated air is limited by
extent to which the subject has acquired CO in his blood from
extraneous sources and by his activity. These considerations
greatly favour the use of biological monitoring.

CO is absorbed by inhalation. The kinetics of absorption and
of desorption are described competently by Antweier in the
proceedings of the Colloquium to which reference has already
been made; more detail can be found in the Annals of the New
York Academy of Sciences 1970 __174__ article 1 pp1-430
(Biological Effects of Carbon Monoxide) and a simple version
of the factors governing absorption and exhalation of CO may
be found in the review 'Carbon Monoxide' published in British
Medical Bulletin, Lawther, 1975 __31__ 3 256-260. In addition to
these useful accounts there have appeared complex mathematical models for the prediction of the ultimate COHb levels
following exposure under various complex conditions. A
detailed review of these matters in this brief essay would be
inappropriate. Suffice it to recall the facts: the COHb
levels in an exposed individual will depend on his initial
COHb, the CO and oxygen content of the air breathed, the

duration of the exposure, and his pulmonary ventilation. At
rest in an atmosphere containing no CO the half life of
COHb in the blood is about 4.5 hours; this is shortened by
hyperventilation and the addition of oxygen to the inspired
air. Figure 1 shows in simple form the rates of increase in
COHb on exposure to four CO concentrations at two levels of
activity assuming COHb = 0 initially (there is always some
COHb present as the result of breakdown of Hb in the body).
The rough values at equilibrium are given as derived from the
Haldane equation. Such a simple diagram, and tables
constructed from such calculations are invaluable for
prediction of the likely COHb values which might follow a
known exposure, but it is rare to have exposure to constant.
ambient concentrations. As they fluctuate, absorption
increases, decreases, or may become negative; the subject
might lose CO gained from smoking or faulty ventilation of
his house or he might, by virtue of his extraneously acquired
CO find himself well advanced along one of the curves
depicted in Fig 1. Little more need be said to extol the
merits of biological monitoring at least as an adjunct to the
prudent monitoring of CO in ambient air.

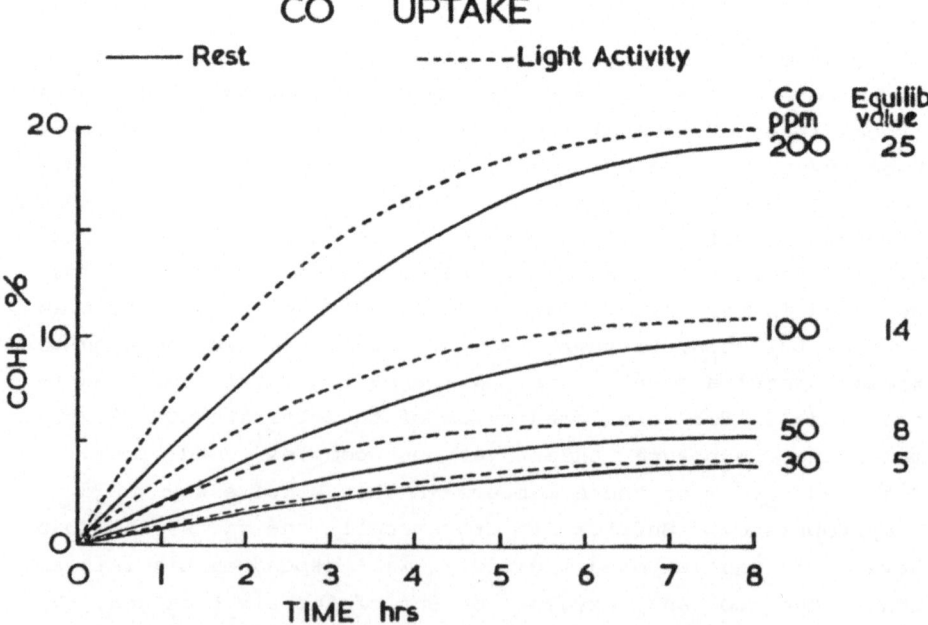

Figure 1   Rates of increase of COHb on exposure to
             carbon monoxide

Many methods are available. Probably the oldest method is
the use of the canary by miners who are likely to encounter
CO underground. Warning of lack of oxygen and the presence
of dangerously inflammable gas mixtures may be given by the
Davy lamp but the fact that a small bird can reach equilibrium with ambient CO much more quickly than does a man with
about 5.5 litres of blood enables ample warning to be given
of CO in certain dangerous ranges. It is said that a canary
will reach equilibrium with ambient CO in about 20 minutes
whereas a resting man might take 6 hours. If the ambient CO
is 2500 ppm a canary will fall off its perch in 4 minutes.
So, in comparatively high concentrations the canary will have
much value to the man carrying it. But a canary can live
happily in a CO concentration of 500 ppm whilst a man will
eventually show marked symptoms from such an exposure. There
are other obvious limitations of the use of canaries.

There is a frequent need to assess the COHb levels in
blood; there is an abundant 'literature' on the effects
on health of chronic exposure to CO either from smoking or
work (some of the published work is of dubious quality) and
calculations based on some estimates of the parameters
mentioned above can only give rough approximations for the
reasons given. It might be trite to state that the human
body is stuffed with a reagent which absorbs CO avidly, has
a 'pump' which requires no external power source, is mobile
and is truly the object of concern. He is his own 'personal'
sampler and it follows that the determination of his COHb by
analysis rather than by calculation is highly desirable in
any assessment of the hazard constituted by exposure to CO.
Strangely, this fact is often forgotten.

Again, as in the case of air monitoring, many methods are
available for the determination of COHb. Again, most are
described by Commins in the proceedings of the CEC Colloquium
to which reference has been made. There is an adequate
bibliography for those who would wish to make their own
assessment of the validity and applicability of any method

to their own problem. Methods for the analysis of COHb by direct examination of blood vary from those in which the CO is extracted from the blood by the addition of reagents and application of vacuum and the subsequent determination of the gas in air by various means to the more convenient and more sensitive spectrophotometric methods. Methods using the mass spectrometer and gas chromatography have much to commend them. Reference ought to be made to a review article such as that by Commins before a method is chosen. (He has written a more extensive review in Ann.Occ. Hyg. 1975 18 69-77.) The choice might depend on the availability of some instrument already in use for the analysis of ambient air if the ranges can be adjusted. There are advantages in using samples of blood obtained by venipuncture but several micro-methods which require only finger-prick samples are convenient and accurate. It cannot be assumed that a subject will prefer a simple finger-prick to the more elaborate procedure for the collection of venous blood. There are, however, many advantages in the determination of COHb by analysis of expired air which has come to equilibrium with the pulmonary blood flow. They are simple and non-traumatic; use can be made of CO analysers already in use for air monitoring; they have a disadvantage in that some assumption must be made of Haldane's affinity factor (M) in the construction of a curve expressing the relationship between CO in the exhaled air and COHb. But they suffice for the purposes of much biological monitoring where calculation of likely blood values would be far too imprecise to be of value.

There are many examples in the literature of the use of all the methods mentioned briefly in this short essay and referred to in the larger review articles, the most convenient of which is that by Commins. This essay has been prepared for a seminar; examples of the application of different techniques in different circumstances can be shown during presentation and subsequent discussion.

CURRENT USE OF AMBIENT AND BIOLOGICAL MONITORING: REFERENCE
WORKPLACE HAZARDS. INORGANIC TOXIC AGENTS - CADMIUM I

R. LAUWERYS (BELGIUM)

Summary

*Cadmium, a naturally occurring element, may be absorbed via
food and tobacco in the case of the non-occupationally exposed person and via fumes and dust in the case of the occupationally exposed person. It is efficiently retained in the
organism, the liver and kidney being the two main sites of
deposition; in man, the biological half-life has been estimated to exceed ten years. Prevention of the acute toxic
effects of cadmium can only be brought about by keeping the
airborne concentration of cadmium below a certain level.
Prevention of the chronic effects of cadmium can be assisted
by reducing inhalation and by better personal hygiene such as
washing the hands. There is no reason to postulate the existence of a relationship between the airborne concentration of
cadmium and the amount absorbed; a biological monitoring programme which includes the determination of cadmium in blood
and in urine offers several advantages over environmental
monitoring. It is suggested that a biological limit value
should be considered as a primary guide for the prevention of
health impairment and a time-weighted average exposure value
for cadmium in air, a secondary or technical guideline.*

Introduction

Cadmium is a naturally occurring element. In non-occupationally exposed persons, food and tobacco consumption represent
the main sources of exposure to cadmium. Exposure in industry is to fumes and dust which enter the organism through
inhalation and ingestion. Cadmium is efficiently retained in
the organism, the liver and the kidney being the two main
sites of deposition. In man, the biological half life has
been estimated to exceed 10 years (for a review, see
Environmental Protection Agency US 1979; Friberg et al. 1974
Lauwerys 1978, 1979a; W.H.O. 1979).

Prevention of acute effects of cadmium

In man, acute excessive exposure to cadmium by the pulmonary or the oral route may cause an inflammatory reaction in
the lungs and in the gastro-intestinal tract respectively. In

animals, acute administration of cadmium can cause toxic
effects in many organs, but the relevance of these effects to
humans is probably limited. In practice, the main acute risk
of cadmium in industry is the occurrence of chemical pneumonitis due to the inhalation of freshly generated cadmium oxide fume. Cadmium dust is less acutely toxic for the lung
than cadmium fume (Lauwerys, 1979 b).

The prevention of the acute toxic effects of cadmium on the
lungs can only be prevented by keeping the airborne concentration of cadmium below a certain level. The local effect
of cadmium does not lend itself to a biological surveillance
programme. A World Health Organisation (WHO) task group (WHO
1980) has concluded that a short term ($<$ 1 h) exposure limit
for cadmium oxide fume and dust of 200 μg Cd/m^3 will
prevent the occurrence of acute lung damage in workers with
normal lung function.

Prevention of the chronic effects of cadmium

In workers, the two main target organs after long term exposure to cadmium are the lungs and the kidneys. Other organs
(bone, liver, haematopoietic system etc.) can also be affected, but in workers, these lesions occur later and less
frequently than renal dysfunction (Lauwerys, 1979 b).

A WHO task group (WHO 1980) has recently concluded that the
epidemiological data concerning the carcinogenic activity of
cadmium in man "are not yet conclusive because of the limited
number of workers involved in the majority of the studies and
the difficulty in some investigations to evaluate the possible role of other carcinogenic agents, like tobacco smoke.
The lack of adequate data precludes presently the consideration of the potential carcinogenic activity of cadmium to
derive a permissible level of exposure."

Some studies among groups of the general population have
implicated cadmium as an aetiologic agent in the development

of cardiovascular diseases, in particular hypertension
(Lauwerys, 1978). Such a relationship has not been established in cadmium workers. In some strains of rats, repeated
administration of cadmium can induce a slight hypertensive
effect (Perry et al., 1979; Ohanian and Iwai, 1979), but the
relevance of these observations for man remains to be
assessed.

It is generally recognised that in workers chronically
exposed to cadmium signs of renal dysfunction occur usually
before significant respiratory impairment.

The lung disturbances found in some workers chronically
exposed to cadmium result probably from a local toxic action
of the metal on the pulmonary tissue. Although individual
factors (lung antitrypsin activity, exposure to other lung
irritants like tobacco smoke etc.) may play a role in the
lung reaction to cadmium, one can logically assume that their
intensity is related to external exposure parameters (amount
of cadmium deposited in the lung and duration of exposure).

A WHO task group (WHO 1980) has concluded that to prevent any
deleterious effect on the respiratory system, the time
weighted average exposure to cadmium fume or to respirable
cadmium dust (aerodynamic diameter $<$ 5 μ) should not exceed
20 to 50 μg Cd/m^3 (duration of exposure: 40 h per week
during the whole professional life).

However, as already indicated above, in long term low level
occupational exposure to cadmium the kidney is more frequently the critical organ than the lungs. It is usually accepted
that renal damage occurs when the amount of cadmium stored in
the organ has reached a critical value (Friberg et al., 1974;
Lauwerys et al., 1979 c).

The recommendation of an atmospheric permissible limit of
exposure may not be sufficient to prevent undue cadmium
absorption and hence the occurrence of renal dysfunction.
Several arguments support this conclusion.

First of all, the pulmonary route is not the only exposure route in industry. Oral absorption may also play a significant role.

The following observation made by Adamsson et al. (1979) illustrates this point. They collected the faeces from 15 cadmium battery workers during the last two days of a normal working week and they measured their cadmium content.

During the same week, cadmium in air was determined by the use of personal samplers. The workers were subdivided in two groups:

- 7 smokers
- 8 non-smokers

Although the average airborne concentration of cadmium to which both groups were exposed was rather similar (7 - 10 $\mu g/m^3$), the faecal excretion of cadmium was 2 to 3 times more important in smokers (x = 619 μg/day) than in non-smokers (x = 268 μg/day). Even in non-smokers the concentration of cadmium in faeces was 30 times higher than that found in the control population (approximately 20 μg/day). Since the workers were exposed to relatively low concentrations of cadmium in air, the amount which could be expected to be transferred from the lung by the mucociliary clearance mechanism to the gastrointestinal tract amounts to less than 75 μg.

The most plausible explanation for Adamsson et al.'s findings is the fact that the workers ingest significant amounts of cadmium (e.g. through contaminated hands). Our results on the intensity of hand contamination in workers from an electric condenser factory support the above explanation (Roels et al., unpublished results). In a few workers exposed to cadmium, we have determined at different times of the day, the amount of cadmium which could be collected after rinsing one hand with 500 ml of slightly acidified water. Even before entering the canteen for lunch, up to 280 μg Cd could be mobilised from one hand (versus less than 7 μg in the controls during work).

These observations demonstrate clearly that in industry, the amount of cadmium which accumulates in the organism does not only depend on the amount of cadmium inhaled but also on the amount ingested.

Even if there exists a relationship between the airborne concentration, the overall dustiness of the workplace and hence the amount of cadmium entering the organism by the pulmonary and the oral routes, one cannot expect that the determination of the airborne concentration of cadmium might allow to estimate the total amount of cadmium absorbed by the workers.

Firstly personal hygiene habits (hand washing, smoking at work, etc.) vary from one person to another. Secondly, it is well known that great individual variation exists in the oral absorption rate of cadmium. For example, a study by Flanagan et al. (1978) indicates, as it was demonstrated previously in animals, that subjects with low iron stores absorb considerably more cadmium (8.9%) through the gastrointestinal tract than persons with normal iron stores (2.4%). A plot of cadmium absorption versus the logarithm of the serum ferritin value shows a correlation coefficient of - 0.68. Oral absorption of cadmium is therefore higher in females than in males.

The results by Flanagan et al. (1978) have recently been confirmed by Shaikh and Smith (1980). Seven male and five female volunteer subjects were given a single dose of 50 μg Cd along with radiolabelled cadmium. The subjects were monitored during the study using a whole body counter. In the males and in 3 of the female subjects, the oral absorption rate ranged from between 1.6% and 3.6%. The absorption in the two iron-deficient females was 7.15% and 8.6% respectively. Furthermore, it should be recognised that slight iron deficiency is not uncommon in the general population.

Even if strict personal hygiene measures could be implemented so as to limit the amount of cadmium ingested to the quantity cleared from the respiratory system by the muco-ciliary clearance mechanism, there is no reason to postulate the existence of a relationship between the airborne concentration and the amount abosrbed. This has been clearly demonstrated for lead (King et al., (1976). Many physico-chemical and biological factors (particle size distribution, solubility of cadmium salts, ventilatory parameters etc.) preclude the existence of such a correlation. Furthermore, in some persons, non-occupational exposure (dietary and smoking habits) may significantly contribute to the cadmium body burden.

From all the above reasons, it is clear that the respect of any concentration of cadmium in air may not necessarily prevent an undue accumulation of cadmium in the critical organ i.e. the renal cortex.

An evaluation of the internal dose of cadmium by (a) biological method(s) might circumvent these difficulties.

It is now possible to measure by neutron activation the amount of the metal which has accumulated in the two main sites of deposition i.e. the liver and the kidney (Ellis et al., 1979, Thomas et al., 1979). Comparison of the results with the estimated critical level allows a direct evaluation of the health risk. However, it is unlikely that evaluation of tissue cadmium in vivo by neutron activation will soon become a routine medical procedure.

But other biological indicators such as cadmium in blood and in urine which are more amenable to routine determination may be used for estimating the internal dose of cadmium and hence the risk of health impairment.

Repeated blood cadmium analyses on newly exposed workers have shown that after the start of exposure, cadmium concentration in blood increases during the first 4 to 6 months and then levels off. The value of the plateau level seems to be proportional to the exposure intensity (Lauwerys et al., 1979 d; Kjellstrom, 1979). This indicates that in occupationally exposed persons cadmium level in blood is a good indicator of the average intake during recent months but not of body burden nor of the most recent exposure. Experimental studies support this conclusion (Bernard et al., 1980).

Cadmium level in urine is influenced by both body burden and exposure, but there is indication that when cadmium exposure is moderate and the body burden has not yet reached the critical level, cadmium concentration in urine is probably more a reflection of the quantity stored in the organism than a reflection of the current exposure (Lauwerys et al., 1979 d). Under these circumstances, the cadmium concentration in urine rarely exceeds 10 to 15 μg/g creatinine. Higher values repeatedly found in workers exposed to cadmium suggest that saturation of the body binding sites is occurring. Cadmium level in urine may then be more influenced by current exposure than by body burden.

Under moderate exposure conditions and before the occurrence of renal dysfunction, the information given by both determinations (cadmium in blood and cadmium in urine) are therefore complementary since the average absorption dose of cadmium during recent months can be estimated by the level of cadmium in blood whereas the amount already stored in the organism can be evaluated by the level of cadmium in urine.

Hence, a biological monitoring programme which includes the determination of cadmium in blood and in urine offers several advantages over environmental monitoring. As already stressed above, the measurement of cadmium in blood takes into consideration absorption by all the routes and not only through the lungs as well as individual differences in the factors conditioning lung deposition, oral intake (personal hygiene habits) and absorption of cadmium.

Furthermore, by combining the determination of cadmium in urine with cadmium in blood not only recent non-occupational

background exposure is taken into consideration but also the
cumulative internal dose (body burden). For a very cumulative toxic such as cadmium with a biological half life
exceeding 10 years this is a very important advantage.

Indeed, for a similar current external exposure, the risk of
health impairment may be markedly different depending on the
amount of cadmium already stored in the organism. Of course,
one can take benefit of all these theoretical advantages of
the biological monitoring programme if at least, meaningful
biological threshold limit values can be proposed for cadmium
in blood and in urine.

Several epidemiological studies on adult male workers chronically exposed to cadmium allow to estimate the critical
levels of cadmium in blood and in urine with the use of a
portable neutron activation system.

Roels et al. (1980) have determined cadmium concentration in
liver and in kidney of approximately 300 Belgian workers
employed in two cadmium smelters. At the same time, cadmium
concentration in blood and in urine as well as their renal
status (total proteinuria, B_2-microglobulinuria, albumin-
uria) were determined. They found that the lowest liver
cadmium concentration above which some workers exhibit signs
of renal dysfunction is 30 ppm and all the workers with a
cadmium concentration in liver exceeding 60 ppm had signs of
renal dysfunction. In workers without signs of renal dysfunction, the corresponding values for cadmium concentration
in renal cortex and in urine were 162 and 221 ppm and 10 and
13.5 μg/g creatinine respectively. This study suggests that
in adult male workers, the critical level of cadmium in urine
above which a certain proportion of subjects may exhibit
signs of renal dysfunction is 10 μg/g creatinine.

This estimate of the critical level of cadmium in urine has
been confirmed in another epidemiological study. Buchet et
al. (1980) have examined the renal function of 148 cadmium

workers and have compared the results with those obtained in
88 control workers. By subdividing the control and the cadmium workers in 4 groups on the basis of the levels of cadmium in urine, they have found that the prevalence of biological signs of renal dysfunction is greater than that found
in the control group mainly when cadmium in urine exceeds 10
μg/g creatinine.

We have indicated that cadmium in blood reflects mainly the
last few months exposure. However, if exposure remains more
or less stable with time, it is logical to find also a dose-
response relationship between cadmium level in blood and the
prevalence of signs of renal dysfunction. The data by Buchet
et al. (1980) suggest that a value of 1 μg Cd/100 ml whole
blood might be proposed as a tentative no-effect level for
long term exposure to cadmium.

In summary, the available data suggest that to prevent renal
dysfunction in adult male workers exposed to cadmium, the
amount stored in the organism should not exceed a value
corresponding to a urinary excretion of 10 to 15 μg/g
creatinine. For blood a value of 1 μg Cd/100 ml whole blood
is proposed as tentative no-effect level for long term
exposure.

Since under moderate occupational exposure to cadmium, kidney
dysfunction occurs usually earlier than lung impairment the
biological limit values proposed on the basis of the above
studies should, in practice, be considered as primary guides
for the prevention of health impairment. If proposed, a
time-weighted average exposure value for cadmium in air
should only be considered as a secondary or technical
guideline upon which one should not only rely to protect the
health of workers.

Finally, it is important to realise that the proposed guidelines are derived from observations made on adult male
workers and therefore these proposals may not necessarily be
valid for other groups of the general population.

References

1. Adamsson, E. Piscator, M., Nogawa, K. Pulmonary and gastro-intestinal exposure to cadmium oxide dust in a battery factory. Environ. Health Perspectives 28, 219, 1979.

2. Bernard, A., Goret, A., Buchet, J.P., Roels, H., Lauwerys, R. Significance of cadmium levels in blood and urine during long-term exposure of rats to cadmium. J. Tox. Environ. Health 6, 175, 1980.

3. Buchet, J.P., Roels, H., Bernard, A., Lauwerys, R. Assessment of renal function of workers exposed to inorganic lead, cadmium or mercury vapor. J. Occupat. Med., 1980.

4. Ellis, K.J., Vartsky, D., Zainzi, I., Cohn, S.H., Yasamura, S. Cadmium: in vivo measurement in smokers and non-smokers. Science 205, 323, 1979.

5. Environmental Protection Agency (US). Health Assessment Document for Cadmium. Preprint. Research Triangle Park, USA, 1979.

6. Flanagan, P.R., McLellan, J.S., Haist, J., Cherian, G., Chamberlain, H.J., Valberg, L.S. Increased dietary cadmium absorption in mice and human subjects with iron deficiency. Gastroenterology 74, 841, 1978.

7. Friberg, L., Piscator, M., Nordberg, G.F., Kjellstrom T. Cadmium in the Environment. 2nd ed. Cleveland, CRC, 1974.

8. King, E., Conchie, A., Hiett, D., Milligan, B. Lead, Particle Size, Solubility and Absorption in Industry. Report ILZRO Venture LH 207. New York 1976.

9. Kjellstrom, T. (project coordinator). Exposure and accumulation of cadmium in people from Japan, USA and Sweden. Report on a 3 year cooperative research project. Environ. Health Perspectives 28, 169, 1979.

10. Lauwerys, R. (rapporteur). CEC - Criteria (Dose/ Effect Relationships) for cadmium. Published for the Commission of the European Communities by Pergamon Press Oxford, 1978.

11. Lauwerys, R. The health effect of cadmium in Trace Metals: exposure and health effects. Research Seminar. Guildford U.K., 10-13 July 1978. Published for the Commission of the European Communities by Pergamon Press (E. Di Ferrante, Editor) 1979 (a).

12. Lauwerys, R. Cadmium in man, Chapter 11 in Chemistry, Biochemistry and Biology of Cadmium (M. Webb, editor). Elsevier/North-Holland, Amsterdam, 1979 (b).

13. Lauwerys, R., Bernard, A., Buchet, J.P., Roels, H. Dose-response relationship for the nephrotoxic action of cadmium in man. P. 19 in International Conference. Management and Control of Heavy Metals in the Environment. CEP Consultants Ltd, Edinburgh 1979 (c).

14. Lauwerys, R., Roels, H., Regniers, M., Buchet, J.P., Bernard, A., Goret, A. Significance of cadmium concentration in blood and in urine in workers exposed to cadmium. Environ. Research 20, 375, 1979 (d).

15. Ohanian, E.V., Iwai, J. Effects of cadmium ingestion in rats with opposite genetic predisposition to hypertension. Environ. Health Perspectives 28, 261, 1979.

16. Perry, H.M., Erlanger, M., Perry, E.F. Increase of the systolic pressure of rats chronically fed cadmium. Environ. Health Perspectives 28, 251, 1979.

17. Roels, H.A., Lauwerys, R.R., Buchet, J.P., Bernard, A., Chettle, D.C., Harvey, T.C., Al-Haddad, I.K. In vivo measurement of liver and kidney cadmium in workers exposed to this metal. Its significance with respect to cadmium in blood and urine.

18 Shaikh, Z.A., Smith, J.C. Metabolism of orally ingested cadmium in humans. Toxicology Letters, Suppl. 1, 81, 1980.

19. Thomas, B.J., Harvey, T.C., Chettle, D.R., McLellan, J.S., Fremlin, J.H. A transportable system for the measurement of liver cadmium in vivo. Phys. Med. Biol. 24, 432, 1979.

20. W.H.O. Environmental Health Criteria for Cadmium, Geneva 1979.

21. W.H.O. Programme on Internationally Recommended Health-Based Permissible Levels for Occupational Exposure to Chemical Agents. Cadmium, Lead, Manganese, Mercury. Geneva 1980.

CURRENT USE OF AMBIENT AND BIOLOGICAL MONITORING: REFERENCE
WORKPLACE HAZARDS. INORGANIC TOXIC AGENTS - CADMIUM II

H.M. Perry and E.F. Perry (USA)

Summary

*Cadmium is apparently accumulated, primarily in the kidney
and the liver, by all human beings by the time that they
reach adulthood but environmental cadmium is generally considered to have no deleterious effects. In contrast workers
with industrial exposure to cadmium have long been known to
develop characteristic toxic manifestations; however, there
is a suggestion that cardiovascular toxicity can arise from
environmental exposure. The possibility that low levels of
environmental cadmium might ultimately be responsible for
some or all of essential hypertension focuses attention on
the present maximum tolerable limits of cadmium exposure. A
major decrease (which at present does not seem to be warranted) would extend the target population from a relatively few
workers in the factory to the entire population in their
normal environment.*

Introduction

Cadmium is an ubiquitous element which all human beings
apparently accumulate, primarily in kidney and liver, by the
time they reach adulthood. In the United States the average
adult body burden accumulated from the environment without
any recognised specific exposure approximates 30 mg. Nonetheless, except where conditions are extreme, as they are in the
"itai-itai" area of Japan, environmental cadmium is generally
considered to have no deleterious effects (1).

In contrast to the usual environmental exposure, specific
industrial exposure to cadmium which can result in a much
larger body burden has long been known to produce characteristic toxic manifestations (2). Industrial exposure can be
either by inhalation or ingestion. With the former, there is
a direct effect on the lung with loss of pulmonary function
(3) which can both incapacitate and kill. Chronic ingestion,
and inhalation as well can lead to very large accumulations
in the kidney where cadmium is sequestered as a result of
binding to a specific protein, metallothionein (4). There is

a threshhold level of about 200 μg of cadmium per gm of renal cortex above which a characteristic "tubular" proteinuria occurs. This proteinuria, however, rarely progresses to renal failure or to symptomatic disease (1).

In addition to the classical toxic manifestations from high exposure, there is a new and disturbing suggestion that the much lower environmental exposure can produce previously unsuspected cardiovascular toxicity. Certainly in rats, chronic ingestion of cadmium, in amounts comparable to what many Americans eat, can induce hypertension and simultaneously decrease cardiac function (5, 6). The hypertension induced in rats is usually mild and associated with no other biological effects, thereby mimicking two important characteristics of human essential hypertension, the cause of which remains unknown despite extensive research. The hypertension induced in rats seems to be an all-or-none phenomenon, with the increase in blood pressure being the same for a fifty-fold range of cadmium exposures, i.e. 0.1 to 5 μg/ml of drinking water (Figure 1) (6). Smaller amounts of cadmium are inert and larger amounts make the rats overtly ill but do not induce hypertension (6, 7). Industrial workers with classic "high exposure" cadmium toxicity apparently fail to develop hypertension, and this failure is mirrored by the failure of rats to develop hypertension following large cadmium intake.

The possibility that low levels of environmental cadmium might ultimately be responsible for some or all of the essential hypertension, which occurs in almost one-third of Americans and which even in its mildest forms at least doubles the risk of myocardial infarction and stroke (8), focuses attention on the present maximum tolerable limits of cadmium exposure in the United States which were designed to prevent toxic manifestations from high industrial exposure (9). A major decrease in tolerable exposure would extend the target population from a relatively few workers in the factory to the entire population in their normal environment.

Such a major change does not presently seem warranted, but the suggestion of an inimical biological effect from environmental cadmium makes it prudent to prevent any further increase in such exposure - which is apparently greater in industrial societies than in less developed countries - while intensively investigating the relationship of cadmium to chronic cardiovascular disease.

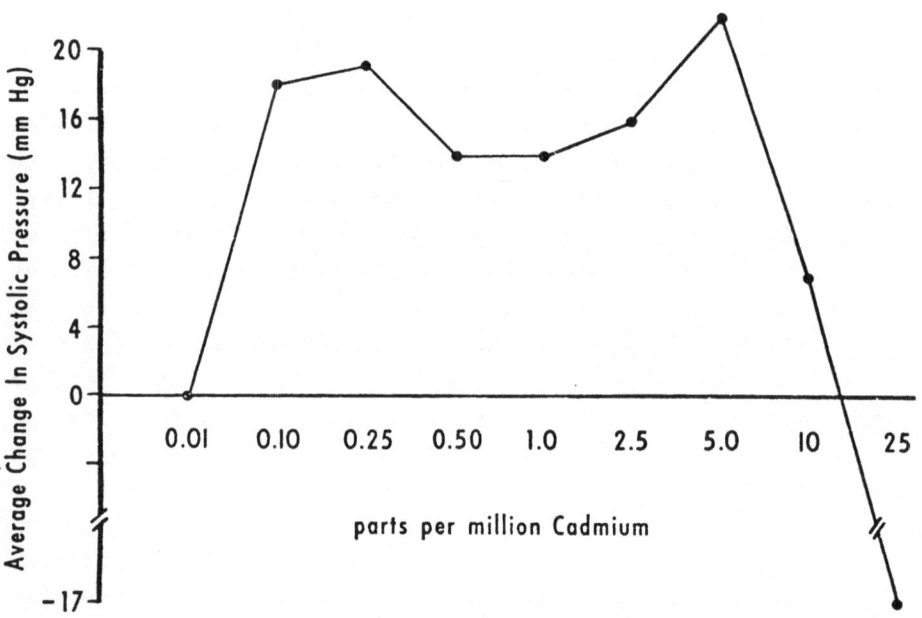

Figure 1   18 months exposure to 0.01 to 25 ppm cadmium

Average changes in systolic pressure induced by nine exposure levels of cadmium for 18 months. At 18 months there were still at least 13 rats in all groups, and the groups exposed to 0.1, 5, and 10 ppm of cadmium each contained more than 30 rats (6).

Biological effects of cadmium

Human toxicity to cadmium, resulting from heavy industrial exposure, was first recognised in 1920 (2). Both acute and chronic toxic effects of cadmium in man have recently been reviewed by Friberg and his colleagues (1). Table 1 outlines reported human toxicity. Acute exposure to cadmium by inges- tion can cause severe but temporary gastroenteritis (10), and by inhalation, severe and sometimes fatal pulmonary oedema (1). Prolonged inhalation of cadmium oxide can result in pulmonary dysfunction (11) and emphysema (12). Prolonged industrial exposure by ingestion and/or inhalation can pro- duce renal dysfunction, characterised by "tubular" protein- uria, glycosuria, and aminoaciduria (13-15); however, pro- gression to azotemia and renal failure occurs very rarely. Other less alarming toxic manifestations have included moderate anaemia, probably in part haemolytic (16), and apparent hepatic dysfunction manifested primarily by hyper- gammaglobulinaemia (1). Finally, a peculiar disease called itai-itai, characterised by severe bone pains and osteomala- cia and involving multiparous middle-aged women living in certain parts of Japan where there is a very high environ- mental exposure to cadmium, has been ascribed to chronic cadmium poisoning in combination with a low intake of calcium and vitamin D (17).

Table 1   Effects of Industrial exposure to Cadmium In man

	Toxic Effect	Explanatory Comment	First Author & Reference
1.	Acute Gastroenteritis	Acid foods In cadmium-plated containers	Cole (10)
2.	Acute Pulmonary Oedema & Interstitial Pneumonitis	Oedema In 24 hours and pneumonitis In 3 to 10 days	Friberg (1)
3.	Chronic Pulmonary Dysfunction		
	a. Decreased Pulmonary Function	Residual volume Increased by 10% after 10 years of Inhaling cadmium oxide	Buxton (11) Lauwerys (3)
	b. Emphysema		Friberg (49) Hirst (12)
4.	Chronic Renal Dysfunction		
	a. Proteinuria	Following 9 years of Inhaling cadmium oxide	Piscator (13)
	b. Glucosuria		Bonnell (14)
	c. Aminoaciduria		Clarkson (15)
5.	Moderate anaemia	Following Inhalation of cadmium oxide	Nicoud (16)
6.	Itai-Itai disease	Osteomalacia In multiparous women over 40 with other dietary deficiences	Hagino (17)
7.	Increased mortality	Death rate In cadmium workers was higher (p 0.01) than expected	Friberg (18)
8.	Possible Carcinogenesis	Possibly Increased prostatic cancer In workers exposed to cadmium oxide	Kipling (19)

Animal toxicity from injected cadmium has included the wide
range of biological effects listed in Table 2. Of these,
the autoimmune, renal, and cardiovascular effects seem to
have the most potential significance for possible human
disease. The earliest effect on the immune system is stimulation followed by inhibition of antibody formation (26);
with continued exposure, increased urinary excretion of
"light chains" occurs (27); and finally with heavy exposure,
there is amyloid deposition (27, 28). Renal dysfunction,
including proteinuria of the "tubular" type (29), glycosuria
(30), and amino-aciduria (31), has occurred with heavy cadmium exposure; however, as in human cadmium poisoning, this
dysfunction in animals has not characteristically progressed
to renal failure. Increased sodium reabsorption by the
proximal tubule suggests a mechanism by which cadmium might
induce hypertension (32); however, the acute hypertension
induced by single small doses of cadmium seems more likely to
result from a direct effect on vascular smooth muscle (35-
38).

Animal toxicity from ingested cadmium can be either obvious
and associated with relatively large doses, or subtle and
associated with smaller doses (Table 3, Part I). The large
doses are presumably comparable to specific and sizable
industrial exposure which involves a small identifiable
population; whereas the lower doses, which do not produce
obvious sickness, seem more likely to be related to effects
of the ordinary environmental exposure which involves
everyone.

Table 2   Effects of Injected Cadmium in Animals

Effect	Animal	Route	Cadmium Exposure			First Author and Reference
			Daily Dose (mg/kg)	Length of Exposure (days)	Total Dose (mg/kg)	
1. Haemorrhage In Nervous Gangila	Rat	sc*	8	1x[+]	8	Gabbiani (20
2. Congenital Malformation	Hamster	iv*	2	1x	2	Holmberg (21)
3. Local Induction of Cancer	Rat	sc	0.2	1x	0.2	Gunn (22)
4. Reproductive System Effects						
a. Testicular necrosis	Rat	sc	1	1x	1	Clegg (23)
b. Placental necrosis	Rat	sc	4.5	4	18	Parizek (24)
5. Anaemia	Rabbit	sc	0.3	130	33	Piscator (25)
6. Autoimmune Effects						
a. Decrease in antibody	Rat	sc	0.6	10	6	Jones (26)
b. Urinary light chains	Rabbit	sc	0.3	22	6	Vigliani (27)
c. Amyloidosis	Rabbit	sc	0.3	250	63	Vigliani (27)
Amyliodosis	Rabbit	sc	1	60	60	Baum (28)
7. Renal Effects						
a. Proteinuria	Rabbit	sc	0.3	130	33	Piscator (29)
Proteinuria	Rabbit	sc	0.3	64	16	Vigliani (27)
b. Glycosuria	Rabbit	sc	0.2	120	46	Axelsson (30)
c. Amino-aciduria	Rabbit	sc	1.5	45	68	Nomiyama (31)
d. Sodium retention	Dog	iv	0.2	1x	0.2	Vander (32)
8. Cardiovascular Effects						
a. Hypertension	Dog	ip*	0.3	180	50	Thind (33)
Hypertension	Rabbit	ip	0.3	50	15	Thind (34)
Hypertension	Rat	ip	2.0	1x	2.0	Schroeder (35)
Hypertension	Rat	iv	0.8	1x	0.8	Perry (36)
Hypertension	Rat	ip	0.2	1x	0.2	Perry (37)
Hypertension	Rat	ia*	0.1	1x	0.1	Perry (38)

*sc, subcutaneous; iv, intravenous; ip, intraperitoneal; ia, intra-arterial.
+ "1x" indicates that cadmium was administered one time.

Table 3   Cadmium-induced effects in animals following exposure simulating human exposure

Part I. INGESTION

| Effect | Animal | Cadmium Exposure | | First Author and Reference |
		Intensity	Duration	
1. Anaemia	Quail	77 ppm in food	28 days	Fox (39)
2. Decreased growth	Rat	50 ppm in water	120 days	Itokawa (40)
3. Decreased growth	Sheep	15 ppm in food	163 days	Doyle (41)
4. Microscopic lung changes	Rat	17 ppm in water	280 days	Miller (42)
5. Microscopic kidney changes	Rat	10 ppm in water	42 days	Nishizumi (43)
6. Hypertension	Rat	5 ppm in water	120 days	Schroeder (44)
7. Diminished myocardial excitability	Rat	1 to 5 ppm in water	450 to 600 days	Kopp (5)*
8. Hypertension	Rat	0.1 to 5 ppm water	90 to 900 days	Perry (7)

Part II. INHALATION

1. Pulmonary oedema interstitial pneumonitis and emphysema	Rats	33 mg/m^3	0.25	Paterson (47)
2. Emphysema	Rat	10 mg/m^3	15 hours	Snider (48)
3. Peribronchial inflammation and emphysema	Rabbits	5 mg/m^3	480 hours	Friberg (49)
4. Peribronchial necrosis and emphysema	Guinea Pigs	0.6 mg$^+$	x 3$^+$	Thurlbeck (50)
5. Emphysema and scarring	Dogs	0.3 mg/m^3	0.5 hours	Harrison (51)

*This reference describes the changes for rats which received 5 ppm cadmium in water for 600 days the same changes were seen in rats receiving 1 ppm cadmium in water for 450 days.

+Thurlbeck and Foley injected 1 ml/kg of a solution containing 0.9 mg cadmium per ml H_2O into the trachea; emphysema was observed following 3 or more injections.

Ingestion of 0.1 to 5 parts per million (ppm) of cadmium in drinking water has produced hypertension in rats (Figure 1) (6, 7, 44); moreover, altered myocardial excitability, morphology, and metabolism have also recently been noted in some of these hypertensive animals (5). Cadmium-induced hypertension in animals resembles human essential hypertension in that it is usually mild and not accompanied by renal dysfunction or other associated changes. On the basis of microgrammes of cadmium ingested per kilogramme of body weight, however, even the lowest animal intake which has consistently induced hypertension (6) is at least an order of magnitude more than the usual American diet which provides approximately 1 μg/kg of body weight, although many Americans certainly ingest as much as the hypertensive rats. Despite the disparity in intake, tissue concentrations in exposed rats are comparable to those in human beings without unusual exposure. Thus, renal cadmium concentration in rats rendered hypertensive by cadmium ranges from 5 to 50 μg/gm (45), while the average American adult has about 30 μg/gm (46).

Animal toxicity from inhaled cadmium is characterised by serial changes in the lung, with the earliest and most acute change being pulmonary oedema (47) followed by proliferative interstitial pneumonitis (47), including necrosis of the alveolar lining and peribronchial inflammation (49). The latest and most chronic anatomic change is emphysema with scarring (48, 50, 51) (Table 3, Part II).

In vitro effects of cadmium are presumed to be primarily associated with inhibition of enzymatic activity resulting from mercaptide formation with cysteinyl residues of many enzymes including alcohol dehydrogenase, glutamic dehydrogenase, glutathione reductase, adenylate kinase, and disulphide reductase. In addition, cadmium, in concentrations of 5×10^{-6} molar, uncouples phosphorylation from oxidation (52), and at ten times this concentration it has been reported completely to inhibit mitochondrial respiration of pulmonary alveolar microphages by binding to components of the respiratory chain (53).

Effect of second metal on cadmium-induced hypertension in rats

Obviously cadmium exerts its influence in concert with other
bodily constituents, and related metals seem most likely to
alter the biological effects of cadmium directly. Thus, it is
not surprising that certain metals can either inhibit or
enhance cadmium-induced hypertension. The pressor effect of
cadmium is inhibited by half as much (on a molar basis)
selenium, fifty times as much zinc, or ten times as much
copper (6). In contrast, equimolar lead augmented the pressor
effect of cadmium, doubling the cadmium-induced elevation in
systolic pressure to an average level as much as 40 mm Hg
(Figure 2) (6).

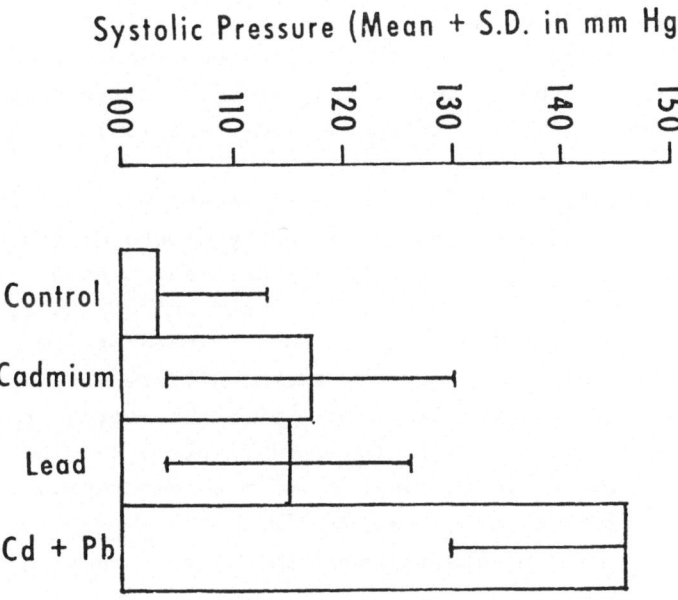

Systolic Pressure (Mean + S.D. in mm Hg)

Figure 2 Augmentation of cadmium-induced hypertension by lead

Average systolic pressures ± standard deviations are
presented for 45 control rats and for groups of 15
rats fed 1 ppm of cadmium and/or lead for three months (6).

Total body burden and critical target organ

The body burden of the average adult American has been estimated to be about 30 mg of cadmium (1), of which 10 mg are in
the kidneys and 5 mg are in the liver. Unlike other "non-
essential" trace elements, cadmium has a specific and unique
pattern of distribution, with the kidney having about ten
times the concentration of the liver which in turn has at
least five times the concentration of most other organs (54).
There is very little renal cadmium in the new-born, and the
metal is accumulated throughout life (Figure 3) (46). Moreover, there are wide geographical differences even among
those without specific exposure, with some groups of Negroid
Africans having significantly less and some groups of Asiatic
Mongoloids having significantly more renal cadmium than
Caucosoid Americans, Europeans and Indians (Figure 3) (46).
These differences seem likely to be primarily environmental,
since in the United States, tissue cadmium concentration is
apparently largely independent of race (54).

Any biological effects of relatively small amounts of
cadmium in man would presumably depend on its distribution
among the organs and within a critical tissue, as well as on
the substances to which it is bound and on the concentrations
of other metals with which it competes. Thus, it may be
significant that there are marked differences in the ratio of
renal to hepatic cadmium, with the average ratios for the
groups of subjects included in Figure 3 ranging from 7 to 25
(46). The ratio of renal cadmium concentration to renal zinc
concentration also varies, with the average ratios for the
groups of subjects included in Figure 3 ranging from 0.25 to
1.0 (46).

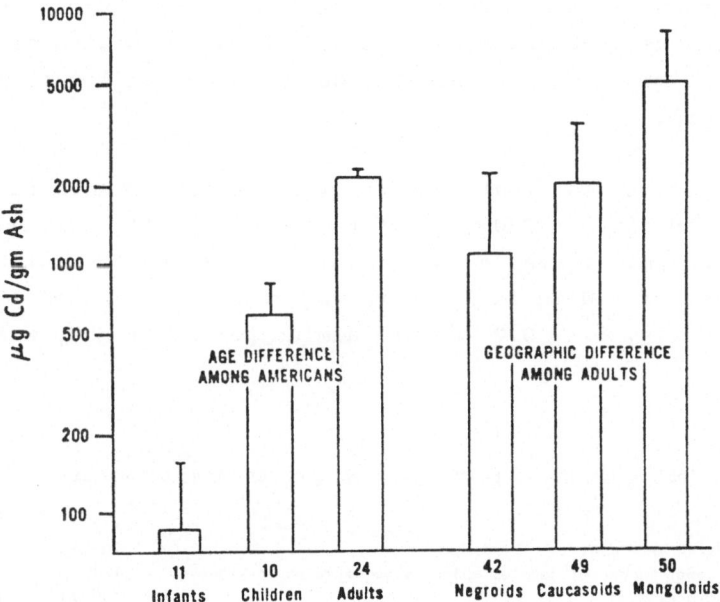

Figure 3   Differences in renal cadmium concentration

Mean   renal   cadmium concentrations and their standard deviations   for six populations of subjects on a logarithmic scale
(46).   The "Americans" in the first panel were all from the
St. Louis   area   and included 10 infants from 45 to 450 days
old,   11   children   from   450 to 4500 days old, and 24 adults
over   45   years   of age.   Both whites and blacks are included
because   there   is   no significant difference between the two
groups.   The "adults" in the second panel included six groups
of   Negroids   from Africa, four groups of Caucasoids from the
United   States,   Switzerland   and   India,   and five groups of
Mongoloids   from   the   Far   East.   Note: Although the mean is
similar,   the   standard   deviation for the "adult" group from
one   geographical   location (St. Louis) is much less than for
the adult "Caucasoids" from three continents.

The kidney is the obvious critical organ in chronic cadmium poisoning. This is true not only for the conventional view which holds that renal dysfunction is the major manifestation of chronic industrial toxicity and proteinuria its benchmark - although with high exposures by inhalation the lung is also a major target organ. The kidney however would also be the target organ if the much smaller environmental exposures do indeed induce hypertension; under these circumstances the heart too might be a target organ despite its low cadmium content. (5).

Friberg postulated that the critical cadmium concentration for proteinuria was 200μg/g of renal cortex (1). Using the assumptions of table 4, he calculated that to accumulate a body burden of 120 mg in 50 years requires <u>retention</u> of 15 of cadmium daily, i.e. 0.2 μg of cadmium per kg of body weight (1).

Table 4 Conditions producing a body burden of 120 mg of Cadmium

Weight of "standard" man:	70 kg
Fraction of body burden of cadmium which is sequestered in kidneys:	1/3
Weight of both kidneys:	300 gm
Ratio of renal cortical cadmium concentration:	50% greater
Critical level in renal cortex for proteinuria:	200μg/gm
Body burden associated with critical level:	120 mg
Absorption of ingested cadmium:	4.5%
Absorption of inhaled cadmium:	25%
Excretion of body burden daily:	0.01%*

*This percentage gives a biological half life of 20 years and assumes that percent excretion of body burden is independent of its size.

[Accepting first the approximation that the excretion rate of the cadmium accumulated in the body does not depend on the size of the body burden and second the more dubious condition that the entire pool of accumulated cadmium behaves similarly, the body burden resulting from the daily <u>retention</u> (i.e. actual transfer into the mucosal cell from the organ lumen) of 1μg cadmium can be calculated under different alternatives for rate of excretion and time of exposure. This calculated body burden can then be corrected for different amounts of retained cadmium.

Thus, asssuming that the daily excretion of accumulated cadmium is 0.01% of the body burden, 6.0 and 8.4 mg of cadmium respectively will have accumulated after 25 and 50 years in the body for each μg of cadmium retained daily. Note that if a renal cortical concentration of 40μg/gm is associated with hypertension, the critical body burden would be lowered from the 120 mg cited in the table to 24μg/gm.

The foregoing calculations are based on the conventional wisdom that proteinuria is the first manifestation of toxicity. If hypertension should prove to be induced by smaller amounts of cadmium, these figures will have to be adjusted downward. Since the pressor effect of cadmium in man is unproven, there are no human data which fix the toxic level for induction of hypertension. In the few available studies, however, normotensive adults have average renal cortical cadmium concentrations which appear to cluster about 25 μg/gm (Table 5), while comparable hypertensive values cluster about 40 μg/gm. The latter concentration may therefore be a first approximation to the level which induces hypertension. If 40 μg/gm is the critical level, the maximum permissible retention would be decreased by a factor of 5, becoming 3 μg per day for "standard man", which represents a daily intake of about 60 μg of dietary cadmium. This intake approximates the level which has been proposed as occurring in the diet of the average American adult (1).

Table 5 Renal cadmium as a function of blood pressure

	No. of Patients	μg/g Tissue Mean	Median	μg/10 mg Ash* Mean	Significance and Author
Hypertensive	17		37[+]	42	$P < 0.005$
Normotensive	117		29[+]	29	Schroeder – U.S. (55)
Hypertensive			49[+]	51	$P < 0.025$
Normotensive	23		27[+]	32	Schroeder – foreign (55)
Hypertensive	12		27	25	Not significant
Normotensive	25		22	25	Morgan – Alabama (56)
Hypertensive	12	36			$P < 0.05$
Normotensive	10	27			Lener – Prague (57)
Hypertensive	39			12	$P \ 0.001$
Normotensive	43			21	Ostergaard – Copenhagen (58)
Hypertensive	11	40			$P < 0.05$
Normotensive	11	26			Perry – U.S. (59)

*The unusual units make the order of magnitude similar for aliquots of ash and wet tissue.
+Personal communication.

Data from six small series that have compared renal cadmium concentrations in hypertensive and "matched" normotensive subjects. Of the comparisons with statistically significant differences, both sets of Schroeder's data and Lener's data show more renal cadmium in hypertensive subjects than in normotensive subjects; whereas Ostergaard's data show the reverse.

Permissible exposure to cadmium

Intake of cadmium from industrial air which would provide a body burden of 120 mg of cadmium has been calculated by Friberg et al using various assumptions (1). The most reasonable set of assumptions is presented in Table 4 and used in setting the exposure limits cited below for industrial air as well as for food, ambient air, and tobacco smoke (1). It is generally assumed that a worker works 225 eight-hour days a year and inhales 10 m^3 air daily. After working 10 years, his renal cortical cadmium concentration will reach 200 μg/gm if the average concentration in the workplace is 25 μg of cadmium per m^3 of air, or if it is 13 μg/m^3 for 25 years.

Cadmium intake from food and drink probably comprises the major part of accumulated cadmium in those without specific exposure. Using the assumptions of Table 4, the necessary cadmium intake to produce a body burden of 120 mg at age 50 has been calculated as 350 μg daily. According to Friberg et al this is far above the usual total daily amount ingested which approximates 50 μg and ranged from 25 to 75 μg. The concentration of cadmium in most foods is less than 0.05 μg/gm; but certain foods, like shellfish and mammalian liver, may contain more than 100 μg/gm. Moreover, when large amounts of cadmium are present in the soil or water as much as 1 μg/gm may accumulate in some plants including staple grains; such concentrations occur in rice from some regions of Japan. In addition, absorption of ingested cadmium may rise from the usual 5% to 10% or more when the diet is deficient in calcium or protein (1).

Cadmium concentration in water is usually less than 1 μg/l (60); however, soft (acidic) water may contain more than 15 μg/l (61), apparently because it tends to dissolve any available cadmium, particularly from galvanised surfaces, e.g. water pipes. Drinking water that has less than 5 μg/l is unlikely to contribute significantly to the total intake

of cadmium, but water with much higher concentrations might
be a significant contributor if regularly used. Hard water
may well have lower amounts of cadmium than otherwise comparable soft water because the cadmium is removed by coprecipi-
tation. In some animal experiments added cadmium was quickly
cleared from hard water with resultant much lower cadmium
accumulations than when the same amounts of cadmium were
added to soft water. Cadmium in hard water also failed to
produce biological effects in exposed rats (62).

Cadmium intake from ambient air is usually responsible for
relatively little of the body burden of cadmium, except in
smokers. Assuming that an average individual inhales 20 m^3
of ambient air during 24 hours, accumulation of a body burden
of 120 mg of Cd would require breathing air with an average
concentration of 3μg/m^3 for 50 years. The usual cadmium
content of air in the United States varies from less than
0.001 to as much as 0.05μg/m^3 (2), although air concentrations as high as 5 μg/m^3 have occurred in areas around
cadmium-emitting factories (14). With this very high concentration, 100μg/day would be inhaled and 25μg absorbed.

Cadmium intake from tobacco smoke, with other cadmium exposure, is unlikely to produce toxicity. One cigarette contains
approximately 0.1μg and Friberg et al. calculated that
almost 30 packs of cigarettes would have to be smoked daily
in order to account for a body burden of 120 mg of cadmium in
50 years. Even assuming a pulmonary absorption of 50% and a
daily excretion rate of 0.005%, ten packs of cigarettes per
day are necessary to produce the "critical" renal cadmium
concentration, although under these conditions a pack a day
could produce half of the body burden suggested as possibly
associated with hypertension. The average smoking rate in
the United States, however, is reported to be only ten
cigarettes - rather than 10 packs -daily (63).

Sources of cadmium

In 1975 the Environmental Protection Agency estimated that in
the United States approximately 1800 MG/year of cadmium
entered the environmental pool. Some recent estimates more
than double this amount. The primary sources of this
cadmium are mining operations, leaching from wastes deposited
in the soil, and fall-out from atmospheric emissions.
General population exposure is greatest from municipal incin-
erators and is said to come primarily from stabilisers for
plastics and cadmium containing paint. Iron and steel production is the second most significant source for total
population exposure because of emissions resulting from
processing of steels coated with cadmium. The next sources
are primary and secondary smelters. Although large segments
of the population receive some exposure from these industrial
sources, exposure outside the workplace seems to be well
within acceptable levels (64).

Excessive exposure to cadmium is most likely to occur in the
workplace. Overexposure to cadmium fumes can develop specifically from three types of processes: (1) burning or welding
of cadmium-plated metals; (2) silver brazing with cadmium-
containing alloys, rods, solders or wires; and (3) heating or
burning of other cadmium containing substances. Because of
cadmium's relatively low boiling point, there is a very high
risk of overexposure from fumes in a worker's breathing zone.
Chronic cadmium inhalation from cadmium dust which can occur
in mining operations and battery manufacture is also of
significance (64).

Monitoring

Industrial and environmental cadmium exposures are currently
difficult to estimate with accuracy, and hence are relatively
insensitive measures of risk. For workers with specific
industrial exposure to cadmium fume or dust, the cadmium
content of air in the workplace can be approximated by the

appropriate use of collection filters. For populations living near major sources of atmospheric pollution, the same techniques for monitoring air borne cadmium are useful.

For the large majority without specific occupational exposure, the major bases for estimating environmental cadmium intake include: (i) Cadmium concentration in frequently used foods, such as cereals, which may have a moderate cadmium content. (ii) Cadmium concentration in less frequently used foods, such as shellfish or liver, which are liable to have a very high content. (iii) Cadmium content of cigarettes.

Body burden of cadmium can be estimated with certainty only by measuring the renal and/or hepatic cadmium concentrations with biopsy or at autopsy. Blood is a poor index of body burden. Since cadmium apparently remains in plasma only during transport, plasma concentrations reflect recent exposure rather than long-term accumulation; in addition they are low and hard to measure. The cadmium contents of hair and nails have not correlated well with body burden, perhaps because of methodological difficulties in preparing samples and because they reflect only the relatively recent past.

Urinary cadmium concentration may provide some measure of cadmium exposure; however, at present, the evidence is only indirect, since urinary and tissue cadmium concentrations have not been compared in the same subjects. Some confirmation of the postulated relationship can be found in the reports that average urinary cadmium concentrations change with age in a manner reminiscent of renal cadmium concentrations. Urinary metallothionein holds promise as an index of body burden but more testing is needed (65). Finally, the high "cross-section capture" of cadmium for thermal neutrons offers a potential method for cadmium assay, but there is need for further standardisation (66).

Currently recommended cadmium standards

Industrial exposure to cadmium should be limited to an average of 40 μg/m^3 of air during a 40-hour work week and to no more than 200 μg/m^3 for any 15-minute period according to the National Insitute for Occupational Safety and Health recommendations designed to protect workers during their working lifetime.

Environmental exposure should be limited to a weekly intake of 400 to 500 μg of cadmium, according to the United Nations Food and Agriculture Organisation (FAO) and the World Health Organisation (WHO), which assumed that renal damage might occurwhen cadmium concentrations in the renal cortex exceeded 200 μg/g.

If hypertension is associated with renal cadmium content of 40 μg/g, these recommended weekly intakes would have to be lowered to 80 to 100 μg/g. For the present, it seems reasonable to recommend avoidance of any further increases in environmental cadmium until there are better human data bearing on whether cadmium induces hypertension or cardiac dysfunction. Finally, intensive research to answer these questions is urgent.

References

1. Friberg, L., Piscator, M., Nordberg, G.F., et al; Cadmium in the Environment, Cleveland, Ohio, CRC Press, Inc. 1974.

2. Stephens, G.A.,: Cadmium Poisoning, J. Ind. Hyg. 2:129, 1920.

3. Lauwerys, R.R., Buchet, J.P., Roels, H.A., Brouwers, J., and Stanescu, D.: Epidemiological Survey of Workers Exposed to Cadmium, Archives Environmental Health 28:145, 1974.

4. Pulido, P., Kagi, J.H.R., and Vallee, B.L.: Isolation and Some Properties of Human Metallothionein, Biochemistry 5:1768, 1966.

5. Kopp, S.J., Perry, H.M.,Jr., Glonek, T., Erlanger, M., Perry, E.F. et al: Cardiac Physiologic-Metabolic Changes After Chronic Low-Level Heavy Metal Feeding, Am. J. Physiol. 239:H22, 1980.

6. Perry, H.M.,Jr., Erlanger, M.W., and Perry, E.F.: Increase in the Systolic Pressure of Rats Chronically Fed Cadmium, Environmental Health Perspectives, 28:251, 1979.

7. Perry, H.M.,Jr., Erlanger, M.W., and Perry, E.F.: Elevated Systolic Pressure Following Chronic Low-Level Cadmium Feeding, Am. J. Physiol. 232:H114, 1977.

8. Kannell, W.B., Gordon, T.: The Framingham Study: An Epidemiological Investigation of Cardiovascular Disease, Section 26: Some Characteristics Related to the Incidence of Cardiovascular Disese and Death, 16 Year Follow-up, Bethseda, National Heart Institute, 1970.

9. Federal Register 39:23543, June 27, 1974.

10. Cole, G.M., and Bair, L.S.: "Food Poisoning" from Cadmium, U.S. Nav. Med. Bull. 43:398, 1944.

11. Buxton, R.St.J.: Respiratory Function in Men Casting Cadmium Alloys, II. Brit. J. Ind. Med. 13:36, 1956.

12. Hirst, R.N.,Jr., Perry, H.M.Jr., Cruz, M.G. et al: Elevated Cadmium Concentration in Emphysematous Lungs, Amer. Rev. Resp. Dis. 108:30, 1973.

13. Piscator, M.: Proteinuria in Chronic Cadmium Poisoning, IV. Gel Filtration and Ion Exchange Chromatography of Urinary Proteins From Cadmium Workers, Arch. Environ. Health 12:345, 1966.

14. Bonnell, J.A., Kazantzis, G., and King, E.: A Follow-up Study of Men Exposed to Cadmium Oxide Fume, Brit. J. Ind. Med. 16:135, 1959.

15. Clarkson, T.W., and Kench, J.E.: Urinary Excretion of Amino Acids by Men Absorbing Heavy Metals, Biochem. J., 62:361, 1956.

16. Nicaud, P., Lafitte, A., and Gros, A.: Les Troubles de L'intoxication Chronique Par Le Cadmium, Arch. Mal. Prof. Med. Trav. Secur. Soc. 4:192, 1942.

17. Hagino, N.: Itai-Itai Disease and Vitamin D., Dig. Sci. Labour. 28:32, 1973.

18. Friberg, L., and Kjellstrom, T.: Unpublished data. In Friberg, L., Piscator, M., Nordberg, G., et al: Cadmium in the Environment, Cleveland, Ohio, CRC Press, 1974.

19. Kipling, M.D., and Waterhouse, J.A.H.: Cadmium and Prostatic Carcinoma, Lancet 1:730, 1967.

20. Gabbiani, G.: Action of Cadmium Chloride on Sensory Ganglia, Experientia 22:261, 1966.

21. Holmberg, R.E., and Ferm. V.H.: Inter-relationships of Selenium, Cadmium and Arsenic in Mammalian Terato-genesis, Arch. Environ. Health 18:873, 1969.

22. Gunn, S.A., Gould, T.C., and Anderson, E.A.D.: Cadmium-Induced Interstitial Cell Tumors in Rats and Mice and Their Prevention by Zinc, J. Natl. Cancer Inst. 31:745, 1963.

23. Clegg, E.J., and Carr, I.: Changes in the Blood Vessels of the Rat Testis and Epididymis Produced by Cadmium Chloride, J. Pathol. Bacteriol 94:317, 1967.

24. Parizek, J.: Vascular Changes at Sites of Oestrogen Biosynthesis Produced by Parenteral Injection of Cadmium Salts. The Destruction of Placenta by Cadmium Salts, J. Reprod, Fertil. 7:263, 1964.

25. Piscator, M.: Haemolytic Anaemia in Cadmium Poisoned Rabbits, Excerpta Med. Int. Congr. Series 62:952, 1963.

26. Jones, R.H., Williams, R.L., and Jones, A.M.: Effects of Heavy Metal on the Immune Response, Preliminary Findings for Cadmium in Rats, Proc. Soc. Exper. Biol. Med. 137:1321, 1971.

27. Vigliani, E.C.: The Biopathology of Cadmium, Amer. Ind. Hyg. Assoc. 30:329, 1969.

28. Baum, J., and Worthen, H.G.: Induction of Amyliodosis by Cadmium, Nature 213:1040, 1967.

29. Piscator, M.: Proteinuria in Chronic Cadmium Poisoning. II. The Applicability of Quantitative and Qualitative Methods of Protein Determination for the Demonstration of Cadmium Proteinuria, Arch. Environ. Health 5:325, 1962.

30. Axelsson, B., and Piscator, M.: Renal Damage After Prolonged Exposure to Cadmium. An Experimental Study, Arch. Environ. Health 12:360, 1966.

31. Nomiyama, K., Sato, C., and Yamamoto, A.: Early Signs of Cadmium Intoxication in Rabbits, Toxicol. Appl. Pharmacol. 24:625, 1973.

32. Vander, A.J.: Cadmium Enhancement of Proximal Tubular Sodium Reabsorbtion, Amer. J. Physiol. 203:1005, 1962.

33. Thind, G.S., Biery, D.N., and Bovee, K.C.: Production of Arterial Hypertension by Cadmium in the Dog, J. Lab. Clin. Med. 81:549, 1973.

34. Thind, G.S., Karreman, G., Stephen, K.F., et al: Vascular Reactivity and Mechanical Properties of Normal and Cadmium-Hypertensive Rabbits, J. Lab. Clin. Med. 76:560, 1970.

35. Schroeder, H.A., Kroll, S.S., Little, J.W. et al: Hypertension in Rats From Injection of Cadmium, Arch. Environ. Health 13:788, 1966.

36. Perry, H.M., Jr., Erlanger, M.W., Yunice, A. et al: Hypertension and Tissue Metal Levels Following Intravenous Cadmium, Mercury and Zinc, Amer. J. Physiol. 219:755, 1970.

37. Perry, H.M. Jr. and Erlanger, M.: Hypertension and Tissue Metal Levels After Intraperitoneal Cadmium, Mercury and Zinc, Amer. J. Physiol. 220:808, 1971.

38. Perry, H.M.,Jr. and Yunice, A.: Acute Pressor Effects of Intra-Arterial Cadmium and Mercuric Ions in Anesthetized Rats, Proc. Soc. Exper. Biol. Med. 120:805, 1965.

39. Fox, M.R., Fry, B.E.G.: Cadmium Toxicity Increased by Dietary Ascorbic Acid Supplements, Science 169:989, 1970.

40 Itokawa, Y., Abe, To., Tabu, R. et al: Renal and Skeletal Lesions in Experimental Cadmium Poisoning, Arch. Environ. Health 23:93, 1971.

41. Doyle, J.J., Pfander, W.H., Grebing, S.E., et al: Effect of Dietary Cadmium on Growth, Cadmium Absorption and Cadmium Tissue Levels in Growing Lambs, J. Nutr. 104:160, 1974.

42. Miller, M.L., Murthy, L., and Sorenson, J.R.: Fine Structure of Connective Tissue After Ingestion of Cadmium, Arch. Path. 98:286, 1974.

43. Nishizumi, M.: Electron Microscopic Study of Cadmium Nephrotoxicity in the Rat, Arch. Environ. Health 24:215, 1972.

44. Schroeder, H.A. and Vinton, W.H.J.: Hypertension Induced in Rats by Small Doses of Cadmium, Amer. J. Physiol. 202:515, 1962.

45. Perry, H.M., Jr.: Review of Hypertension Induced by Chronic Ingestion of Cadmium: Trace Elements in Human Health and Disease, Vol. 2, 1975, Pg. 417.

46. Perry, H.M.,Jr., Tipton, I.H., Schroeder, H.A. et al: Variation in the Concentration of Cadmium in Human Kidney as a Function of Age and Geographic Origin, J. Chron. Dis. 14:259, 1961.

47. Paterson, J.R.: Studies on the Toxicity of Inhaled Cadmium. III. The Pathology of Cadmium Smoke Poisoning in Man and in Experimental Animals, J. Ind. Hyg. Toxicol. 29:294, 1947.

48. Snider, G.L., Hayes, J.A., Korthy, A.L., et al: Centri-lobular Emphysema Experimentally Induced by Cadmium Chloride Aerosol, Amer. Rev. Resp. Dis. 108:40, 1973.

49. Friberg, L.: Health Hazards in the Manufacture of Alka-line Accumulators With Special Reference to Chronic Cad-mium Poisoning, Acta Med. Scand. 138: (Suppl 240) 1950.

50. Thurlbeck, M.W., and Foley, F.D.: Experimental Pulmonary Emphysema. The Effect of Intratracheal Injection of Cadmium Chloride Solution in the Guinea Pig, Amer. J. Pathol. 42:431, 1963.

51. Harrison, H.E., Bunting, H., Ordway, N.K., and Albrink, W.S.: The Effects and Treatment of Inhalation of Cadmium Aerosols in the Dog, J. Indust. Hygiene and Toxicol, 29:302, 1947.

52. Jacobs, E.E., Jacob, M., Sanadi, D.R. et al: Uncoupling of Oxidative Phosphorylation by Cadmium Ion, J. Biol. Chem. 223:157, 1956.

53. Mustafa, M.G., Cross, C.E., and Tyler, W.S.: Interfer-ence of Cadmium Ion With Oxidative Metabolism of Alveo-lar Macrophages, Arch. Intern. Med. 127: 1050, 1971.

54. Tipton, I.H., and Cook, J.J.: Trace Elements in Human Tissue. II. Adult Subjects From the United States, Health Physics 9:103, 1963.

55. Schroeder, H.A.: Cadmium as a Factor in Hypertension, J. Chron. Dis. 18:648, 1965.

56. Morgan, J.M.: Tissue Cadmium Concentration in Man, Arch. Intern. Med. 123:404, 1969.

57. Lener, J. and Bibr, R.: Cadmium and Hypertension, Lancet 1: 970, 1971.

58. Ostergaard, K.: Cadmium and Hypertension, Lancet 1:677, 1977.

59. Perry, H.M.,Jr.: A Preliminary Examination of the Renal and Hepatic Cadmium and Zinc in Normotensive and Hypertensive Men From St. Louis, Joint World Health Organization/ International Atomic Energy Agency Research Program on Trace Elements in Cardiovascular Diseases, Vienna, Austria.

60. Hem, J.D.: Chemistry and Occurrence of Cadmium and Zinc in Surface Water and Ground Water, Water Resources Research 8:3, 1972.

61. Schroeder, H.A., and Balassa, J.J.: Abnormal Trace Metals in Man: Cadmium, J. Chron. Dis. 14:236, 1961.

62. Perry, H.M.,Jr., Erlander, M.W., and Perry, E.F.: Inhibition of Cadmium-Induced Hypertension in Rats, The Science of the Total Environment 14:153, 1980.

63. Beese, D.H.: Tobacco Consumption in Various Countries, Res. Paper #6, Tobacco Research Council, London, 1972.

64. Niosh Criteria for a Recommended Standard Occupational Exposure to Cadmium, US Dept. HEW Aug. 1976.

65. Tohyama, C., Shaikh, Z.A., Ellis, K.J., and Cohn, S.H.: Urinary Metallothionein as a Biological Indicator of Occupational Cadmium Exposure, Third International Cadmium Conference, Miami, 1982 180-2.

66. Ellis, K.J., Vartsky Italo Zani, D., Cohn, S.H. and Yasumura, S.: Cadmium: In Vivo Measurement in Smokers and NonSmokers, Science 205:323, 1979.

CURRENT USE OF AMBIENT AND BIOLOGICAL MONITORING: REFERENCE
WORKPLACE HAZARDS.   INORGANIC TOXIC AGENTS - DISCUSSION OF
CARBON MONOXIDE AND CADMIUM*

W. SUNDERMAN (USA)

Summary

*Workers vary in susceptibilities to specific toxic agents as
a consequence of individual variations in work practices,
personal habits, predisposing conditions, and genetic
factors.   In order to safeguard workers' health, ambient
monitoring of toxic agents must oftimes be supplemented by
biological monitoring.   To illustrate the current status of
biological monitoring of toxic inorganic agents, carbon
monoxide and cadmium are discussed as reference hazards in
the workplace.   Attention is focused particularly upon (a)
selection, standardisation, and interlaboratory comparison
comparison of analytical procedures, (b) applications of non-
invasive instrumental techniques to estimate body burdens,
(c) diagnostic tests for organ-specific toxicity, and (d)
problems in interpretations of analytical results owing to
confounding factors such as cigarette smoking and mixed
exposures to toxic agents. In the multidisciplinary approach
to protection of workers' health, clinical pathologists play
an important role by developing and supervising biological
monitoring procedures and by helping to interpret the
analytical results.*

* Supported by Grant No. ES-01337 from the National Institute
  of Environmental Health Sciences and Grant No. EV-03140
  from the US Department of Energy.

Introduction

Ambient monitoring of toxic agents in the workplace has become an indispensable facet of health protection programmes for workers. Nonetheless, as the papers in this session amply demonstrate, ambient monitoring procedures often need to be supplemented by biological monitoring procedures. To safeguard the health of exposed workers, it frequently is necessary to measure concentrations of toxic agents and their metabolites in body fluids and excreta, and also to perform diagnostic tests for organ-specific toxicity (e.g. blood leukocyte counts, urine protein determinations). Such biological monitoring procedures identify persons with propensity for toxicity from specific workplace hazards, as a consequence of individual variations in (a) work practices (e.g. mixed exposure to toxic agents, failure to observe safety precautions), (b) personal habits (e.g. smoking, alcohol), (c) predisposing disease (e.g. anaemia, emphysema), and (d) genetic factors (e.g. slow acetylation phenotype, erythrocyte NADH dehydrogenase variant). The organisers of this International Seminar have selected carbon monoxide (CO) and cadmium (Cd) as reference workplace hazards upon which to focus the considerations of inorganic toxic agents. I am elaborating upon selected topics introduced by previous speakers that pertain to the biological monitoring of CO and Cd and am sketching the role of clinical pathologists in the multidisciplinary approach to protection of workers' health.

Analysis of CO in blood

Gasometric methods for analysis of blood CO content by the Conway microdiffusion cell, the Scholander-Boughton syringe, or the Van Slyke-Henderson apparatus are cumbersome, time-consuming, imprecise, and insensitive; they are now outmoded. At present, gas chromatography is the reference procedure for analysis of CO in blood and tissues. In my laboratory, blood CO content is currently measured by a modification of the gas chromatographic procedure of Rodkey and Collison (1). Blood is injected into a septum vial that contains potassium ferricyanide-citric acid-Sterox reagent to release CO into the head-space. The evolved gas is swept by a stream of helium on to a train of chromatographic columns, including calcium chloride (to remove H_2O vapour), soda lime (to remove CO_2), molecular sieve 5A (to separate CO), and nickel catalyst (to convert CO to CH_4); the CH_4 is measured by a hydrogen flame ionization detector. Like other gas chromatographic techniques for CO analysis (2-7), this procedure has the advantages of being precise, sensitive, and specific; it has the disadvantages of being relatively time-consuming and requiring an analyst with specialised skills.

Numerous spectrophotometric methods have been described for analysis of CO in blood. Most of these procedures were developed for forensic analysis of blood obtained post-mortem; only a few of the procedures are suitable for analysis of blood carboxyhaemoglobin (COHb) in the range from 0.5 to 20 % saturation that generally pertains to biological monitoring of workers. Heinemann _et al_. (8) evaluated five commonly used spectrophotometric methods and found that three of the procedures were insufficiently sensitive and precise for measurements of blood samples with COHb saturation near the normal range. The two acceptable procedures were the five-wavelength method of Commins and Lawther (9) and the three-wavelenth "CO-Oximeter" method of Malenfant _et al_. (10). Results obtained by these two procedures were in close agreement; both techniques yielded within-run precision values of less than 5% (coefficient of variation) for blood samples with 2 to 6% COHb saturation. Another method that is well suited for biological monitoring of blood COHb satura-tion has recently been reported by Rodkey _et al_. (11), based upon dilution of blood approximately 10000-fold in sodium hydrosulphite solution and spectrophotometric measurements in the Soret region (420 and 432 nm). This procedure, which requires only 3 μ of blood, yields results that correlate closely with the results of gas chromato-graphic analyses of blood samples with 0.5 to 12% COHb saturation (11).

There is reasonable agreement among reported values for blood COHb saturation in healthy nonsmokers who do not have occupational exposures to CO; McCredie and Jose (3), Coburn et al. (12), and Collison et al. (4) reported means (+SD) for blood COHb saturation in nonsmokers of 0.87 + 0.29%, 0.88 + 0.11%, and 0.85 + 0.26%, respectively. Smokers have significantly higher values for blood COHb saturation. For instance, McCredie and Jose (3) found that blood COHb saturation averaged 4.13 (SD + 1.99%) in 23 chronic smokers. Therefore, data about workers' smoking habits are essential for interpreting measurements of blood COHn saturation. Measurements of blood haemoglobin concentration and packed cell volume are advisable in conjunction with analyses of blood HbCO saturation, since chronic exposures to low concentrations of CO (e.g. in cigarette smoke) may induce compensatory erythrocytosis (13-15), and since persons with anaemia have increased susceptibility to CO toxicity. Analyses of methaemoglobin (MetHb) concentrations in blood should be performed in conjunction with HbCO analyses in blood of workers who have combined exposure to nitrates and CO. Such workers may develop reduced O_2-carrying capacity of blood owing to simultaneous occurrence of mild elevations of MetHb and COHb. The same problem can result from familial methaemoglobinaemia, owing to genetic variants of erythrocyte NADH dehydrogenase. Measurements of COHb and MetHb can be performed concurrently in microsamples of blood by the spectophotometric procedure of Rodkey et al. (11).

Analysis of CO in breath

The partial pressure of CO in end-expired breath approximates that in alveolar air (Paco), and is directly related to the COHb saturation of venous blood. Based upon analyses of CO in end-expired breath of human subjects following breath-holding for 20 seconds after maximum inspiration, Jones et al. (16) documented close correlation between Paco and blood COHb saturation. They concluded that CO concentration in end-expired breath can serve as a reliable index of CO exposure. Stewart et al. (17) used a portable electrochemical CO analyser to measure CO concentrations in end-expired breath of fire-fighters. This procedure has not been widely adopted for biological monitoring in the workplace, since sampling of end-expired breath after breath-holding requires training of the subjects. Moreover, the technique is invalid in persons with pulmonary insufficiency. Rawbone et al. (18) and Rees et al. (19) showed that Paco can be reliably estimated from analysis of CO concentration in mixed-expired breath, provided that a suitable allowance is made for deadspace. To provide a sample of mixed-expired breath, the subject merely breathes tidally for 10 to 20 breaths through a one-way valve. The expired air is passed through a canister of soda lime and calcium chloride to absorb CO_2 and H_2O vapour, and the CO concentration is measured with a portable infra-red CO analyser(19). Rees et al. (19) demonstrated that smokers can be discriminated from nonsmokers by analysis of CO in mixed-expired breath; Paco values ranged from 0.8 to 1.6 Pascals in 49 nonsmokers, versus 1.9 to 4.2 Pascals in 31 persons who smoked 21 to 30 cigarettes per day. Analysis of CO in mixed-expired breath has the following advantages for biological monitoring of CO expousres in the workplace: (a) blood samples are unnecessary; (b) the procedure can be completed in approximately one minute; (c) the equipment is portable and moderately priced, and (d) prior training of the subjects is unnecessary.

Endogenous CO production xenobiotic metabolism

Observations by Stewart et al. in 1972 (20) provided the initial evidence that CO poisoning can result from metabolism of dichloromethane. They found sustained elevations of blood COHb saturation in subjects who inhaled dichloromethane in atmospheric concentrations from 500 to 10000 ppm for 1 to 3 hours. These findings were confirmed by Fodor and Roscovanu (21). Carboxyhaemoglobinaemia from metabolism of dichloromethane has been reported to induce myocardial infarction (22). Since dichloromethane is widely used as a paint remover and

industrial solvent, the metabolism of dichloromethane to CO
has practical importance in the workplace; monitoring of
blood COHb saturation is valuable for surveillance of
workers exposed to dichloromethane. Studies in experimental
animals demonstrate endogenous production of CO from metabolism of other haloalkanes and of various methylenedioxy-
phenyl compounds (27). Although the mechanisms of CO-
generation have not been elucidated in detail, the endogenous
production of Co from these xenobiotics occurs in hepatic
microsomes and requires NADPH, cytochrome P-450, and glutathione (25,27). Phenobarbital markedly stimulates the metabolism of bromoform to CO (24). Endogenous formation of CO
from the metabolism of xenobiotics is a surprising phenomenon, since endogenous CO production was formerly believed to
derive exclusively from (a) the activity of haeme oxygenase,
a microsomal enzyme that cleaves -methen bridge of haeme to
liberate CO, iron, and biliverdin (28,29), and (b), the
perodixation of microsomal lipids (30).

Analysis of Cd in body fluids

Biological monitoring of Cd exposure in the workplace rests
primarily upon analyses of Cd concentrations in whole blood
and urine. Colorimetric dithizone methods and emission
spectrographic techniques, formerly employed for analysis of
Cd in body fluids, lack sufficient sensitivity, specificity,
and reproducibility; they have been discarded by clinical
laboratories. Electrothermal atomic absorption spectrophotometry and anodic stripping voltametry are now the preferred
methods for determination of Cd concentrations in biological
materials (30,31). Although techniques for Cd analysis in
blood and urine have advanced considerably during the past
decade, there is serious need for further improvement.
Interlaboratory surveys of blood Cd analyses conducted by
Lauwerys et al. (33) Paulev et al. (34) and Stoeppler and
Tonks (personal communication) have revealed poor correlations among the results obtained by participating laboratories. Many techniques that are used for analyses of Cd in

body fluids rely upon "standard additions" or "internal standardisation" to compensate for interferences by various constituents of the biological matrices. Such approaches are subject to analytical errors that are particularly trouble-some since they are often unsuspected. Cd concentrations obtained by rapid, direct methods should be validated by comparisons with results obtained by a reference method of established accuracy. The Subcommittee on Environmental and Occupational Toxicology of Cadmium of the International Union of Pure and Applied Chemistry (IUPAC) is currently developing reference procedures for analysis of Cd in blood and urine by electrothermal atomic absorption spectrophotometry and by anodic stripping voltametry. These reference procedures will be the basis of an international effort for collaborative harmonization of analyses of Cd concentrations in body fluids. This effort is vitally important for biological monitoring of workers' exposures to Cd compounds in industries throughout the world.

Results of recent analyses of Cd concentrations in body fluids of healthy subjects without known occupational exposures to cadmium compounds are listed in Table 1. The tabulated mean values for Cd concentrations in whole blood of nonsmokers vary 6-fold from 0.5 μg/litre (35) to 3.3 μg/litre (31). Despite this variability, mean Cd concentrations in blood of tobacco smokers were consistently higher than the corresponding values in blood of nonsmokers. Therefore, data about workers' smoking habits are equally essential for interpreting biological indices of occupational exposures to Cd as they are for interpreting biological indices of occupa-tional exposures to CO.

Table 1   Concentrations of Cd in whole blood and urine
          of healthy persons without known occupational
          exposures to Cd compounds

Authors	Date	No. of Subjects	Cd concentra-tions blood	(μg/litre)* urine
Ulander & Axelson (35)	1974	45 nonsmokers 45 smokers	0.5 (0.2-1.2) 2.1 (0.5-7.6)	
Beevers et al. (36)	1976	35 nonsmokers 35 smokers	1.8 + 0.8 3.2 $\mp$ 1.6	
Miller et al. (37)	1976	22[+]		1.1($<$0.5-2.5)
Christensen & Angelo(31)	1978	67 nonsmokers 114 smokers	3.3 (0.6-6.7) 5.5 (0.6-9.6)	
Ward et al. (38)	1978	16 nonsmokers 7 smokers	1.8 + 0.7 3.8 $\mp$ 1.2	
Pleban & Pearson (39)	1979	61 nonsmokers 50 smokers	0.7 (0.3-2.1) 1.5 (0.3-4.2)	
Ellis et al. (40)	1979	8 nonsmokers 12 smokers	1.6 + 0.8 2.5 $\mp$ 1.1	1.7 + 1.0 2.7 $\mp$ 1.3
Lagesson & Andrasko (41)	1979	12[+]	1.5(0.7-3.8)	1.6 (0.5-3.2)
Allain & Mauras (42)	1979	10[+]	0.7 + 0.3	0.5 + 0.3
Bernard et al. (43)	1979	77[+]	1.8 (0.2-4.9)	0.8 (0.1-1.8)#

* Mean (and range) or mean + standard deviation

+ Smoking habits unspecified

Cd concentration expressed as μg/g creatinine

Neutron activation Analysis of Cd burdens in vivo

Several investigations have shown that Cd concentrations in
human organs can be estimated by in vivo neutron activation
analysis (IVNAA) (40,43-47). The IVNAA technique involves
irradiation of the targeted organ (e.g. liver, left kidney)
with a collimated neutron beam; Cd atoms in the organ emit
prompt gamma-rays (559 keV) that are quantitated with a
Ge(Li) detector. Prior to 1979, clinical applications of
IVNAA were limited by use of a cyclotron as the neutron
source. The recent introduction of isotopic neutron sources
(e.g. $^{238}Pu/Be$, $^{241}Am/Be$) has resulted in transportable
IVNAA instruments for biological monitoring of Cd burdens in
healthy smokers versus nonsmokers. They found that the
geometric mean content of Cd in left kidneys of 12 healthy
smokers was 5.8 (SD $\pm$ 1.7) mg/organ (P< 0.05 versus 3.1 $\pm$ 2.0
mg/organ in nonsmokers). They also observed that the
geometric mean concentration of Cd in livers of 12 healthy
smokers was 4.1 (SD $\pm$ 1.6) mg/kg (P < 0.05 versus 2.3 $\pm$ 1.6
mg/kg in nonsmokers). The IVNAA instrument used by Ellis et
al. (8) has a Cd detection limit of 2.5 mg/kidney or 1.5
mg/kg of liver, with a localised radiation dose of 0.067 rad.
Roels et al. (47) employed IVNAA to estimate Cd burdens in
309 workers in two cadmium-producing plants. In 231 workers
with normal renal function, Cd burdens in renal cortex
averaged 200 mg/kg (5th and 95th percentiles = 87 to 248
mg/kg); Cd burdens in liver averaged 39 mg/kg (5th and 95th
percentiles = 17 to 48 mg/kg). In 78 workers with renal
dysfunction, Cd burdens in renal cortex did not differ significantly from the corresponding values in workers with normal
renal function. Roels et al. (47) speculated that Cd burdens
in renal cortex decrease progressively after the onset of
kidney damage; they estimated that the critical concentration
of Cd in renal cortex that induces renal damage lies between
200 and 250 mg/kg. Roels et al. (47) employed an IVNAA instrument described by Thomas et al. (45) that has a detection
limit of 10 mg/kg of liver with a measurement time of 10
minutes, and a localised radiation dose of 0.05 to 0.07 rem.

Since IVNAA is the only direct, noninvasive method to estimate Cd burdens in target organs, this technique is valuable as a research tool to test possible correlations between Cd burdens in liver and kidney and concentrations of Cd in blood, urine, and other body fluids. Applications of IVNAA should help to elucidate the toxicokinetics of Cd in man and the possible influence of Cd burdens in liver and kidney on the occurrence of hypertension, cancers, and other disease. However, because of the drawbacks of radiation exposures, time-consuming procedures, and costly, complex instrumentation, IVNAA is not yet suitable as a routine technique for biological monitoring of Cd burdens in industrial workers.

Proteinuria as an index of Cd nephrotoxicity

Proteinuria is the earliest biochemical sign of chronic cadmium intoxication (48-53). Nephrotoxicity from chronic inhalation or ingestion of cadmium compounds induces three forms of proteinuria: (a) "tubular-type" proteinuria with increased urinary excretion of beta-2-microglobulin, retinol-binding protein, and other proteins with low molecular weight (40,000 daltons); (b) "glomerular-type" proteinuria with increased urinary excretion of albumin, transferrin, and other proteins with high molecular weight (40,000 daltons); and (c) "mixed-type" proteinuria, which is a combination of the other two types. Bernard and coworkers (52,53) studied the urinary excretion of proteins in 42 Cd-exposed workers with blood Cd concentrations $> 10 \mu g$/litre and urine Cd concentrations $> 10 \mu g$/g creatinine. Abnormal electrophoretic patterns of urine proteins were observed in 15 (36%) of the Cd-exposed workers. Four of the Cd-exposed workers had tubular-type proteinuria with increased renal clearance of beta-2-microglobulin and normal albumin clearance; three of the Cd-exposed workers had glomerular-type proteinuria with increased renal clearance of albumin and normal beta-2-microglobulin clearance; five of the Cd-exposed workers had mixed-type proteinuria, with increases of both beta-2-micro-

globulin and albumin clearance. Proteinuria of the tubular,
glomerular, and mixed types, as well as lysosomal enzymuria
(beta-galactosidaseuria), were chiefly observed in workers
with 25 years of Cd-exposure. No single abnormality of
urine protein excretion developed systematically before the
others (52,53). Bernard et al. (54) investigated the urinary
excretion of proteins in rats following long-term oral
administration of $CdCl_2$; glomerular or mixed type protein-
urias predominated in the rats. The observations of Bernard
et al. (52-54) agree with the conclusions of Friberg et al.
(48) that urinary excretion of low-molecular weight proteins
(e.g. beta-2-microglobulin) is insufficient to reflect the
general status of Cd-induced proteinuria. To evaluate proteinuria in Cd-exposed workers, Friberg et al. (48) recommended electrophoretic fractionations of urine proteins and
quantitation of urine total proteins and beta-2-micro-
globulin. In my laboratory, measurements of urine total
protein, beta-2-microglobulin, and N-acetyl-beta-D-
glucoseaminidase activity are used routinely to monitor
workers in a Ni-Cd battery plant and in electroplating shops
for metal-induced nephrotoxicity. Urine total protein is
measured by the biuret procedure of Savory et al. (55); urine
beta-2-microglobulin concentration is measured by the radioimmunoassay of Horak and Sunderman (56); and N-acetyl-beta-D-
glucoseaminidase activity is measured by the spectrophotometric assay of Horak et al. (57). When abnormal results are
obtained in one or more of these assays, electrophoretic
fractionations of urine proteins are performed by the
cellulose acetate technique of Savory et al (58) to classify
the proteinuria a "glomerular", "tubular" or "mixed type".

A recent report by Iannaccone et al (59) suggests that diminished urinary excretion of kallikrein activity might serve as
a sensitive biological index of Cd-exposure. In Cd-exposed
workers and in experimental animals (rabbits), Iannaccone et
al. (59) found that Cd-induced nephrotoxicity is associated
with marked diminution of urine kallikrein activity. This
interesting observation deserves further investigation.

Role of clinical pathologists in biological monitoring

Major topics for consideration at this International Seminar
are the roles of individual disciplines (e.g. the nurse, the
industrial hygienist, the occupational physician, the
epidemiologist, the engineer, the analytical chemist, etc.)
in the multidisciplinary approach to health protection and
disease prevention by monitoring in the workplace. In this
context, the organisers of the seminar asked me to mention
the expanding role of the clinical pathologist in the
occupational arena. As the focus of monitoring toxic agents
in the workplace has shifted from ambient to biological
indices, clinical patholgists have become involved in
formulating monitoring protocols, in developing and
supervising haematological, biochemical and ctyological
tests, in establishing reference ranges and critical values,
and in helping to interpret analytical results. The
expertise of clinical patholgists is particularly valuable in
identifying genetic factors and predisposing conditions that
contribute to indiviudal variatons in susceptibility to
chemical toxins in the workplace.

References

1.   Rodkey, F.L., Collison, H.A. An artifact in the analy-
     sis of oxygenated blood for its low carbon monoxide
     content. Clin. Chem. 1970; 16:896-899.

2.   Ayres, S.M., Criscitiello, A., Giannelli, S., Jr.
     Determination of blood carbon monoxide content by gas
     chromatography. J. Appl. Physiol. 1966; 21:1368-1370.

3.   McGredie, R.M., Jose, A.D. Analysis of blood carbon
     monoxide and oxygen by gas chromatography. J. Appl.
     Physiol. 1967; 22:863-866.

4.   Collison, H.A., Rodkey, F.L., O'Neal, J.D.
     Determination of carbon monoxide in blood by gas
     chromatography. Clin. Chem. 1968; 14:162-171.

5.   Dahlms, T.E., Horvath, S.M. Rapid accurate technique
     for determination of carbon monoxide in blood. Clin.
     Chem. 1974; 20:533-537.

6.   Dubowski, K.M., Luke, J.L.   Measurement of carboxyhaemo-
     globin and carbon monoxide in blood. Ann. Clin. Lab.
     Sci. 1973; 3:53-65.

7.   Griffin, B.R.   A sensitive method for the routine deter-
     mination of carbon monoxide in blood using flame
     ionization gas chromatography. J. Anal. Toxicol. 1979;
     3:102-103.

8.   Heinemann,   G.,   Loschenkohl,   K.,   Schievelbein, H.
     Comparative evaluation of different spectrophotometric
     methods for the determination of small amounts of
     carboxyhaemoglobin.   J.   Clin.   Chem.   Clin.   Biochem.
     1979; 17:647-651.

9.   Commins, B.T., Lawther, P.J.   A sensitive method for the
     determination of carboxyhaemoglobin in a finger prick
     sample of blood.   Brit. J. Ind. Med. 1965; 22:139-143.

10. Malenfant, A.L., Gambino, S.R., Waraksa, A.J., Roe, E.I.
     Spectrophotometric determination of haemoglobin concen-
     tration and percent oxyhaemoglobin and carboxyhaemo-
     globin saturation.   Clin. Chem. 1968; 14:789.

11. Rodkey,   F.L.,   Hill,   T.A.,   Pitts,   L.L.,   Robertson, R.F.
     Spectrophotometric measurements of carboxyhaemoglobin
     and methaemoglobin in blood.   Clin. Chem. 1979; 29:1388-
     1393.

12. Coburn, R.R., Danielson, G.K., Blakemore, W.S., Forster,
     R.E.   Carbon monoxide in blood: Analytical method and
     sources of error.   J. Appl. Physiol. 1964; 19:510-515.

13. Isager,   H., Hagerup, L.   Relationship between cigarette
     smoking and high packed cell volume and haemoglobin
     levels. Scand. J. Haemat. 1971; 8:241-244.

14. Sagone, A.L. Jr.   Balcersak, S.P.   Smoking as a cause of
     erythrocytosis.   Ann. Intern. Med. 1975; 82:512-515.

15. Smith,   J.R.,   Landaw,   S.A.   Smokers' polycythemia.   New
     Engl. J. Med. 1978; 298:6-10.

16. Jones,   R.H.,   Ellicott,   M.F.,   Cadigan, J.B.,   Gaensler,
     E.A.   The relationship between alveolar and blood carbon
     monoxide concentrations during breatholding.   J. Lab.
     Clin. Med. 1958; 51:533-564.

17. Stewart,   R.D.,   Stewart,   R.S.,   Stamm, W.,   Seelen, R.P.
     Rapid estimation of carboxyhaemoglobin level in fire
     fighters.   J. Amer. Med. Assn. 1976; 235:390-392.

18. Rawbone, R.G., Coppin, C.A.,, Guz, A.   Carbon monoxide
     in alveolar air as an index of exposure to cigarette
     smoke.   Clin. Sci. Mol. Med. 1976; 51:495-501.

19. Rees, P.J., Chilvers, C., Clark, T.J.H. Evaluation of
     methods used to estimate inhaled dose of carbon
     monoxide. Thorax 1980; 35:47-51.

20. Stewart, R.D., Fisher, T.N., Hosko, M.J., Petersen,
     J.E., Baretta, E.D., Dodd; H.C. Carboxyhaemoglobin
     evaluation after exposure to dichloromethane. Science
     1972; 176:295-296.

21. Fodor, G.G., Roscovanu, A. Increased blood CO-content
     in humans and animals by incorporated halogenated
     hydrocarbons. Zbl. Bakt. Hyg. I Abt., Orig B. 1976;
     162:34-40.

22. Stewart, R.D,, Hake, C.L. Paint-remover hazard. J.
     Amer. Med. Assn. 1976; 235:398-401.

23. Kubik, V.L., Anders, M.W., Engel, R.R., Barlow, C.H.,
     Caughey, W.S. Metabolism of dihalomethanes to carbon
     monoxide. I In vivo studies. Drug Metab. Dispos. 1978;
     6:556-560.

24. Anders, M.W., Stevens, J.L., Sprague, R.W., Shaath, Z.,
     Ahmed, A.E. Metabolism of haloforms to carbon monoxide.
     II In vivo studies. Drug. Metab. Dispos. 1978; 6:556-
     560.

25. Stevens, J.L., Anders, M.W. Metabolism of haloforms to
     carbon monoxide. III Studies on the mechanism of the
     reaction. Biochem. Pharmacol. 1979; 28:3189-3194.

26. Ahmed, A.E., Kubic, V.L., Stevens, J.L., Anders, M.W.
     Halogenated methanes: metabolism and toxicity. Fed.
     Proc. 1980; 39;3150-3155.

27. Yu, L-S, Wilkinson, C.F., Anders, M.W. Generation of
     carbon monoxide during the microsomal metabolism of
     methylenedioxyphenyl compounds. Biochem. Pharmacol.
     1980; 29:1113-1122.

28. Tenhunen, R., Marver, H.S., Schmid, R. Microsomal
     haeme oxygenase: Characterization of the enzyme. J.
     Biol. Chem. 1968; 244:6388-6394.

29. Sunderman, F.W.,Jr. Effects of xenobiotics on haeme
     oxygenase activity. Dev. Clin. Biochem 1980; 2 : 221-
     35.

30. Wolff, P.G,, Bidlack, W.R. The formation of carbon
     monoxide during peroxidation of microsomal lipids.
     Biochem. Biophys. Res. Commun. 1976; 73:850-857.

31. Christensen, J.M., Angelo, H. A rapid direct
     determination of cadmium in blood by anodic stripping
     voltametry. Scand. J. Clin. Lab. Invest. 1978; 38:655-
     658.

32. Stoeppler, M., Brandt, K. Contributions to automated trace analysis. V. Determination of cadmium in whole blood and urine electrothermal atomic-absorption spectrophotometry. Fresenius Z. Anal. Chem. 1980; 300:372-380.

33. Lauwerys, R., Buchet, J-P., Roels, H., Berlin, A., Sweets, J. Intercomparison program of lead, mercury and cadmium analysis in blood, urine and aqueous solutions. Clin. Chem. 1975; 21:551-557.

34. Paulev., P-E., Solgaard, P.M., Tjell, J.C. Inter-laboratory comparison of lead and cadmium in blood, urine and aqueous solutions. Clin. Chem. 1978; 24:1797-1800.

35. Ulander, A,, Axelson, O. Measurement of blood-cadmium levels. Lancet 1974; 1:682-683.

36. Beevers, D.G., Campbell, B.C., Goldberg, A., Moore, M.R., Hawthorne, V.M. Blood-cadmium in hypertensives and normotensives. Lancet 1976; 2:1222-1224.

37. Muller, G.J., Wylie, K.J., McKeown, D. Cadmium exposure and renal accumulation in an Australian urban population. Med. J. Austral. 1976; 1:20-23.

38. Ward, R.J., Fisher, M., Tellez-Yudilevich, M. Signifi-cance of blood cadmium concentrations in patients with renal disorders or essential hypertension and the normal population. Ann. Clin. Biochem. 1978; 15:197-200.

39. Pleban, P.A., Pearson, K.H. Determination of cadmium in whole blood and urine by Zeeman atomic absorption spectroscopy. Clin. Chem. Acta 1979; 99:267-277.

40. Ellis, K.J., Varsky, D., Zanzi, I., Cohen, S.H., Yasumura, S. Cadmium: in vivo measurements in smokers and nonsmokers. Science 1979; 205:323-325.

41. Lagesson, V., Andrasko, L. Direct determination of lead and cadmium in blood and urine by flameless atomic absorption spectrophotometry. Clin. Chem. 1979; 25:1948-1953.

42. Allain, P., Mauras, Y. Microdetermination of lead and cadmium in blood and urine by graphite furnace atomic absorption spectrophotometry. Clin. Chem. Acta 1979; 91:41-46.

43. McLellan, J.S., Thomas, B.J., Fremlin, J.H., Harvey, T.C. Cadmium - its in vivo detection in man. Phys. Med. Biol. 1975; 20:88-95.

44. Vartsky, D., Ellis, K.J., Chen, N.S., and Cohn, S.H. A facility for in vivo measurement of kidney and liver cadmium by neutron capture prompt gamma ray analysis. Phys. Med. Biol. 1977; 22:1085-1096.

45   Thomas, B.J., Harvey, T.C., Chettle, D.R., McLellan,
      J.S., Fremlin, J.H. A transportable system for the
      measurement of liver cadmium in vivo. Phys. Med. Biol.
      1979; 24:432-437.

46.   Al-Hiti, K., Slaibi, S., Al-Kayat, T. Portable system
      for detecting cadmium in the human liver. Int. J. Appl.
      Radiat. Isot. 1979; 30:55-60.

47.   Roels, H., Bernard, A., Buchet, J.P., Goret, A.,
      Lauwerys, R., Chettle, D.R., Harvey, T.C., Al-Haddad, I.
      Critical concentration of cadmium in renal cortex and
      urine. Lancet 1979; 1:221.

48.   Friberg, L., Kjellstrom, T., Nordberg, G., Piscator, M.
      Cadmium. In "Handbook on the Toxicology of Metals" (L.
      Friberg, G.F. Nordberg, V.E. Vonk, Eds). Elsevier/North
      Holland Biomedical Press, 1979; 355-381.

49.   Carruthers, M., Smith, B. Evidence of cadmium toxicity
      in a population living in a zinc-mining area. Lancet
      1979; 1:845-847.

50.   Sandifer, S.H., Wilkins, R.T., Whitlock, N.H., Virella,
      G., Loadholt, C.B., Leitner, T.C. Urinary protein
      excretion in workers exposed to low doses of cadmium.
      Bull. Environ. Contam. Toxicol. 1979; 23:129-135.

51.   Iwao, S., Tsuchiya, K., Sakurai, H. Serum and urinary
      beta-2-microglobulin among cadmium-exposed workers. J.
      Occup. Med. 1980; 22:399-402.

52.   Bernard, A., Buchet, J.P., Roels, H., Masson, P.,
      Lauwerys, R. Renal excretion of proteins and enzymes in
      workers exposed to cadmium. Eur. J. Clin. Invest.
      1979; 9:11-22.

53.   Roels, H., Bernard, A., Buchet, J.P., Lauwerys, R.,
      Masson, P. Urinary excretion of beta-2-microglobulin
      and other proteins in workers exposed to cadmium, lead
      or mercury. Path. Biol. 1978; 26:329-331.

54.   Bernard, A., Goret, A, Buchet, J.P., Roels, H.,
      Lauwerys, R. Characterization of the proteinuria
      induced by long-term administration of cadmium in rat.
      Soc. Toxicol. Abst. 1980; 19:A94, No 280.

55.   Savory, J., Pu, P.H., Sunderman, F.W.,Jr. A biuret
      method for the determination of protein in normal urine.
      Clin. Chem. 1968; 14:1160-1171.

56.   Horak, E., Sunderman, F.W., Jr. Radioimmunoassay of
      beta-2-microglobulin in body fluids. In: "Proteins and
      Proteinopathies" (F.W. Sunderman, Ed). Institute for
      Clinical Science, Philadelphia, 1977; 99-110.

57   Horak,   E.,   Hopfer,   S.M.,   Sunderman,   F.W., Jr.
      Spectrophotometric   assay   of   N-acetyl-beta-D-
      glucosaminidase activity in urine. In: "Laboratory
      Diagnosis and Monitoring of Disorders of the Kidney"
      (F.W. Sunderman, Ed).   Institute for the Clinical
      Sciences, Philadelphia, 1980; 157-170.

58.   Savory,   J.,   Sunderman, F.W.,Jr., Pu, P.H. Methods for
      measurement and fractionation of proteins in urine and
      serum.   In: "Laboratory Diagnosis of Kidney Disease"
      (F.W. Sunderman and F.W. Sunderman Jr., Eds). W.H.
      Green, Inc., St. Louis, Mo. 1970; 496-503.

59.   Iannaccone, A., Porcelli, G., Boscolo, P.   The urinary
      kallikrein activity in cadmium exposure.   Adv. Exp.
      Biol. Med. 1979; 1208:683-684.

CURRENT USE OF AMBIENT AND BIOLOGICAL MONITORING: REFERENCE
WORKPLACE HAZARDS. ORGANIC TOXIC AGENTS - BENZENE I

B. D. GOLDSTEIN (USA)

Summary

*Benzene is a potent haematotoxin capable of causing aplas-
tic anaemia and acute myeloblastic leukaemia. Surveillance
of workers potentially exposed to benzene is focused on
detecting evidence of bone marrow toxicity. A particularly
thorough haematological evaluation should be conducted upon
entrance to the workforce at risk. This should be followed
by at least quarterly surveillance using the routine complete
blood count as the major monitoring technique. Attention
should also be placed on increases in the mean corpuscular
volume and decreases in the lymphocyte count as possible
early indicators of benzene toxicity. No single finding or
constellation of findings is pathognomic of benzene haematotoxicity and all findings must be carefully interpreted in
terms of the individual or group at risk. Basic research
into the mechanism of benzene haematotoxicity is a
prerequisite to developing improved means of protecting
potentially exposed workers.*

Introduction

Benzene is an important and inherent component of our chemical era.   Its toxicity to man has been recognised since the
nineteenth century.   The major adverse effect of benzene is
on the haematological system, although at very high concentrations ($>$ 1,000 ppm) acute central nervous system effects
will also occur.

The subject of benzene haematotoxicity has been extensively
reviewed in recent years. (1-4) The two major serious haematological disorders clearly caused by benzene exposure in man
are aplastic anaemia and acute myeloblastic leukaemia. Benzene produces a dose-dependent peripheral blood pancytopenia
in animals and man which in its severe form is associated
with complete bone marrow aplasia. This does not appear to

be an idiosyncratic effect; anyone exposed to a sufficient
benzene dose will become pancytopenic. Individual variability in susceptibility presumably does occur and there is some
suggestive, but inconclusive, evidence that women may be more
susceptible than men, that there is a familial tendency
toward susceptibility, and that age, obesity and pre-existing
haematological disease may also be factors. (5-7) In milder
forms of benzene toxicity individual cytopenias may occur;
i.e. anaemia, leucopenia and thrombocytopenia.

The causal relation of benzene exposure to human acute myeloblastic leukaemia and its variants is supported by evidence
obtained from a number of different approaches. These include the many case reports from different countries and with
different exposure conditions in which the only common denominator is benzene. The case reports are also notable for
the frequency in which an individual with benzene-induced
pancytopenia is followed through a preleukaemic phase into
frank acute myeloblastic leukaemia, and the relatively high
incidence of the erythroleukaemic variant. (1) A number of
different epidemiological approaches have also led to evidence supporting the causal role of benzene in leukaemia.
These include studies centred on case detection such as the
recent efforts of Aksoy and his colleagues in Turkey (8-10)
and the extensive series of studies by Vigliani, Forni, Saita
and colleagues in Italy. (11-13) In these investigations
there was a clear temporal relation between benzene and
leukaemia. In contrast to such studies where the number of
individuals with haematotoxicity (i.e., the numerator) is
relatively certain but the denominator is open to question,
the more classic epidemiological approach of evaluating a
relatively well defined workforce has been used by Infante et
al. (14) In this approach an increased incidence of deaths
due to leukaemia was observed by the indirect approach of
obtaining death certificates. Yet a third approach has been
employed by Girard and his colleagues who found that patients
with acute myeloblastic leukaemia were far more likely to
have a history of benzene exposure than suitable control

groups. (15) Unfortunately, none of these studies provide convincing information concerning the dose relationship between benzene exposure and leukaemia.

Benzene exposure has also been associated with a number of other haematological neoplasms and paraneoplastic disorders including chronic myelogenous leukaemia, acute and chronic lymphocytic leukaemia, lymphomas, myelofibrosis and myeloid metaplasia, and paroxysmal nocturnal haemoglobinuria. These cases are summarised and tabulated in a recent review. (1) For none of these is the evidence as convincing as it is for acute myeloblastic leukaemia and its variants (including erythroleukaemia, myelomonocytic leukaemia and acute promyelocytic leukaemia).

The major question in benzene toxicology is the relation of pancytopenia to benzene-induced acute myeloblastic leukaemia. The question can be phrased as to what extent, if any, is benzene-induced pancytopenia a necessary prerequisite for acute myeloblastic leukaemia? Haematologists recognise the general relationship between these two entities. Patients with idiopathic aplastic anaemia have a higher risk of developing acute myeloblastic leukaemia, as apparently do individuals with chloromycetin or phenylbutazone-induced aplastic anaemia. It has been suggested that leukaemogenesis is due to some error in the repair process instigated originally by non-mutagenic damage to haematopoietic stem cells. Of interest in this regard is that benzene itself has not been found to be mutagenic. However, it must be emphasised that there is no conclusive evidence for this or any other mechanism linking pancytopenia and acute myeloblastic leukaemia. Review of the literature reveals no case about which it can conclusively be stated that there was no evidence of benzene induced pancytopenia prior to the development of acute myeloblastic leukaemia. On the other hand, it would be extremely difficult to obtain evidence favouring such a case. The presence of one normal blood count would not rule out the possibility of there having been abnormal blood counts at

some other time during or subsequent to benzene exposure.
Only with routine monthly surveillance in which there had
been repeatedly normal blood counts could one reasonably
infer the absence of an overt pancytopenic effect of
benzene.

Determination of the relation, if any, of pancytopenia to
acute myeloblastic leukaemia is hampered by the lack of an
animal model of benzene-induced acute myeloblastic leukaemia,
and by lack of understanding of which metabolite(s) of benzene is responsible for its bone marrow effects. Until such
time as this information is available, the more prudent
approach has been to assume that benzene leukaemogenesis
conforms to the model of radiation and other carcinogens for
which it is believed that no threshold exists. This question
of whether leukaemogenesis can occur at benzene levels not
producing overt cytopenia is of course very pertinent to the
problem of surveillance.

Another unanswered question about benzene-induced leukaemia
is whether it represents an idiosyncratic response in which
only a few particularly susceptible individuals may be at
risk. This possibility is suggested by the relative infre-
quency of leukaemia in work forces in which a high percentage
of individuals have been noted to have benzene-induced pancytopenia. (15) Elucidation of any such mechanism responsible
for benzene-induced leukaemogenesis would obviously point the
way toward future screening techniques capable of prevention
of this disorder in the workplace.

General considerations

Laboratory monitoring data obtained on a work force can, and
should, be used in two ways. In the first the major consideration is surveillance and protection of the workforce as a
whole. In the second, the aim is to detect affected individuals. These two approaches must be clearly distinguished as
they require different statistical techniques and in part

reflect different occupational situations. In the former case, consider that moderately toxic levels of benzene are spread rather diffusely in the workplace affecting all workers roughly equally. Observable haemological affects due to benzene would be expected to begin as relatively mild decreases in total blood counts. In view of the wide range of normal values, it is unlikely that these early changes of benzene haematotoxicity will be recognised as significant effects in individual workers. Rather, it would be necessary to utilise standard statistical approaches to evaluate the entire work force at risk in relation to previous counts in that population. Obviously, a temporal variation in blood counts could also reflect changes in laboratory technique; e.g. a new technician or recalibration of the cell counter. Accordingly, it is necessary simultaneously to obtain laboratory data on groups of individuals who would not be suspected to be exposed to benzene, such as management or clerical workers. A decrease in cell counts that was limited to the potentially exposed subgroup would then be of significance. It would lead at the least to careful industrial hygiene monitoring of the affected area and cessation of work exposure until the problem was rectified.

The second type of situation is one in which the individual members of the work force are particularly likely to develop adverse effects, due perhaps to a point source, or to individual work habits, e.g. the sloppy worker syndrome. In this case, surveillance for benzene toxicity must be aimed at detecting those who have a fall in blood counts greater than would be expected by chance variation alone. Obviously, this would also identify an individual with a hypersusceptibility to the pancytopenic effects of benzene, if such should exist.

A very important aspect in the consideration of haematological surveillance is the wide range of normal in the routine blood counts. This is particularly true for the white blood count in which the normal is usually 5,000-10,000 per cu mm, and the platelet count for which the normal is often quoted as 150,000-350,000 per cu mm. Even in the case of haemo-globin, haematocrit, and the red blood cell count, the varia-tion between the accepted higher and lower limits of normal is about 30%. These relatively wide ranges of normal compli-cate detection of early benzene toxicity. As an extreme ex-ample, consider the individual whose true platelet count is 300,000 but because of exposure has had a decrease in plate-let count to 150,000, a 50% decrease, but still within the range of normal. Obviously, screening based solely on detecting abnormal counts would not find this individual. However, he or she could be singled out in a surveillance programme which followed each individual as their own control.

Another complication to detecting early benzene toxicity is the relatively extensive bone marrow reserve. From studies of patients with haemolysis, it has been estimated that the bone marrow is capable of making perhaps six times as many red cells as it normally does. Furthermore, it is recognised clinically that patients previously treated with haemato-toxins for malignant disease not infrequently may have normal or low normal peripheral cell counts despite an obviously diminished bone marrow reserve. It is conceivable that a similar effect occurs with benzene, thereby obscuring a sig-nificant degree of haematotoxicity. If so, a normal peri-pheral blood count cannot be automatically assumed to indi-cate no evidence of bone marrow toxicity due to benzene. This of course is particularly pertinent to arguments con-cerning the basis of benzene leukaemogenesis.

Surveillance procedures

The usual thorough medical evaluation of all entering the work force is indicated. If potential exposure to benzene is expected it is important to obtain a more thorough than usual haematological evaluation. The purpose is to establish a baseline useful for differential diagnosis between benzene related and unrelated haematological changes detected in

future surveillance efforts. This is particularly important
due to the fact that many common disorders impact on the
haematological system. Incoming workers should have a
complete blood count, reticulocyte count, direct and indirect
bilirubin, serum iron and total iron binding capacity, serum
lactate dehydrogenase, and stools for guaiac.

The usual surveillance procedure for haematological disorders
is the routine complete blood count. With any reasonably-
sized work force this most likely will be performed by automatic equipment and will consist of the red blood cell count,
haematocrit, haemoglobin, and the white blood cell count.
This approach provides very useful information and should be
sufficient for the average workplace. A decrease in white
cell count or in the red cell parameters should be considered
as possibly indicative of benzene effect and lead to appropriate measures to further confirm the diagnosis. The limitations of this approach both in terms of sensitivity and
specificity are described above. Important information can
also be obtained from the complete blood count by computing
the red cell indices. A number of studies have identified an
increase in the mean corpuscular volume (MCV) as an early
sign of benzene toxicity.(16) An increase in the MCV also
occurs in various other disorders including megaloblastic
anaemia, hypothyroidism, and liver disease. Of note, is that
an increase in the MCV has also been reported as an early
sign of alcoholism even in the absence of folic acid deficiency, and has been suggested to be useful in the early
detection of the alcoholic in the work force.(17) As both
alcoholic liver disease and megaloblastic processes might
also be associated with low peripheral blood counts, it is
important to interpret with care the findings in each patient
before ascribing alterations in the complete blood count
simply to benzene toxicity.

A decrease in the platelet count is also observed in classic
benzene haematotoxicity. Some investigators have suggested
that thrombocytopenia may be more prominent than either

anaemia or leukopenia in benzene affected groups. Bleeding due to benzene-induced platelet abnormalities not infrequently occurs in more severe cases. However, I am unaware of any such symptomatic effects in the absence of a decrease in either the white count or haematocrit.

Lymphocytopenia has also been reported to be a relatively early indicator of benzene haematotoxicity in man and in rats and mice subjected to a long-term repetitive inhalation of benzene.(18-19) However, one must be cautious in utilising the absolute lymphocyte count computed from a routine white count and differential in the screening process. This is in part because of the wide range of normal in the lymphocyte count, as well as the fact that lymphocyte number is subject to variation by a wide variety of processes including minor viral infections. Another major factor compounding interpretation of the lymphocyte count is the wide variation inherent even in the most accurate counting of 100 cells at random under the microscope. Even when counting 200 cells to determine the percentage of lymphocytes a large degree of variation persists. This problem may possibly be overcome by the use of automatic cell counting equipment if such instruments are successfully developed, otherwise the amount of technician time required to reduce this random variation precludes routine use of the lymphocyte count in the surveillance of individuals. However, determination of the lymphocyte count can be useful in certain situations where there is a question of benzene haematotoxicity, and may also be of value for surveillance of the entire work force.

Other laboratory tests which have been suggested to be useful in screening for benzene haematotoxicity are the reticulocyte count and serum bilirubin. However, the tendency for a low reticulocyte count in aplastic processes is of little diagnostic or screening value. An elevated reticulocyte count occurs in response to haematinics or in haemolytic states. The latter also results in an increase in serum indirect bilirubin. Although a decrease in red cell survival has been

suggcotod to occur in relatively severe cases of benzene
haematotoxicity, there is no reason to believe that these
two tests would be useful in surveillance of a work force for
early disease, nor in diagnosis of overt benzene haematotoxicity. They are of value in obtaining a differential
diagnosis in individuals with haematological variations which
may or may not be due to workplace exposure to benzene and
baseline values should be obtained at least once.

Exposure to benzene clearly results in qualitative as well as
quantitative changes in circulating blood cells. Such
changes in the constitution or function of red cell, white
cell, or platelets might conceivably be exploitable in surveillance for benzene haematotoxicity. One example is the
use of the mean corpuscular volume described above. Other
red cell changes include recent studies in this laboratory
which have demostrated that a prolongation in the glycerol
haemolysis time occurs in mice exposed to 100 ppm or 300 ppm
benzene 6 hours daily five days weekly.(20) The prolongation
of the glycerol haemolysis time occurred when a decrease in
haematocrit became manifest after about three weeks of exposure. However, there was less overlap in the glycerol haemolysis time between exposed and control mice than there was in
the haematocrit. Reported qualitative white cell abnormalities include changes in phagocytic function, osmotic fragi-
lity, nuclear fluorescence, and a decrease in leukocyte alkaline phosphatase.(21-24) The latter particularly merits
further evaluation as a surveillance test. Changes in serum
levels of immunoglobulins and of various enzymes have also
been suggested as early indicators of benzene toxicity,(25-
27) but confirmatory studies are required.

A difficult question concerns the feasibility and utility of
performing cytogenetic studies as a routine surveillance
method to detect the toxicity of benzene, or other workplace
hazards. It is clear that individuals with significant benzene haematotoxicity have various chromosomal changes.(28-30)
However, two major questions need be answered. Are tech-

niques sufficiently reliable to provide defined endpoints pertinent to benzene haematotoxicity and, if so, would the identification of affected workers obtainable from these relatively expensive tests not be available from other surveillance methods?

Benzene exposure can also be determined by monitoring the urinary output of its metabolites. The usual approach is to measure the excretion of phenol, a relatively major metabolite of benzene. This can be very helpful in circumstances in which there is a question concerning the presence or extent of recent benzene exposure. However, routine monitoring for benzene should best be done with a combination of air measurements and blood studies.

A major problem in surveillance programmes of this type is the lack of specificity of the manifestations of benzene haematotoxicity. No absolute criteria can be given which will completely distinguish benzene effects from other primary and secondary haematological disorders, many of which are very common. This is particularly true for the early manifestations of benzene haematotoxicity. Each case must be evaluated individually and, where indicated, more thorough studies performed including a bone marrow aspiration and many of the tests described above. In view of potential leukaemogenesis, suspicion of benzene toxicity should be sufficient to remove the worker from exposure.

Additional points about surveillance for benzene exposure also relate to the individual at risk. As with other compounds, the identification of one worker with benzene haematotoxicity should be an automatic signal for intensive surveillance of the work force and workplace. Finally, it must be kept in mind that leukaemia associated with benzene has been reported to occur many years following cessation of exposure. Accordingly, where possible individuals should continue under some degree of surveillance following retirement or change in jobs for at least two years, particularly when benzene-induced cytopenias have been observed.

References

1. Goldstein B.D. Haematotoxicity in Man, Chapter 7 In: Benzene Toxicity, a Critical Evaluation. Sidney Laskin and Bernard Goldstein (Eds.) J.Tox.Environ. Health 1977; Suppl. 2: 69-105.

2. Snyder R, Lee E.W., Kocsis J.J., and Witmer C.M. Bone marrow depressant and leukaemogenic actions of benzene. Life Sci. 1977; 21:1709-1721.

3. Recommended Standard for Occupational Exposure to Benzene. U.S. Dept. of Health, Education and Welfare, Washington, D.C. NIOSH 1974;74-137.

4. United States Environmental Protection Agency. Assessment of Health Effects of Benzene Germane to Low-Level Exposure. EPA-600/1-78-061 1978.

5. Aksoy M., Erdem S., Erdogan G., Dincol G. Acute leukaemia in two generations following chronic exposure to benzene. Hum Hered 1974; 24:70-74.

6. Ito T. Study on the sex difference in benzene poisoning. Report 1. On the obstacles in benzene workers. Showa Igakukai Zasshi 1962; 22:268-272.

7. Doskin T. A. Effect of age on the reaction to a combination of hydrocarbons. Hygiene and Sanitation 1971; 36:379-384.

8. Aksoy M, Dincol K, Erdem S, Dincol G. Acute leukaemia due to chronic exposure to benzene. Am. J. Med. 1972; 52:160-166.

9. Aksoy M., Erdem S., Dincol G. Types of leukaemia in chronic benzene poisoning. A study in thirty-four patients. Acta Haematologica 1976; 55:65-72.

10. Aksoy M., Erdem S., Dincol G. Leukaemia in shoe-workers exposed chronically to benzene. Blood 1974; 44:837-841.

11. Vigliani E.C., Forni A. Benzene and Leukaemia. Env. Res. 1976; 11:122-127.

12. Vigliani E.C., Saita G. Benzene and Leukaemia. N. Engl. J. Med. 1964; 271(17):872-876.

13. Forni A., Vigliani E.C. Chemical leukaemogenesis in Man. Ser Haemat 1974; 7:210-223.

14. Infante P.F., Rinsky R.A., Wagoner J.K., Young R.J. Leukaemia in benzene workers. Lancet 1977; 2:76-78.

15. Girard R., Revol L. La frequence d'une exposition benzenique au cours des hemopathies graves. Nouv. Revue Fr. Hemat. 1970; 10:477-484.

16. Goldwater L.J. Disturbances in the bloodfollowing exposure to benzene (benzol). J. Lab. Clin. Med. 1941; 26:957-973.

17. Unger K.W., Johnson D.,Jr. Red blood cell mean corpuscular volume: A potential indicator of alcohol usage in a working population. Am. J. Med. Sci. 1974; 267:281-289.

18. Aksoy M., Dincol K., Akgun T., Erdem S., Dincol G. Haematological effects of chronic benzene poisoning in 217 workers. Brit. J. Industrial Med. 1971; 28:296-302.

19. Snyder C.A., Goldstein B.D., Sellakumar A., Wolman S.R., Bromberg I., Erlichman M.N., Laskin S. Haematoxicity of inhaled benzene to Sprague-Dawley rats and AKR mice at 300 rpm. J. Toxicol Environ. Health 1978; 4:605-618.

20. Goldstein B.D., Rozen M.G., Snyder C.A. Prolonged red cell glycerol haemolysis in mice inhaling benzene. Proceedings of the Society of Toxicology Annual Meeting 1980; A39.

21. Koslova T.A., Volkova A.P. Blood picture and phagocytic activity of leucocytes in workers having contact with benzene. Gig Sanit 1960; 25:29-34.

22. Kolesar D., Ballog O. Studies by fluorescent microscopy of the effect of occupational benzene exposure on leucocyte nuclei changes. Bratislavaske Lekarske Listy 1965; 4511 (4):212-219.

23. Pollini G., Colombi R. Changes in the osmotic resistance of the leucocytes in persons exposed to benzene. Lavoro Umano 1964; 16(4):177-184.

24. Girard R, Mallein M.L., Bertholon J., Coeur P.,Cl. Evreaux J. Etude de la phosphatase alcaline leucocytaire et du caryotype des ouvriers exposes au benzene. Arch. Mal. Prof. 1970; 31(1-2):31-38.

25. Lange A., Smolik R., Zatonski W., Szymanska J. Serum innumoglobulin levels in workers exposed to benzene, toluene and xylene. Int. Arch. Arbeitsmed 1973; 31:37-44.

26. Hanke J. Z. Preliminary investigations of prolonged occupational exposure to toxic substances on the level of some serum exzymes. Arch. Hig. Rada. 1964; 15:57-66.

27. Lob M. L'action du benzene sur les thrombocytes et sur certaines activities enzymatiques. Archives des Maladies Professionnelles 1963; 24(4-5):371-374.

28. Forni A., Pacifico D., Limonta A. Chromosome studies in workers exposed to benzene or toluene or both. Arch. Environ. Health 1971; 22:373-378.

29. Tough I.M., Smith P.G., Court Brown W.M., Harnden D.G. Chromosome studies on workers exposed to atmospheric benzene. Europ. J. Cancer 1970; 6:49-50.

30. Wolman S.R. Cytologic and cytogenetic effects of benzene, Chapter 6 In: Benzene Toxicity, a Critical Evaluation. Sidney Laskin and Bernard Goldstein (Eds.) J. Tox. Environ. Health 1977; Suppl. 2:63-68.

CURRENT USE OF AMBIENT AND BIOLOGICAL MONITORING: REFERENCE
WORKPLACE HAZARDS. ORGANIC TOXIC AGENTS - BENZENE II

E. FOURNIER (FRANCE)

Summary

*The discovery of the clinical effects of benzene relates to
two types of blood disorder - medullary insufficiencies and
certain forms of leukaemia. There can be a time lapse of 2-
15 years between the beginning of exposure to benzene and the
appearance of diseases making it extremely difficult to
reconstitute a history of exposure during a working life;
however some systematic surveys have been carried out; there
are also associated factors such as age and sex of the
individual concerned. It is now difficult to improve our
knowledge of occupational benzene poisoning since for
instance, there has been a considerable reduction in use of
benzene in the workplace in the last ten years. New parameters of measurement are being developed and the most recent
contribution to defining the effect of small doses relates to
chromosomal alterations. Theories on the action of benzene
and tests linked to benzene metabolism are also discussed.*

Introduction

Publications on the monitoring of benzene in the workplace
environment and on studies of systematic biological
monitoring show that very different parameters are used
depending on the date of the study, the detection methods
chosen and the thinking which lies behind the choice of
preventive systems in occupational medicine.

A quick glance at the historical record is enough to remind
one that the discovery of the clinical effects of benzene
relates to two types of blood disorder.
  i) Medullary insufficiencies. These may either be
     general or relate to one or more of three types of
     cell (granulocytes, thrombocytes and erythrocytes).
     These develop in isolation or in association with
     proliferative and/or dysplastic blood disorders.
     Santessom of Stockholm reported nine cases of chronic
     poisoning with anaemia and purpura at the Moscow
     Congress in 1897.

ii) <u>Certain forms of leukaemia</u>. The most frequent form
is acute leukaemia, the first case of which was
described by Delore and Borgomano (Lyon) in 1928.
Apart from this form, cases of chronic myeloid
leukaemia and chronic lymphoid leukaemia have been
observed.

With less certainty, the schools of haematology
regard many anomalies which are less well classified
but which affect the haematopoietic organs (dysglo-
bulinamias, lymphomas, myeloid, splenomegaly and
Osler-Vaquez disease) as possibly resulting from
exposure to benzene. This theory would make it
necessary completely to revise our ideas about
benzene-related disease, for malignant diseases of
the lymphatic organs are quite frequently found.

The limitations of research, and to some extent the impossibility of reaching logical conclusions in human clinical
medicine, arise from the probable time-lapse between the
beginning of exposure and the appearance of the diseases
- three to ten years for aplastic anomalies, two to fifteen
years for proliferative myeloid syndromes, twelve or so years
for malignant diseases (leukoses) in inadequately protected
working conditions which correspond to exposure of between 50
and 100 ppm or more. Even if one accepts such approximations, it remains impossible to reconstitute a history of
exposure during a working life, except for perfectly
identified groups of workers, and these according to the
latest publications, are the exception. The authors
frequently try to explain <u>a posteriori</u> what they were unable
to foresee on the basis of measurement and observation, by
adducing for example the high turnover of workers or the
uncertainty of certain measurements.

Limitations of the epidemiological approach

In the Paris Region a systematic survey between 1957 and 1962
covered all the cases of occupational blood disease notified
under the preventive legislation (1947) (A. Cavigeaux et al.)

Out of a total of 2,650,000 wage-earners, 28,000 patients were examined and 8,000 found to be suffering from occupational disease, of whom 375 had toxic blood diseases.

Benzene was thought to be the cause in most of the cases, and this was confirmed in 20 cases per year (between 13 and 28 depending on the year), including:

leukopenia with neutropenia:	78 cases,
serious anaemia:	9 cases,
slight anaemia:	17 cases,
purpura:	1 case,
leukosis:	10 cases.

The research for the industrial product causing the disease showed that many preparations such as thinners and paint strippers contained between 1.4% and 31% benzene at the time.

In a survey covering 15 years (1947 to 1962), 45 deaths by occupational benzene poisoning (3 per year) were recorded (10 women, 35 men), including:

acute leukosis:	15 cases,
lymphoid leukosis:	2 cases,
myeloid leukosls:	6 cases,
medulloid aplasia:	28 cases.

In a joint study of cases of serious medullary aplasia observed in France between 1971 and 1977, Najean notes 22 cases of benzene-related aplasia (14.1% of toxic aplasia cases, 5.7% of all aplasia cases, with benzene coming first among the proven causes).

In a group of leukaemia cases, earlier exposure to benzene was found in 12% of cases (Girard 1970) whereas the same type of exposure was found in only 4% of non-leukaemic patients, which gives some information on the rise in frequency related to exposure in the 1950s.

Such data may lead one to conclude that the increase in frequency of non-lymphoid malignant blood diseases - which are

fairly rare - has been proved only for obvious exposure related to pre-1960 technology, and that it is rather unrealistic
to hope to obtain statistically useful clinical information
for exposure levels of less than 50 ppm, and particularly for
those of 10 ppm advocated since 1971.

The risk of occupational malignant disease can no longer be
picked out from that of spontaneous disease and especially of
diseases of different origin.

The studies by Thorp and by Fischbech did not provide results
for levels of the order of 20 ppm, but they must be related
to the number of workers exposed, the duration of exposure
and the time-lag before the study, in order to have any
epidemiological value.

Associated factors

In occupational pathology, standard associated factors have
been noted, even at the most recent meetings. Analysis of
them remains difficult and complicates statistical studies.

The following are considered as predisposing factors:
  i)   Age: the susceptibility of very young people and
       elderly people appears greater than that of the
       intermediate age group. At all events, it is espe-
       cially necessary to protect young people against a
       risk of cancer.
  ii) Sex: women appear to be more susceptible during preg-
       nancy and lactation. Even if these are coincidences
       resulting from the employment of women in very poor
       working conditions, the same specific protection rule
       must apply, because of the risk of mutagenesis.
  iii) Earlier blood disorders (Marchiafava-Micheli syn-
       drome, thalassaemia).
  iv) Some dietary deficiencies, physical exhaustion or
       acute episodes of infection.
  v)   Chronic liver and kidney diseases.

vi)   Chronic alcoholism, an important co-factor in pri-
      mary blood disease.

vii) Hereditary factors (a connection with blood group A
      has been accepted).

Conversely, other factors such as intake of substances which
stimulate enzyme adaptation appear to have had a protective
effect in experiments, e.g. the inhalation of vapours
(toluene) interferes with benzene metabolism.

Because the chronic toxicity of benzene was demonstrated so
long ago, because the circulating blood cells are easy to
study and because access to the elementary cells is extremely
difficult, it is difficult to improve our knowledge of
occupational benzene poisoning.

Moreover, research conditions have now become very uncertain
for obvious practical reasons. The considerable reduction in
the use of pure benzene in industry, apart from handling
not involving contamination of human beings, has been an
established fact for more than 10 years. The restrictions
imposed on the benzene content of industrial solvents, especially products for dissolving grease and paint, have thus
limited the number of potential poisonings in industry,
though without eliminating domestic risks in cases where
benzene is still tolerated as a household solvent.

In the industrial pathology of solvents, other subjects for
concern or study have arisen, such as the connection between
chronic kidney disease and solvents, between peripheral nervous disorders and petroleum products, and between central
nervous disorders and the handling of paint. These have
tended to overshadow research on benzene.

The strict haematological monitoring of most of the workers
still exposed to benzene, and the possibility of precise detection of benzene traces in the air at the workplace, have
helped to reduce the specific risk.

However, some anomalies of blood composition continue
to be observed in occupational groups exposed to solvents
not containing benzene, and diseases (usually leukopenia or
thrombopenia) are still observed in spraygun painters.

In France, benzolism - a term covering the occupational blood
diseases caused by benzene - which was fourth on the list of
notifiable diseases in 1946, has ceased to be a priority
subject for research because of the low frequency of blood
disorders observed since the statutory limitation of the
benzene content of solvents and thinners to 1%, proposed by
the International Convention on Benzene in 1971, has reduced
the benzene content of the atmosphere.

Parameters

The biological reference parameters remain blood cell counts
of erythrocytes, granulocytes and thrombocytes, using automated counting methods, and statistical variations.

The introduction of new parameters, such as chromosomal
alterations in bone marrow cells and in circulating leuko-
cytes, was done on a research basis, as were studies on
thrombocyte aggregation, the biology of haem including the
red cell absorption of iron, alkaline leukocyte phosphatase
(reduced), changes in immuniglobulins (increase in IgG and
IgA, reduction in IgM). These parameters have an indicative
value and are not very specific, but lead one to devote
particular attention to lymphocyte disorders. In experimental conditions, a myelocytic depression effect appears in
rats after they have inhaled air containing 50 ppm benzene
for 600 hours. In mice the changes begin at about 10 ppm.
In man, it is thought that anomalies of blood composition
would be very frequent for an exposure of 200 ppm, and the
frequency of acute leukoses would reach 130×10^{-6} after an
average exposure of 10 years. The increase in frequency
would be substantial for an exposure of more that 25 ppm.

The main recent contribution to defining the effect of small doses relates to <u>chromosomal alterations</u>. Between 5 and 25 ppm, studies of chromosomal anomalies sometimes appeared to show significant changes and at other times no changes. Above 25 ppm the effect seems unquestionable. The most recent joint epidemiological studies showed no changes for exposures of up to 20 ppm, and some authors drew from this the hasty conclusion that the anxiety aroused by the benzene risk was unjustified.

From this group of occupational or epidemiological studies it emerges that the most recent descriptions do not indicate any significant progress in clinical detection beyond the tables and lists drawn up in all the industrialised countries. No new renal, hepatic, nervous or neonatal disease is described.

When devising procedures for screening its workers, each country has thus to work out its own counting methods and ascertain the variations within an ethnic group and the variations from one ethnic group to another.

<u>Recent exposure rates</u>

The most recent measurements relate to benzene content ascertained by gas chromatography.

Results are checked by standardised methods, of which the most simple consists of e.g. a Chromosorb W support and an Apiezon or tricyano-ethylpropane stationary phase, with a flame ionisation detector. In conditions where these methods are accurate and inexpensive, they could be generally adopted to reduce the risk involved in handling solvents containing benzene. International Labour Convention No. 136 (convention on benzene, 1971) already limited the benzene content of the air to a maximum of 25 ppm ($80mg/m^3$) and the equipment is sensitive enough to measure a level of less than 1 ppm. In the last ten years, the most important discussion meetings and reference works such as that by J.K. Piotrowski on "Exposure tests for organic compounds in industrial toxicology" (1977) take stock of the essential conclusions on the subject reached on the basis of studies carried out throughout the world.

Two other papers, by R. Lauwerys and by H.S. Cohen, M.L. Freedman and B.D. Goldstein, to which this paper frequently refers, sum up the situation in Europe and America up to 1978 and expand the question to cover environmental protection.

Paired studies

A group of complementary studies, in the best traditions of occupational pathology, seeks to link clinical cases with levels measured in workshop atmospheres. The frequency of spontaneous chromosomal phenomena, the appearance of one and, even more, of a number of cases of blood anomalies in a workshop, should cause one to look for benzene in the atmosphere, particularly if the cases are concentrated in one area of the workshop. It is in this way that levels which are very probably dangerous have been defined.

Most of the groups of paired epidemiological studies do not seem to have detected anomalies in cell counts for exposures less than 20 to 25 ppm - a figure much higher than the exposure currently advocated.

The much quoted study by M. Berlin, K. Fredga et al. (1975), which used cytogenetic methods, shows the difficulty of interpretation. Drivers of road tankers showed changes regarded as significant for an exposure to benzene estimated at 1.3 ppm over a long period, whereas the increase is not significant for workers exposed to 10 ppm. In spite of such uncertainties, however, most of the works on this subject mention an increase in chromosome and chromotide aberrations exceeding 2% of cells, whereas the reference value is normally less than 1%. It is not stated whether the anomaly was found in all the subjects studied is generally too low to attain this level of discrimination.

Here again, it is quite certain that a general reduction of the acceptable level to a guaranteed figure of less than 10 ppm will remove any chance for future epidemiological studies based on karyotype anomalies to be demonstrated in practice. However, their contribution to the decision to reduce the level has been very useful.

Theories on the action of benzene

The other limitation of the study is that the mechanisms by which benzene acts are inadequately demonstrated, because there is no precise determination of the reactive metabolite content and of the sites at which benzene reacts with the blood constituents.

The reason for this difficulty is obviously linked with the virtual impossibility of carrying out biochemical research on the elementary cells of bone marrow and the total impossibility of doing so in the working environment.

Briefly, the general effect of benzene on bone marrow would appear to be, first, a stimulation of medullary proliferation, followed by a blockage comprising a "colchicine" effect (cessation of mitosis during the metaphase), and a "radiation" effect (modifications to the nuclei in the stage preceding the prophase), effect on chromosome formation and the anaphase (deletion, trisomy) which would explain the karyotype anomalies and potentially malignant mutations.

The biochemical mechanism of the action of benzene presupposes the involvement of its oxidated derivatives, abnormal consumption of sulphate, and glutathione and vitamin C depletion. All this is presented as an explanation of the haemotoxic effect.

The discovery of a benzene epoxide due to the action of the microsomal system (mixed function oxidase) on the benzene marks an important stage in the research, since this metabo-

lite has considerable affinity for biological macromolecules
including DNA (Harper et al. 1973). However, no demonstration of the actual formation in situ of a DNA-epoxy benzene
intermediate substance has been presented.

The overall reaction is said to be a physico-chemical effect
of the aromatic structure of benzene and of the oxygenated
metabolic substituents at the lipophilic sites of the DNA.

Recent studies relate to different cellular models (particularly normo-blasts and reticulocytes).

Measurement of benzene levels

The benzene level in the blood ought to be a good toxico-
kinetic test. In practice, determination of the level is
difficult and above all lacking in sensitivity. Traditional
methods do not permit measurement of levels lower than 250
micrograms per litre - a level which is far too high for the
detection of mild absorption. However, during the observation of occupational poisoning in the 1950s (probable
reference value 100 ppm in the atmosphere), a level of
between 500 and 3,000 micrograms per litre was discovered in
half of the exposed subjects.

It would be desirable to resume this research using modern
methods, for, since the benzene concentration in bone marrow
is high - about 10 to 20 times the concentration in the blood
- the measurement of benzene in the blood would serve as an
indicator of concentration which could be used experimentally
on medullary cells. For practical reasons, the benzene level
in expired air, theoretically equal to the level in the
blood, is used more at present. The determination of benzene in bone marrow - a very traditional method - is capable
of showing the presence of benzene several weeks after the
end of exposure. It would probably be currently the best way
of demonstrating human intake of benzene from the environment
in a group of victims of fatal road accidents.

Tests linked to benzene metabolism

Athird approach seeks to measure the movement of benzene in
the human organism and its metabolic consequences. Since
benzene epoxide is not measured the theory based on this
intermediate substance cannot be verified. Some other metabolites can be measured, the most simple being the sulphuric
and glucuronic conjugates of phenol, which are most abundant-
ly found in the urine.

Elimination would appear to take 24 to 48 hours, and can
therefore be easily monitored in the working environment.

So much research has been done on this that there is no need
to give the results in detail. Moreover, the methods described have nearly all fallen into desuetude after the recommendation by the National Institute for Occupational Safety
and Health (NIOSH) in the USA and by the European group
(Truhaut and Murray, 1978) that 10 ppm be the maximum
tolerable level in air. From the 1960s onwards the recommended method of gas chromatography made it possible to
determine an average level of urinary phenol in non-exposed
subjects, the specificity of measurement being guaranteed.

The results fall within a range of 1 mg/l to 14 mg/l in
subjects not occupationally exposed, with an average of 7
mg/l per day. Reference to urinary creatinine facilitates
statistical calculations. For an exposure of 100 ppm, the
levels are in the region of 40 to 60 mg/l. The variation
around the normal figure (+ 7mg/l) is therefore of the order
of 10 - 20 ppm. An accepted overall conclusion is that a
urinary phenol level of 20 mg/l very probably implies exposure to low concentrations of benzene. But for a worker
whose spontaneous excretion of phenol is low, a level of
20 mg/l would correspond to approximately 50 ppm.

There appears to be no interference with tobacco smoke -
although benzene is present in cigarette smoke, and this

should therefore be checked - with phenacetin, caffeine, saccharin, aspirin or salycylic acid, but it is accepted that there are interferences with skin preparations containing phenol, the ingestion of phenylsalicylate, and the degradation by intestinal bacteria of tyrosine and tryptophan - another point which needs to be checked (see Lauwerys, op. cit.).

Chronologically more precise methods (post-shift urine sample) would make the test more sensitive; the published graphs do not show this clearly. The relatively specific metabolite of benzene epoxide (S[1.2 dihydro 2 hydroxyphenyl] acetyl L cysteine mercapturic acid) does not appear to have been studied in any specialised published work.

Other biological tests relate to the direct action of benzene on cells. They have been described by H.S. Cohen, M.L. Freedman and B.D. Goldstein under the title 'Molecular considerations' (1978), with some references to the levels used by experimenters to obtain effects on RNA, DNA, protein synthesis and the polyribosomes of nucleate cells of bone marrow. According to these authors, the minimum concentration of benzene needed to inhibit the protein synthesis of reticulocytes is 4.38 g/l (0.056 M) (Forte et al.).

A change in liver polyribosomes is observed for doses of injected benzene between 0.52 and 5.63 mM (0.04 to 0.43 g for an animal approx 200 g) (Tryfiates).

Freedman's experiment uses benzene at 0.113 M (approx. 8 g/l) to inhibit haem synthesis.

One is therefore justified in wondering to what extent these studies can have a current industrial application, given that the more serious situation of the 1950s and earlier did not permit observation of benzene levels

higher than 3 mg per litre of blood, or medullary levels
higher than 30 mg/l for atmospheric concentrations of the
order of 100 to 300 ppm. The term 'molecular', often associated in the mass media with research making all previous
studies obsolete, can be used here only with caution, for it
is not certain whether at these concentrations the general
physical effect of lipophilic derivatives may not be the
dominant factor.

On the other hand, research specifically orientated towards
the levels which are believed to be active - of the order of
1 milligram of benzene per litre - would show the toxic
effect of benzene at the levels at present under discussion,
between 1 and 10 ppm in the ambient air.

Finally, the benzene level in expired air can be regarded as
a practical toxicokinetic test.

It is the absorption index most suited to working conditions,
and has become usable as a result of the work of Sherwood and
Cuter, who demonstrated that elimination took place according
to three compartmental parameters, after inhalation ended:
        - rapid (lasting approx. half a hour);
        - long (a few hours);
        - very long (approx. 3 days).
The level for the following morning in exposed workers would
thus belong to the second phase. However, according to R.
Lauwerys, even if the results may suggest that eight hours of
exposure to 10 ppm would produce a benzene concentration of
0.12 ppm in expired air 12 hours after the end of exposure,
these results would be modified by accumulation in the event
of repeated exposure.

The normal level for non-exposed subjects is given as 0.04
ppm or less. The presence of benzene in cigarette smoke (47
to 64 ppm) is said to constitute a significant risk of error
(Egle and Gochberg, 1976). One can conclude from this group
of results that it is possible to detect a benzene level of

25 ppm with certainty using biological parameters, that it is highly probable that exposure to a level of 10 ppm can be detected, and that it is impossible to detect lower levels by an indirect method.

For levels of 1 to 2 ppm, only direct measurement of expired air would then be significant and the test conditions would have to be <u>strict</u>. Clinical sensitivity is possible only for levels higher than 25 ppm, but the risk of blood disease must be clarified by the continuation of promising research such as that on human cytogenetic changes.

New methods relating to other metabolites of benzene epoxide should improve our knowledge of the subject. The main conclusion to be drawn is that protection against the benzene risk is now the result of a compromise between medical and biological data which are difficult to improve upon, technological limitations, and the ecological systems of industrial and post-industrial civilization.

CURRENT USES OF AMBIENT AND BIOLOGICAL MONITORING: REFERENCE
WORK-PLACE HAZARDS. ORGANIC TOXIC AGENTS - AROMATIC AMINES I

V. FOA (ITALY)

Summary

*From a chemical standpoint there are difficulties in defining
aromatic amines and a recent Italian definition of aromatic
amines may be in respect of over 4,000 products. They can
penetrate the organism principally through the skin and by
inhalation; there appears to be little or no importance
attached to the digestive route. The carcinogenic effect of
aromatic amines causes the most concern and as regards
carcinogenicity, aromatic amines can be divided into different categories according to degrees of evidence. On the
basis of all available toxicological data the Italian
Ministry of Labour has issued technical regulations for the
prevention of risk in the use of aromatic amines.*

*The paper describes procedures for environmental monitoring,
health surveillance and biological monitoring of aromatic
amines; and of procedures for analysis. It concludes with
proposals aimed at safeguarding health in working
environments.*

Introduction

In any approach to the problem of environmental and biological monitoring of a group of chemical compounds like aromatic
amines, one cannot avoid starting with some general considerations before specific treatment of the topic.

What is an aromatic amine in fact? Its chemical definition
alone poses difficulties. Faced with the necessity of issuing regulations, in Italy recently it was agreed to define
aromatic amines as "derivatives of ammonia with mono- and
polynuclear aryl groups that can be condensed or non-
condensed, or substituted, and their salts". A definition of
this type, or any others of equal merit that could be
suggested, means that a vast series of substances will be
covered (some speak of over 4,000 products) with physical and
chemical characteristics on the one hand and toxicological
properties on the other that are extremely different.

This fact cannot be ignored when dealing with problems of surveillance of a working environment: if for the great majority of aromatic amines, •the guidelines that can be suggested are simply a repetition of what can be defined as "good industrial hygiene practice", it is quite clear that for some of these compounds environmental and medical surveillance must be more specific.

Thus, for the purposes of prevention in the working environment, it would be appropriate to either restrict the definition of aromatic amines to more homogeneous groups of compounds or, what would have more practical meaning, draw up a list of substances on which attention should be focused; such list would be open and subject to revision.

Absorption of aromatic amines

Aromatic amines can penetrate the organism via the three classical absorption routes. In occupational exposure the most important routes are without doubt the skin, which is the main route for many of the liposoluble compounds of this series, and the inhalation route. The digestive route, however, appears to be of little or no importance.

Aromatic hydrocarbon amino-derivatives are one of the most important classes of chemical compounds in industry that can cause cyanosis. In addition to this effect, which is the clinical manifestation of excessive methaemoglobin formation, chronic exposure can also lead to haemolytic anaemia, skin sensitisation and contact dermatitis. It has been proved experimentally that aromatic amino compounds can cause liver damage; however, in practice, there has been no confirmation of this effect in man, even though isolated reports of cases have appeared in the literature.

But what causes most concern is the carcinogenic effect that a number of aromatic amines have been shown to have on both experimental animals and humans. Environmental conditions in

modern industry have undoubtedly improved to the point that a
worker handling amino-compounds would not be expected to
absorb gross amounts of the substance such as would produce
acute effects like cyanosis, for instance, unless by accident. This means that environmental concentrations are
generally low; but it is just these low concentrations that
come into the argument when dealing with potentially carcinogenic substances, since in the field of chemical carcinogenesis, no one has yet supported the existence of a threshold dose for carcinogens below which there would be no risk
whatsoever.

Categories of carcinogenicity

Aromatic amines can be divided into different categories of
carcinogenicity according to the evidence of risk obtained
from human observations and experimental data.

According to the International Agency for Research into
Cancer (IARC), the degrees of evidence can be defined as
sufficient, limited, or inadequate on the basis of human epidemiological data and experimental data in various animal
species, and also negative if, within the limits of the
experimental test used, the substance under study is not
found to be carcinogenic.

In the IARC classification, the chemical substances and the
industrial processes for which published human data existed
suggesting a relationship between exposure and human cancer
were divided into three groups.

Eighteen substances of industrial processes have been
classified under the first group covering substances or processes for which sufficient evidence exists of a causal
relationship between exposure and human cancer. Another 18
substances or industrial processes were considered as
probably carcinogenic for man (group 2) and further 18 (group
3) could not be classified due to inadequate data on human

carcinogenicity. Out of all these substances thus classified, there are 6 aromatic amines or industrial processes
involving aromatic amines classified under group 1 (4-
aminobiphenyl, manufacture of auramine, benzidine, N,N-
bis(2-chloroethyl)-2-naphthylamine, 2-naphthylamine), one
classified under group 2 (auramine), and one under group
3 (N-phenyl-2-naphthylamine).

To these 8, 3-3'-dichlorobenzidine and o-toluidine must be
added which were not taken into consideration by the IARC
working group because although sufficient evidence of carcinogenicity in laboratory animals exists, the human data
were not considered adequate enough to make a conclusive
evaluation of carcinogenic risk.

It should be pointed out that the IARC working group could
classify only 14% of the 442 chemical substances covered in
the first 20 volumes of the monographs published by the
agency, that is, only those substances for which some human
data exist; whereas the aromatic amines that have exhibited
carcinogenic potential in laboratory animals at various
degrees of evidence number over 60, including dyes and
pigments.

There are also aromatic amines that have been tested and, at
least under the experimental conditions used, have not proved
carcinogenic for animals. These number about 20.

Hence, of all the aromatic amines in use, only about 100 have
been studied for carcinogenic potential and the experimental
results cannot always be considered adequate for a correct
evaluation. All the other numerous aromatic amines produced
and/or used in industrial processes have yet to be studied,
consequently no experimental and/or human data are available
on their possible carcinogenicity.

Bearing this in mind, and also the fact that a fair percentage of the chemical substances known to be human carcinogens

that have been extensively studied can be classified under
the aromatic amine family, one can appreciate the extreme
caution of regulations issued for the prevention of aromatic
amine risk in industry, as is the case in Italy. Fortunately,
however, on the basis of occupational health experience and
epidemiological evidence it can be reasonably assumed that no
other aromatic amine presently used in industry has such a
high carcinogenic potential as has been demonstrated for
benzidine or 2-naphthylamine.

In view of the fact that relatively few aromatic amines have
been submitted to toxicological evaluation, the attempts to
predict a correlation between physical and chemical features
of the individual amines, their biological behaviour and
toxicological properties also seem justified. For example,
as regards the possibility of skin absorption, compounds
with a high n-octanol/water distribution coefficient are
more liposoluble and relatively insoluble in water and thus
easily penetrate the skin. Conversely, compounds with a low
n-octanol/water distribution coefficient are not normally
absorbed through the skin to any appreciable extent.

As can be seen in Table 1, the substitution of a methyl-or
ethyl-group or chlorine atoms on the benzene ring of amino-
compounds leads to the formation of a more liposoluble chemical compound than those with groups like -OH, -SO$_3$H, -COOH.

Table 1 - n-octanol/water distribution coefficient of some
aromatic amines

Sulphanilic acid	< 0,01
Chloroaniline	< 1
3-aminophenol	1.4 - 1.5
p-aminobenzoic acid	4.78
aniline	7.9 - 9.5
o-toluidine	13.5
p-nitroaniline	4.6

Absorption via the respiratory tract appears to be less dependent than skin absorption on the degree of lipo- or hydrosolubility of the compound. Water soluble compounds such as p-nitrophenol are rapidly absorbed via the lungs.

Amino-compounds with a high vapour pressure and those existing in the form of a fine powder can be absorbed in large quantities via the inhalation route.

Even though not universally applicable, it would therefore appear important to examine the chemical and physical properties of each aromatic amine in order to make an initial evaluation of risk.

Thus, on the basis of all available toxicological data on aromatic amines, but also taking into due consideration both the numerous doubtful aspects of the problem and, in many cases, the absolute absence of data permitting an evaluation, the Italian Ministry of Labour issued technical regulations for the prevention of risk in the use of aromatic amines. According to the regulations, factories or factory departments in which aromatic amines are manufactured and/or used are divided into different zones of risk, with definitions adapted from the regulations for the control of radiation risk. These zones are:
- controlled zone where there are aromatic amines that are known human carcinogens, or industrial processes in which they are involved
- zone under close surveillance where aromatic amines are handled that have been shown to be carcinogenic in laboratory animals
- zone under surveillance where there are aromatic amines for which carcinogenicity has not been studied or demonstrated.

The question that arises here is whether it is right to place as yet unstudied aromatic amines in the same category as those which have been tested and have failed to show a carcinogenic effect in one or more animal species.

For each of the above zones there is a series of technical/ engineering requirements and instructions concerning organisation and procedure such as to avoid the operators coming into direct contact with aromatic amines as far as possible.

The required frequency of medical examinations and biological monitoring is also related to the zonal divisions, i.e., to the type of aromatic amine used and the results of environmental monitoring. These regulations went into force in June 1979; they have led to a further development in environmental and biological monitoring techniques and methods and have undoubtedly given impetus to research in the field.

Environmental monitoring

It is first of all important to remember that in the case of liposoluble amines, which can easily penetrate the skin barrier, control of the atmospheric concentration alone is not sufficient for the purposes of good industrial hygiene practice. Obviously, account must also be taken of contamination of surfaces with which workers come into contact. Bearing the above in mind, the methods for sampling and analysis of aromatic amines can be described as follows.

Analysis of the environment samples is usually performed using two techniques: spectrophotometry and chromatography. The selected spectrophotometric technique is based on the reaction between amines and p-dimethyl amino benzaldeyde. For thin layer chromatography (TLC) detection, development of colour after elution with solvent was used: the primary amines are detected by diazo coupling, the secondary and tertiary amines by coupling.

Tables 2 and 3 give sensitivity limits obtained in measuring a series of products with these two techniques. In our opinion, the limits adequately justify the selection of techniques.

Table 2   Spectrophotometric method: general principles and detection limits

$$R-NH_2 + \text{(4-dimethylaminobenzaldehyde)} \longrightarrow \text{(Schiff base)} + H_2O$$

2,5-dichloroaniline	0.8	mcg/cc
2-amino-4-chlorophenol	0.18	"
4-nitroaniline	0.2	"
2-amino-4-nitrophenol	0.15	"
2-amino-5-nitrophenol	0.3	"
2-amino-6-nitrophenol-4-sulphonic acid	0.4	"
aniline	0.1	"
2-aminophenol	0.1	"
sulphanilic acid	0.15	"
2-aminophenol-4-sulphonic acid	0.28	"
chloro-p-phenylenediamine sulphate	0.15	mcg/cc
4-nitro-1,3-phenylenediamine	0.13	"
3-phenylenediamine	0.05	"
2-aminophenol-4-sulphonamide	0.25	"
o-trifluoroethylaniline	0.5	"
o-aminobenzoic acid	0.15	"
2-chloro-4-toluidine	0.12	"
2-chloro-4-aminotoluene-5-sulphonic acid	0.24	"
5-amino-2 chlorotoluene-4-sulphonic acid	0.46	"
4-toluidine	0.1	"
p-anisidine	0.13	"
4-amino acetanilide	0.12	"
2-methoxy 5 methylaniline	0.2	"
4-amino-phenylsulphoethylenoxy-sulphonic acid	0.22	"
3,4,6-trimethylaniline	0.3	"
1-naphthylamino-6-(7) sulphonic acid	0.3	"
1-naphthylamino-4-sulphonic acid	0.26	"
1,2-naphthylamino-sulphonic acid	0.2	"
6-amino-1 naphthol-3-sulphonic acid	0.2	"
2-amino-8-naphthol-6-sulphonic acid	0.2	"
2-naphthylamino-4,8-disulphonic acid	0.2	"
1-amino-8-naphthol - 3,6-disulphonic acid	0.5	"
4-amino-4'-nitro-azobenzene	0.36	"
4-amino-4-nitrophenylamine-2-sulphonic acid	0.2	"
4,4'-diaminoazobenzene	0.008	"
diaminobenzoilanilide	0.08	"
2-amino toluene-4-sulphanide	0.38	"

Table 3   Thin layer chromatography method: detection limits

2-nitro-4-chloroaniline	mcg totali	2
2-chloro-4-nitroaniline	"	2
p-dichlorosulphanilic acid	"	2
2,4-dinitroaniline	"	2
2-amino-5-nitrobenzene sulphonic acid	"	2
2-cyano,4-nitroaniline	"	2
3-nitrotoluidine	"	2
N-ethyl,-N-oxyethylaniline	"	4
N-cyanoethyl, N-ethylaniline	"	2
1-amino-2-bromo, 4-hydroxy-anthraquinone	"	8
1-amino,-2-sulphonic,-4-bromoanthraquinone	"	4
1-chloro,5-amino-anthraquinone	"	2

Analysis is simple to perform and there are very few variables that can have a negative influence on the determination. The quantitative identification of spots in TLC is sometimes difficult and should be done by a trained expert.

These methods can also be recommended for use in continuous environmental monitoring. The analysis must be performed within relatively short time limits. We did not think it worthwhile using liquid-liquid and gas chromatography at this stage because no complex mixtures are present in the workplaces we studied.

Sampling

Both static and personal samplers were used. In both cases the filter holders (50 and 37 mm diameter respectively) were double cone type with an input air speed of 1.2 m/sec, and the filters were in cellulose nitrate with 0.45 μ pore size. In the fixed positions, samples were taken at both high flow aspiration (18-20 l/min) and low aspiration (3.5 l/min).

In the working environment studied there was not elevated
dust concentration: the aromatic amines were poured from
sacks into depressurised reactors through the upper opening.
The produce is often damp, and is always granular or in
chips. When the sacks are opened there is a dispersion of
fine, almost invisible dust. The operation lasts from 15 to
60 min.

Several indications can be derived from the above sampling
experience.

i) 0.45 μm pore cellulose nitrate membranes seem to be
   suitable for samplings (15 min) provided there are
   no particularly volatile amines present or provided
   that the production cycles are not such as to render
   the amines volatile. In such cases samples must be
   taken on absorbent solids or in liquid.

ii) For samples of short duration, the total weight of
    the dust collected (mg/m^3) offers poor reliability
    unless analytical balances accurate to the 6th or
    7th decimal figure are available. Particular atten-
    tion is necessary in weighing the 37 mm membrane.
    The dust concentration is anyway usually within
    reasonable limits. Conditioning is better done at
    temperatures below 70-80°C to avoid weight loss
    due to amine volatility which often reaches not
    negligible levels.

iii) Determination of the amine/s present appears to be
     sufficient by itself, bearing in mind the limited
     dust pollution where adequate ventilation systems
     are provided.

iv) Recovery of amines from the cellulose filters is
    not always satisfactory; with heat conditioning of
    the membrane at 80-85°C, recovery rates of up to
    65-75% can be obtained. The recovery rate increases
    when conditioning is omitted.

v) Sampling carried out with personal samplers at 3.5
   l/min permit both higher dust concentrations and
   higher amine concentrations to be determined than

those performed in the same position but at an 18
l/min flow. The increase was very high and for some
amines was at times as much as 100-200%.

Health surveillance and biological monitoring

The regulations referred to above require that health measures comprise a pre-employment and a periodic medical examination. The pre-employment medical examination must be combined with a series of biochemical tests which have the dual
function of detecting hypersusceptible subjects (such as
those with constitutional enzymatic erythrocyte diseases and
of furnishing fundamental data on the function of the target
organs of the action of aromatic amines, before the worker is
exposed. In addition to a medical examination, subsquent
periodical checks require performance of a series of tests
which make up biological monitoring. These tests can be considered partly indicators of internal dose and partly indicators of effect. I say "can be" because at the present moment
we do not know if any correlation exists for aromatic amines
between internal and external dose or between dose and
effect. In any case, such indicators of internal dose, both
a specific (total urinary amino-compounds) and particularly
specific (determination of some carcinogenic aromatic amines
and their metabolites in the urine) can provide an acceptable
evaluation of the quantity of these compounds absorbed during
work, provided the analytical method is correct.

Method at present under assessment in Italy

The method chosen is an application of the Bratton-Marshall
reaction (J. Biol. Chem., 1939, 128, 537-550): primary aromatic amines are determined by spectrophotometry after diazo-
tising and coupling with N(1 naphthyl) ethylendiamine. The
calibration curve is done with aniline. The results of analysis are expressed in mg/litre aniline. The Lambert-Beer
law is satisfied up to 75 mg/l aniline.

Before the diazotisation and diazo-coupling reaction, acid hydrolysis must be performed to release the amine groups from the acetylated and glucuroninated derivatives.

The method was adapted to make it easier to perform in normal laboratory routine and it proved to be reproducible and rapid. The method was also tested on an Autoanalyser and a comparison between manual and automatic methods gave identical results.

Nevertheless, with this method, one also measures acetylated and glucuroninated compounds formed in protein metabolism (especially kinurenine, which is formed from catabolism of tryptophan, with concentrations up to about 10 mg/l).

In addition, products such as sulphonylamide, acetanilide and phenacetin, which are contained in commonly used drugs (analgesic, anti-allergic and antihypertensive drugs) have a strong influence on the result. Lastly, although many primary aromatic amines give rise to diazotisation and diazo-coupling products in the chosen analytical conditions, the molar extinction coefficients of compounds thus obtained are subject to considerable variation and some amines (for example, 1,3 diamino-2,4,6 trinitrobenzene and o-phenylene-diamine) do not react at all.

This method requires some improvement in order to be reliable and studies are already under way for this purpose. For example, a purification method is needed that eliminates protein catabolism products from the urine, especially kinurenine. Protein catabolism products are already present in the urine in quantities in the order of several mg and thus it is not possible to detect small variations following occupational absorption of aromatic amines.

For some aromatic amines, for example those considered as having greater carcinogenic potential, feasibility studies are under way on more specific methods of determination, using gas chromatography and also liquid-liquid chromatography.

The recommended indicators of effect are:

>measurement of methaemoglobinaemia, particularly when new technological processes are being put into operation, blood count, liver function test, urine analysis, and cytological examination of the urinary sediment with the Papanicolaou method.

Conclusions

Safeguarding of health in working environments where aromatic amines are handled consist of several procedures.

>i) Abolition of production, use and importation of benzidine, 2-naphthylamine, 4-aminobiphenyl, and their respective salts. There is now sufficient evidence of a causal relationship between occupational exposure to these substances and human cancer. Regulations are also needed concerning the acceptable percentage of these amines if present in other products as impurities formed in the manufacture of the former.

>ii) Provision of differential rules regarding technical engineering, organisation and procedure measures required in the production and use of aromatic amines according to the level of knowledge attained on their carcinogenic potential. For the compounds that have not yet been studied, caution must be used in the rules until sufficient data of negative evidence become available.

>iii) Information to operators about the possible risks involved in their jobs and training in the necessary hygiene rules.

>iv) Environmental monitoring through control of dispersion in the air and in the dust deposited on surfaces with which the workers come into contact.

>v) Health surveillance through pre-employment and periodical medical examinations complete with various laboratory tests according to the group of amino-compounds involved.

It is therefore clear, especially considering (ii) that further research is necessary to provide firstly basic toxicological data for every aromatic amine used; then information on their metabolism and biotransformation in the human organism, particularly in the case of aromatic amines dyes and pigments and lastly to establish, if possible, a correlation between external and internal dose and between dose and effect.

CURRENT USE OF AMBIENT AND BIOLOGICAL MONITORING: REFERENCE
WORKPLACE HAZARDS. ORGANIC TOXIC AGENTS - AROMATIC AMINES II

L. FISHBEIN (USA)

Summary

*Highlights of the principal analytical methodologies (gas
chromatographic, high pressure liquid chromatographic, and
spectrophotofluorimetric) were reviewed for the analysis of
benzidine and its congeners (principally 3,3'-dichloro-,
3,3''-dimethyl-, and 3,3'-methoxy benzidines) as well as a
number of their azo dyes. Emphasis was focused on the
determination of these agents in environmental and biological
samples. Additional monitoring techniques discussed involved
the utility of chromogenic and fluorescent derivatives of
aromatic carcinogenic amines.*

Introduction

The aromatic amines represent a category of considerable
importance in terms of their broad industrial utilisation per
se as well as intermediates in the manufacture of a wide
variety of dyes which have been extensively used to colour
textiles, leathers, rubber, printing inks, paints, lacquers,
metal finishes, plastic and paper products as well as in
permanent and semi-permanent colouring products. The
exposure to these agents, a number of which are carcinogenic
and/or mutagenic can occur via skin contact, inhalation and
ingestion and can cover the spectrum of segments of the occupational and the general public.

The epidemiology of aromatic amine carcinogenesis is essentially the epidemiology of human bladder cancer of industrial
origin. The most important members of the aromatic amines
from the standpoint of industrial epidemiology are benzidine,
3,3'-dichlorobenzidine, 3,3'-dimethylbenzidine (o-tolidine),
and 3,3'-dimethoxybenzidine (o-dianisidine) as well as azo
dyes derived from these amines (1-6). These compounds are of

considerable importance as precursors in the production of 85
dyes and pigments that are commercially available in the
United States, e.g., 22 - benzidine-based dyes, 34 -dianis-
idine-based dyes, 22 - o-tolidine-based dyes, 5 -dichloro-
benzidine-based pigments and 2 - dianisidine-based pigments.
It should be noted that although there are only 85 such dyes
and pigments currently on the US market the technology exists
for producing more than 450 dyes and pigments that are based
on benzidine, or one of its three congeners e.g., 3,3'-
dichlorobenzidine, o-tolidine, and dianisidine (6).

The benzidine-based dyes produced or imported in the USA in
1978 totalled almost 2 million pounds while for the o-
tolidine and o-dianisidine-based dyes the production and
import total during this period was 1 million and at least
1.3 million pounds respectively (7).

Although the Occupational Safety and Health Administration
(OSHA) has regulated benzidine as a human carcinogen since
1974 (8) only recently has there been evidence that
benzidine-based dyes may also cause cancer. A recent health
hazard alert bulletin prepared by OSHA and the National
Institute for Occupational Safety and Health (NIOSH) listed
more than 100 benzidine, o-tolidine and o-dianisidine dyes
manufactured or imported by 22 firms in the US (9). The two
agencies in the alert reported that there is evidence that
some benzidine-based dyes were carcinogenic in experimental
animals and that the dyes were converted in animals to
benzidine (10). These dyes were identified as Direct Black
38, Direct Blue, and Direct Brown 95 (Figure 1). Additionally, the agencies reported that there is evidence that dyes
based on o-tolidine and o-dianisidine may be converted
metabolically to the parent precursor. There are at least
eight o-tolidine based and nine o-dianisidine-based dyes
produced currently in the US. According to the alert, NIOSH
estimated that about 79,000 workers in 63 occupations were
potentially exposed to benzidine-based dyes between 1972-1974
(7, 9). The advisory strongly recommended that these

benzidine-based dyes be handled in the workplace as if they were human carcinogens since NIOSH field studies showed that humans working with these same dyes also excrete higher than expected levels of benzidine in the urine. The advisory also recommended that commercial use of benzidine, o-tolidine and o-dianisidine-based dyes be stopped and appropriate substitutes found.

DIRECT BLUE 6

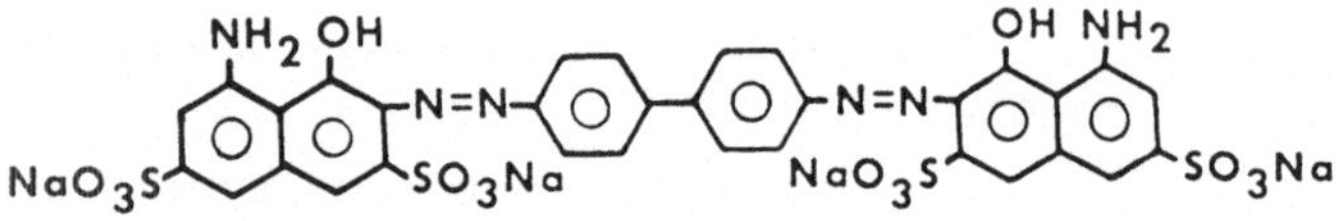

DIRECT BLACK 38

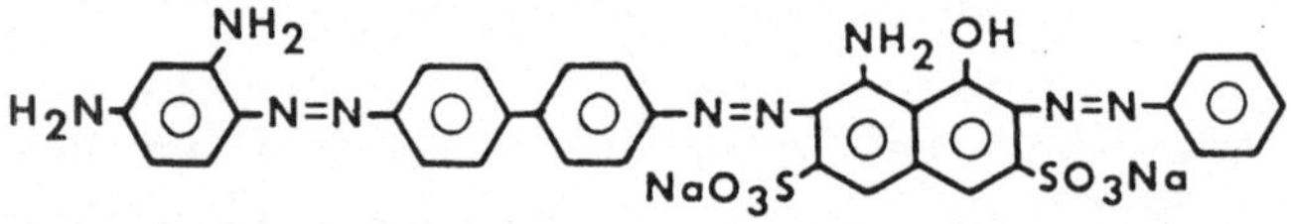

DIRECT BROWN 95

COPPER COMPLEX DERIVED FROM

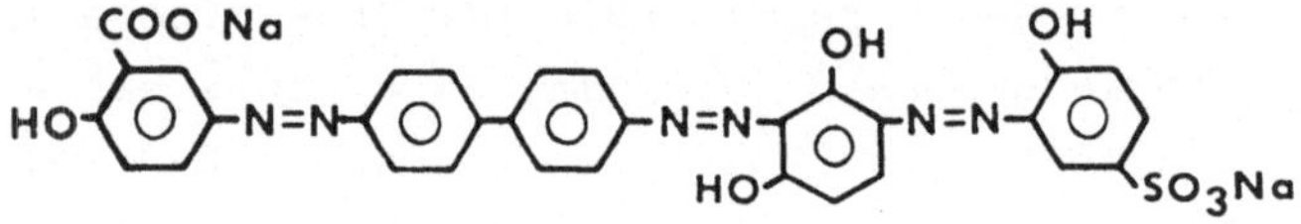

Figure 1   Benzidine derived dyes (10)

It should be noted that not only are segments of the labour force at risk by direct exposure of these agents during production and formulation, but consumers may be in contact with these derived dyes (as well as unreacted aromatic amine precursor) in clothing and through the use of packaged retail products such as dyes for home use and art and craft supplies as well as in hair dyes (6). Additionally, the potential exists for the release of benzidine and congeners, as well as benzidine and congener-based dyes and pigments discharged into waters from primarily dye manufacturing facilities (6, 11, 12).

This overview will principally focus on a number of the recently applied methodologies, e.g., gas-liquid chromatography (GLC) high pressure liquid chromatography (HPLC) and spectrophotofluorimetry (SPF) for the analysis of benzidine and its congeners as well as a number of their derived dyes with emphasis on their determination in environmental and occupational samples.

Analysis of benzidine and congeners

The analysis of samples of waste water containing benzidine, 3,3'-dimethoxybenzidine, diphenylamine and 1-naphthylamine in the ppb range has been reported by Jenkins and Baird (13). A Perkin-Elmer Model 900 gas chromatograph was utilised equipped with flame-ionisation detection and a dual 6 ft x 1/8 in i.d. glass column packed with a mixture of OV-17 (4.7%), QF-1 (5%) and DC-200 (0.5%) on 80/100 mesh Gas Chrom Q. Although programmed thermal operation gave decreased sensitivity for benzidine when compared with isothermal analysis (e.g., 0.5 mg/l compared to 0.1 mg/l), resolution was improved and complete separation of benzidine, 3,3'-dimethoxybenzidine, diphenylamine and 1-naphthylamine was obtained. The procedure for pretreatment of sample prior to analysis by GLC, TLC or colorimetry is shown in Figure 2.

Bowman and his colleagues (14-20) recently described a number of analytical procedures used to augment a variety of investigations involving short-term and chronic low dose feeding of benzidine, 3,3'-dimethyl-, 3,3'-dimethoxy, 3,3'-dicholorobenzidines as well as 4-aminobiphenyl and 2-acetyl-aminofluorene (2-AAF) to experimental animals. Hence, requisite analytical methodology for these compounds was required to: (a) verify purity, proper dosages and chemical stability of the compounds administered in drinking water and feed; (b) monitoring of clothing, work areas and urine of personnel to signal any accidental spillage or exposure to these agents; (c) monitoring of waste water resulting

from decontamination of the test areas; and (d) the
development of methods for decontamination.

SAMPLE PRETREATMENT

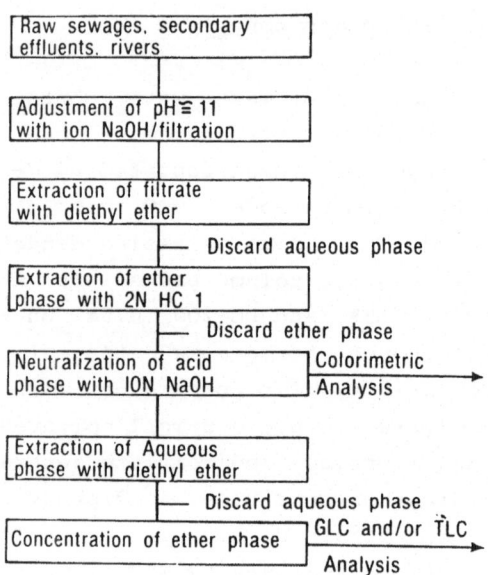

Figure 2   Procedure for pretreatment of sample prior to
analysis by GLC. TLC. or colorimetry (13)

The trace analysis of 3,3'-dichlorobenzidine and its
dihydrochloride salt in animal feedstuffs, waste water and
human urine by three gas-chromatographic procedures was
described by Bowman and Rushing (18). The major features of
the method of these carcinogens in feedstuffs are: extraction of the residues as the free amine and a clean-up via
acid-base liquid-liquid partitioning with benzene, followed
by passage over a silica gel column. With waste water and
human urine, residues were absorbed by percolating the

sample through a column of XAD-2 resin eluted with acetone
and cleaned up with acid-base partitioning and a silica gel
column. Residues were then assayed by GLC either as the free
amine or after conversion to the pentafluoropropionyl (PFP)
derivative by using an electron capture or a rubidium-
sensitised thermionic-type (N/P) detector. Minimum detectable residues in feedstuffs, waste water, and human urine are
about 18 ppb, 18 parts-per-trillion (ppt), and 60 ppt respectively, as determined by electron capture GLC of the
pentafluoropropionyl derivative. Typical electron capture gas
chromatogram of pentafluoropropionyl (PFP), trifluoroacetyl
(FTA) and heptafluorobutyryl (HFB)-derivatives of 3,3'-
dichlorobenzidine are shown in Figure 3. The PFB- and HFB-
derivatives of 3,3'-dichloro-benzidine are shown in Figure 3.
The PFB- and HFB-derivatives gave about equal responses, the
TFA-dichlorobenzidine was about half as sensitive, while the
PFB derivative enhanced detector responses about 300 fold.
Figure 4 illustrates gas chromatograms of underivatised
extracts of animal feedstuffs, waste water and human urine,
compared with standards of 3,3'-dichlorobenzidine and PFB-
dichlorobenzidine. Minimum amounts of dichlorobenzidine
detectable in urine, based on twice background were about
0.060 ppb by electron-capture GLC of the PFB derivative and
1.8 by thermionic type (N/P)-GLC (18).

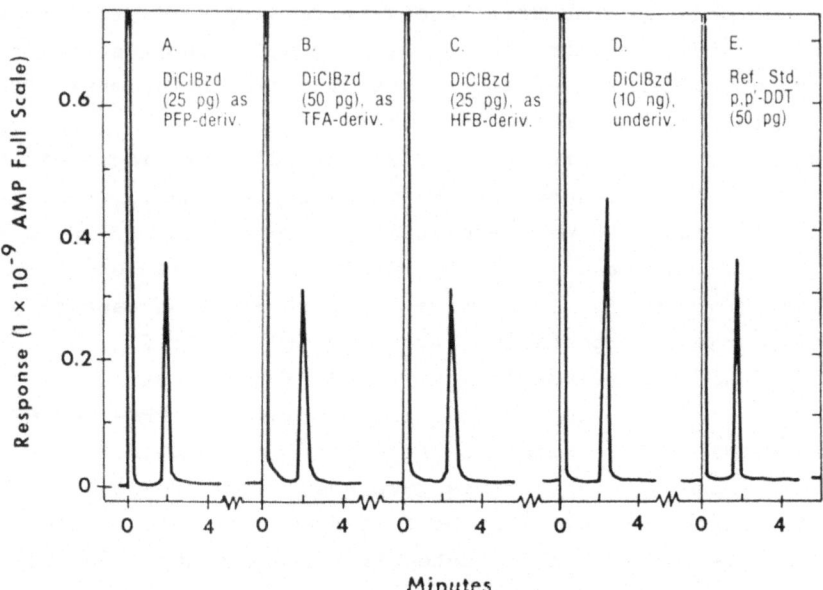

Figure 3. Electron capture gas chromatograms of PFP, TFA, and HFB derivatives of 3,3'-dichlorobenzidine (18)

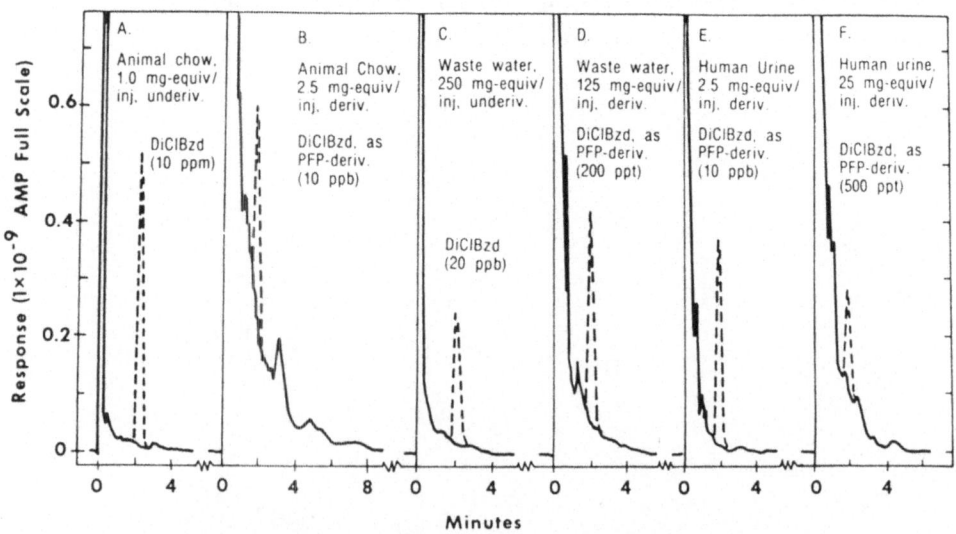

Figure 4 Gas chromatograms of underivatized extracts of animal chow, waste water and human urine compared with standards of 3,3'-dichlorobenzidine (18)

Spectrophotofluorimetric   (SPF)   methods were described by
Bowman   and   co-workers   for   the   trace   analysis   of
benzidine,   3,3'-dimethylbenzidine,   3,3'-dimethoxy-
benzidine (14), 4-aminobiphenyl, 2-napthylamine and their
hydrochloride salts (16) in waste water, potable water,
human   urine   and   rodent blood.   The salient features of the
methods   for   these   known   or   suspected   carcinogens are:
extraction of the residues as the free amine with benzene,
rapid cleanup on an alumina column, and quantification of the
free amine in methanol via SPF. Potable water solutions of
the   salts   are   diluted   with   buffer (pH 4) and quantified
directly by SPF.   Spectrophotofluorimetry is based on the
measurement of fluorescence radiation emitted by a sample
previously   excited   by u.v. or visible light. The intensity
of the emission is proportional to both the concentration of
the analyte and the intensity of the exciting radiation.
Hence, SPF is inherently extremely sensitive, under favour-
able conditions, it can be four orders of magnitude, more
sensitive than molecular absorption spectrophotometry (21).
SPF is potentially important as an analytical method for
benzidine   and   its   congeners   since   these   compounds emit
distinctive fluorescent spectra by which each can be identified and quantified. The detection limits of the amines and
their salts were 2 ng/ml and 10 ng/ml respectively.

Quantitative   determination of benzidine and its congeners in
admixture is somewhat difficult because of spectral overlap
and a large differences in relative intensities. It should
be noted however, that the importance of this deficiency
depends, on the composition and type of the sample to be analysed, for in many instances it is not significant. Figure 5
illustrates   the   SP   excitation   and   emission spectra and
standard   curves   for   benzidine   and   benzidine-2HCl. The
relative   intensities of the free amines in methanol were as
much as five to seven times greater than the corresponding
hydrochloride salts in 0.01 NH_4Cl solutions. In these
solvents, the limit of detection, expressed as twice background, were about 1-2 and 2-5 μg/ml for the free amines
salts respectively.

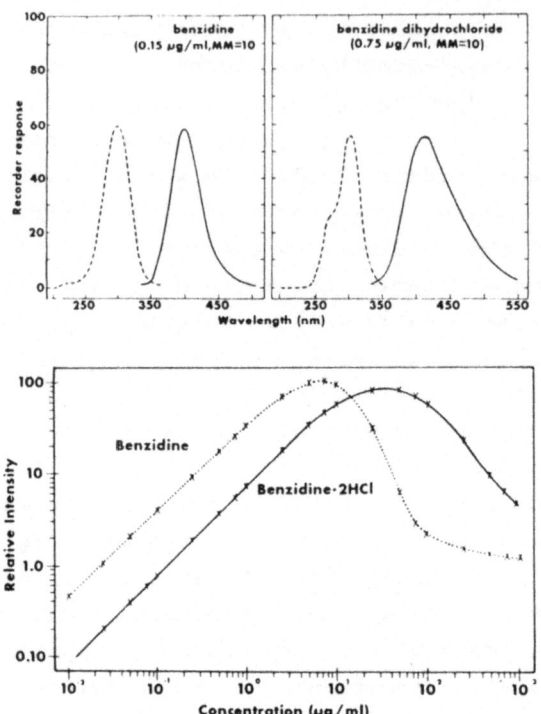

Figure 5. SPF excitation and emission spectra and standard
curves for benzidine and benzidine 2HCl (14)

Spectrophotofluorimetric techniques were found to be quite
useful for the monitoring of work areas such as cages,
floors, benches, apparatus, etc., suspected of being
contaminated with the above carcinogenic amines or their
salts. Background fluorescence, generally equivalent to 0.10
μg of the salt, are readily detected and the identity of the
agent confirmed by its characteristic excitation and emission
maxima (15, 16).

A number of procedures utilising high pressure liquid chromatography (HPLC) for the determination of a number of carcinogenic aromatic amines have been reported (22-28). Riggin and
Howard (27) describe an HPLC method for the determination of
benzidine, 3,3'-dichlorobenzidine and 1,2-diphenylhydrazine
in aqueous media and in municipal sewage. These compounds
can be assayed either by direct injection, or by solvent extraction or resin desorption of the aqueous sample prior to
analysis with detection limits of less than 1 μg/litre. The
system used in this study was assembled from modular components consisting of an Altex Model 110A Liquid Chromatographic
Pump, a Rheodyne 7010 injector with a 50- μl loop, a 4.6 mm
i.d. x 25 cm stainless steel column packed with Lichrosorb
RP-2 (5-um particle diameter) and an electrochemical detector
(Model LC-2A) equipped with a thin-layer glassy carbon elec-
trode (Mode 7L5). The mobile phase consisted of 50/50
acetonitrile/pH 4.7, 0.1 M sodium acetate buffer. Of the
three analytical approaches, e.g., direct injection, solvent
extraction and resin absorption which were applied to actual
waste water and/or surface water samples, direct injection
while more susceptible to interferences, is very rapid and
has a detection limit of approximately 1 μg/l. Solvent
extraction serves to cleanup and concentrate the sample to
give a detection limit of approximately 100 ng/l and offers
some degree of cleanup. The primary advantages of resin
absorption are its speed and the fact that this technique can
be used in the field. This eliminates the need to preserve
dilute aqueous solutions of compounds of interest and also
avoids the emulsion problems frequently encountered during
solvent extraction of certain waste water samples.

Morales et al (28) described air sampling procedures for
benzidine, 3,3'-dichlorobenzidine and their salts. Air is
drawn through a glass-fibre filter followed by a bed of
silica gel to collect these substances as either particles or
vapours. The compounds are extracted with triethylamine in
methanol from the sampler and analysed by HPLC with
sensitivities in the range of 3 μg/m3 for 48-litre air

sampler. The methods were evaluated in the laboratory with test aerosol atmospheres and found to be unaffected by temperature or humidity of the environment. Figure 6 illustrates the probe containing sampler stages.

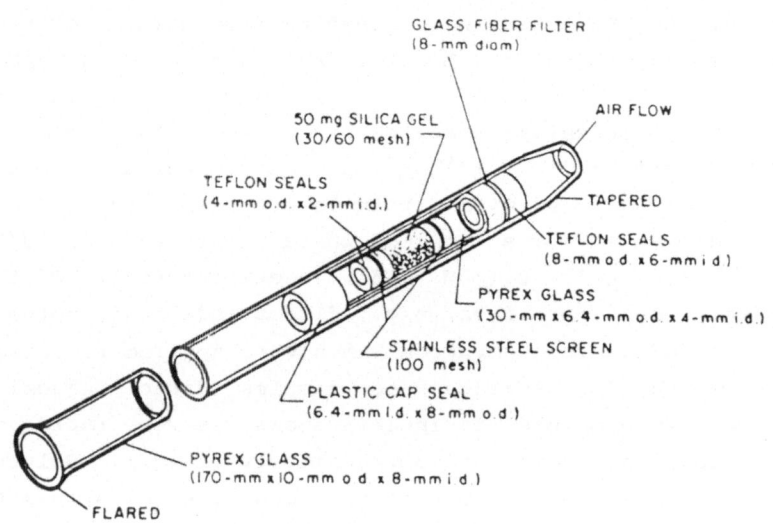

Figure 6 Probe containing sampler stages (28)

The liquid chromatograph utilised was a Waters Model ALC 202/401 equipped with a U.V. detector at 254 nm and a 30 cm x 4.0 mm i.d. u-Bondapa C_{18} column maintained at room temperature (23°C). Mobile phases were methanol/water (3/2,V/V) for benzidine and acetonitrile/water (7/3) for 3,3'-

dichlorobenzidine. At a flow rate of 1.5 ml/min both compounds were eluted in about 3 minutes (K^1=1.4). Calculated efficiencies were 2,800 theoretical plates for benzidine and 3,900 theoretical plates of 3,3'-dichlorobenzidine. Injection volumes were 10 μl for benzidine and 15 μl for 3,3'-dichlorobenzidine.

Tests of precision, sample stability and separation from interferants indicated that the method of Morales et al (28) should provide reliable results for personal monitoring procedures. In regard to possible interferants, one compound was found to interfere in each case, e.g., aniline in the analysis of benzidine and 4,4'-methylenebis(2-chloroaniline) in the analysis of 3,3'-dichlorobenzidine. Relative standard deviations (RSD) of mean air concentrations were calculated for each group of samples. These values varied between 2.26% and 5.21% for benzidine and between 3.81% and 6.38% for 3,3'-dichlorobenzidine. The precision values of S_p were 4.19% for benzidine and 5.05% for 3,3'-dichlorobenzidine. When coupled with sampling pump error of 5%, the precision of the method would be 6.5% and 7.1% for benzidine and 3,3'-dichlorobenzidine respectively. These precision levels should approximate those encountered in field sampling.

As noted previously, since benzidine and 3,3'-dichlorobenzidine are regulated as carcinogens, it is vital that an air sampler provide an accurate assessment of exposures. In most industrial operations it is considered probable that these amines would be present as aerosols although it also seems likely that in certain situations, particularly those that involve elevated temperature the vapours of the free amines would be present. A field-sampling version of the experimental prototype of Morales et al. is shown in Figure 7. The authors note that the only apparent disadvantage of their air sampling and analytical procedures is the relative instability of benzidine and its salts on the sampler stage. However, by keeping samples cold (-15°C) and analysing them within a few days of collection, the procedure should be satisfactory.

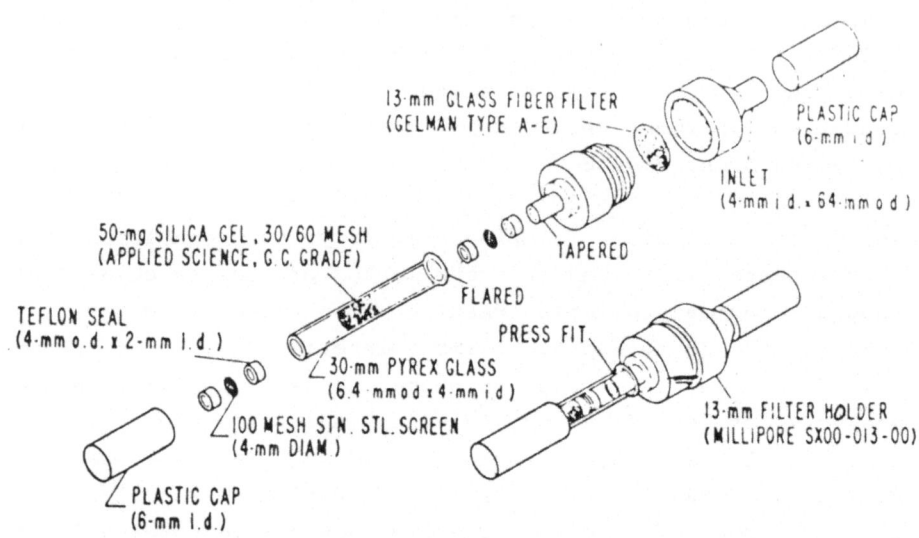

Figure 7   Prototype personal sampler suggested for field use. (28)

Since benzidine is primarily a human bladder carcinogen, urine is by far the most commonly analysed biological medium. The various procedures utilised are those wherein the urinary benzidine is extracted in a solvent (e.g., ether-benzene, 3:2) and thereafter frequently determined colorimetrically by procedures based on diazotization and coupling reactions (29-33). The sensitivity of these methods generally range from 0.5 to 0.1 μg of benzidine per litre of urine. A more generally used colorimetric procedure involves the formation of a yellow meriquinodal complex with chloramine-T (CH$_3$-C$_6$H$_4$-SO$_2$NNaCl) which offers a convenient means for a rapid quantitation determination (34-38). However, the colour reaction is not specific for benzidine as all p,p'-diamino-diphenyl derivatives form the yellow oxidation product to some degree. The reaction is also photo-sensitive, requiring rapid reading of the samples to prevent inaccurate results.

In addition to the procedures of Bowman et al (14,18) described above for the determination of benzidine and congeners in urine involving GLC and SPF analysis, Rice and Kissinger (39) determined benzidine and its mono and diacetyl metabolites in urine by HPLC. The procedure requires 2.0 ml of urine and involves extraction of the compound(s) followed by quantitation via HPLC with electrochemical detection. While this procedure shows considerable promise for use in assaying urine samples containing benzidines and its acety- lated metabolites to levels as low as 10 ppb, quantitation of levels below 10 ppb would probably require fluoroacylation and electron capture-GC. As shown earlier by Bowman and Rushing (18) and Nony and Bowman (20), the EC/GC methods for dichlorobenzidine and benzidine have minimum detection levels in urine of about 60 ppt (pg/ml) pentafluoropropionyl derivative.

Analytical chemical procedures were recently described by Nony and Bowman (40,41) for determining trace levels of poss- ible metabolites of two azo compounds, Direct Black 38 and Pigment Yellow 12 (derived from benzidine and 3,3'-dichloro- benzidine respectively) in hamster urine and to monitor the urine from workers who may be occupationally exposed during the manufacture or use of the dye and pigment. These methods were required for metabolism studies designed to assess the hazards that may occur if the two compounds are converted _in vivo_ mechanism to potential carcinogens. Ger- mane features of the procedure are: extraction of the free aromatic amines and neutral compounds, alkaline hydrolysis of the aqueous phase and extraction of any hydrolysed conjugates as free amines and the analyses of the free amines and acety- lated metabolites directly by HPLC or by electron capture-GC following the conversion of the amines to their respective heptafluorobutyryl derivatives. Residues of metabolites in hamster and human urine were determined at levels as low as 1 ppb. Structural formulas of C.I. Direct Black 38 and Pigment Yellow 12, their possible metabolites in urine from hamsters and humans and their heptafluorobutyryl (HFB) derivatives are shown in Figures 8 and 9 respectively. The scheme for extraction, separation and analysis of benzidine, monoacetyl benzidine, diacetyl benzidine and alkaline hydrolysable conjugates in urine is shown in Figure 10.

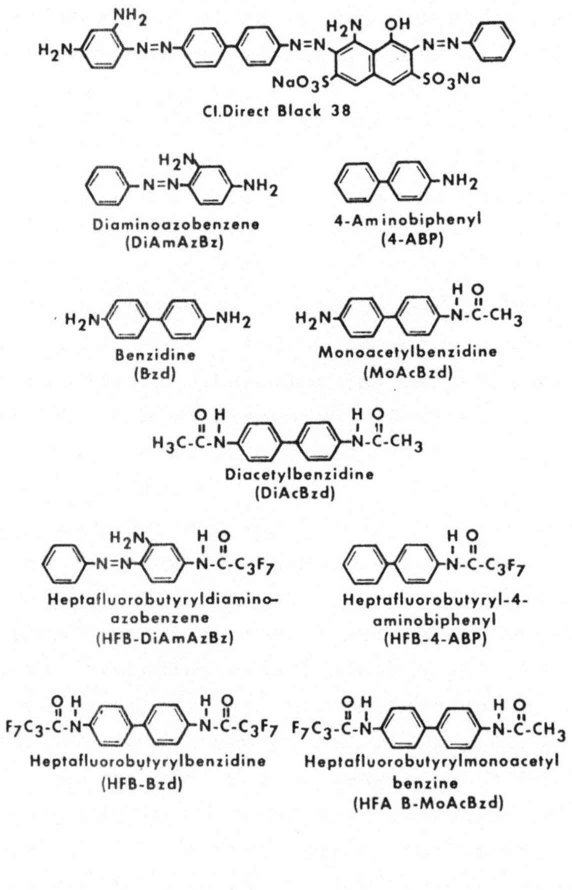

Figure 8   Formulas of Direct Black 38, its metabolites in urine from hamsters, and their heptafluorobutyryl (HFB) derivatives. (40,41).

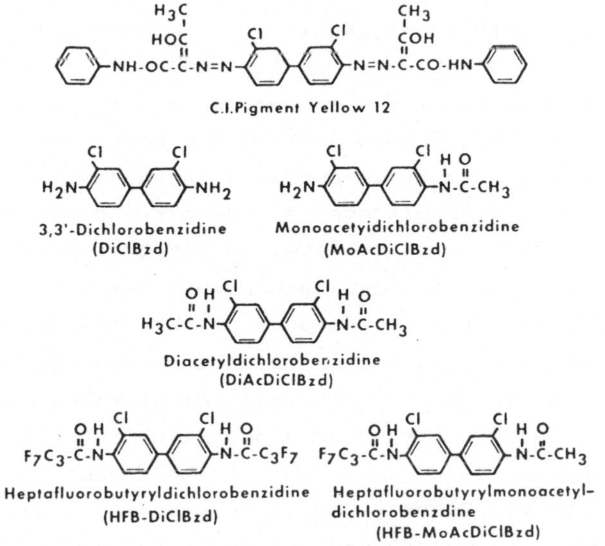

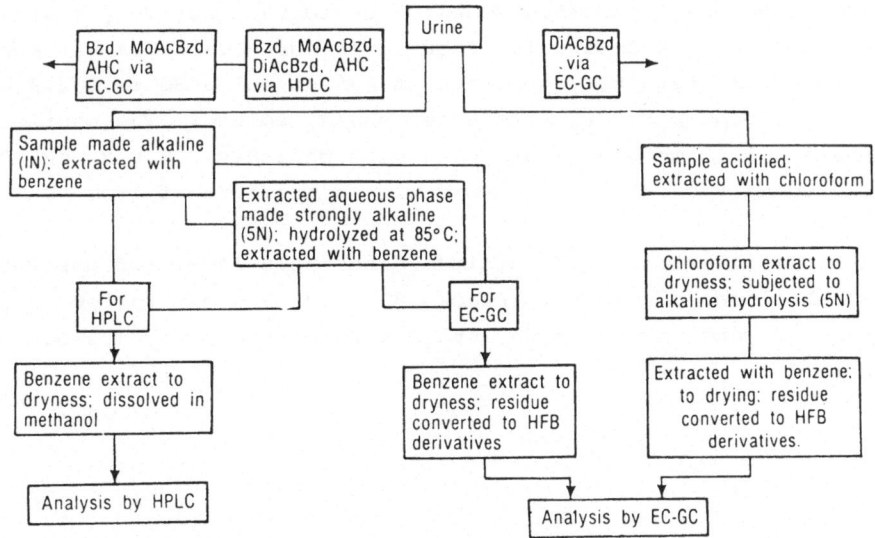

Figure 9   Formulas of Pigment Yellow 12. Some of its possible metabolites in urine from hansters and their heptafluorobutyryl (HFB) derivatives (40,41)

Figure 10   Scheme for extraction, separation, and analysis of benzidine (Bzd), monoacetylbenzidine (MoAcBzd) diacetylbenzidine (DiAcBzd), and alkaline hydrolyzable conjugates in urine. (40,41)

Gas chromatographic analyses were performed using a Hewlett Packard Model 5750B instrument equipped with a [63]Ni detector and a 6 ft glass column (4 mm i.d.) containing 5% Dexsil 300 on 90/100 mesh Anakrom Q conditioned at 300°C for 72 hr prior to use, operated isothermally at 220°, 260° and 280°C with nitrogen as the carrier gas at 160 ml/min. The detector, operated in the DC mode, was set at 300°C and the injection port temperature was 20°C higher than the column oven. Because of the wide difference in retention time (t_R) values for the various HFB derivatives, monoacetyl benzidine, monoacetyl dichlorobenzidine were analysed at 280°C, then benzidine, dichlorobenzidine and diaminoazobenzene were analysed at 260°C and 4-aminobiphenyl at 220°C. Diacetylbenzidine and diacetyldichlorobenzidine must be hydrolyzed and converted to their corresponding free amines prior to derivatization with heptafluorobutyricanhydride (HFBA).

High-pressure liquid chromatographic assays were carrried out with a Waters Associates Model 6000A solvent delivery system, a Model U6K septumless injector, a Tracor Model 970A variable wavelength detector operated at 295 nm and a 30 cm x 3.9 mm i.d. u-Bondapak C_{18} (reverse phase) column. The mobile phase, 50% methanol-50% potassium phosphate (0.01M, pH6.0) flowed at the rate of 1 ml/min with a pressure of 1600 psi.

Table 1 illustrates the minimum detectable levels of possible metabolites of Direct Black 38 and Pigment Yellow 12 in hamster and human urine obtained by electron capture-GC and HPLC.

Table 1. Minimum detectable levels of possible metabolites of
direct black 38 and pigment yellow 12 in hamster and
human urine (40).

| Compound | Minimum detectable level (ppb) by method indicated (twice background) | | |
| | EC/GC[a] | | HPLC |
	Hamster	Human	Hamster
Benzidine (Bzd)	3	1	180
Monoacetylbenzidine (MoAcBzd)	70	2	210
Diacetylbenzidine (DiAcBzd)[b]	2	0.2	260
2,4-Diaminoazobenzene (DiAmAzBz)	5	1	850
4-Aminobiphenyl (4-ABP)	4	2	870
3,3'-Dichlorobenzidine (DiClBzd)	8	c	525
Monoacetyldichlorobenzidine (MoAcDiClBzd)	48	c	660
Diacetyldichlorobenzidine (DiAcDiCl2Bzd)[b]	7	c	600

[a]Assayed as the HFB derivatives.
[b]Assayed as the HFB derivative after alkaline hydrolysis to the
free amine.
[c]Not determined.

Sensitive chemical spot tests employing a "swipe" technique
have been developed by Weeks and co-workers (42,43) for
detecting a variety of carcinogenic primary aromatic amines
and related compounds (e.g., those compounds which are readily transformable to aromatic amines, 4-nitrobiphenyl and
4-dimethylaminoazobenzene) on painted metal and concrete
surfaces. For most of the compounds and surfaces studied,
limit of detection values were obtained at the level of less
than 200 nanograms of material per cm^2 of surface. The
tests in which fluorescent derivatives were formed were
generally more sensitive than those relying upon highly
coloured substances. While chromogenic tests are frequently
not as sensitive as the fluorogenic, positive chromogenic
tests were obtained at concentration levels where quenching
may obviate the fluorescence tests. By utilising both
chromogenic and fluorogenic derivatization techniques as

complementary methods, the analytical derivatization techniques as complementary methods, the analytical confidence of
a test series was enhanced. Figure 11 illustrates the relative detection range of chromogenic and fluorogenic reagents.
While the fluorogenic detection limit is the lower of the
two methods (e.g., of the order of ng/cm^2) it also has an
upper limit due to fluorescence quenching and other secondary
effects. Although the chromogenic test limit of detection
values are generally of the order of tens or hundreds of
$nanograms/cm^2$, there are no effective upper limits (43).
Figure 12 illustrates diagrammatically how these chromogenic
and fluorogenic tests may be used to determine the presence
or absence of primary amines. Only in the case when both the
chromogenic and fluorogenic tests are negative can one
suspect that the subject agents are likely absent at the
respective limits of detection of the systems employed.

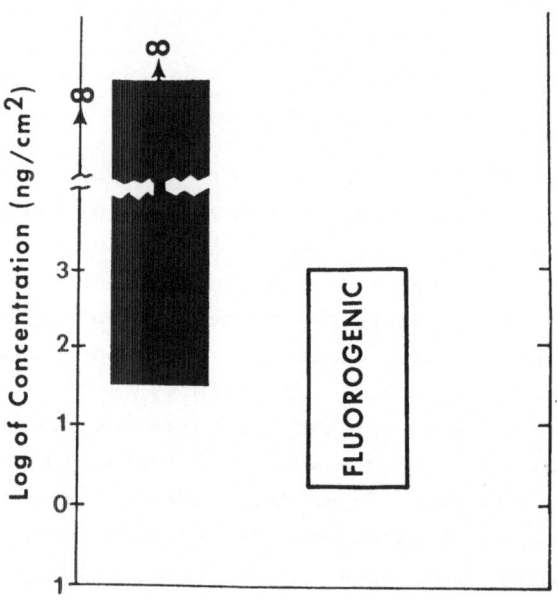

Figure 11. Typical Relative Detection Range for Chromogenic
and Fluorogenic Reagents (42,43)

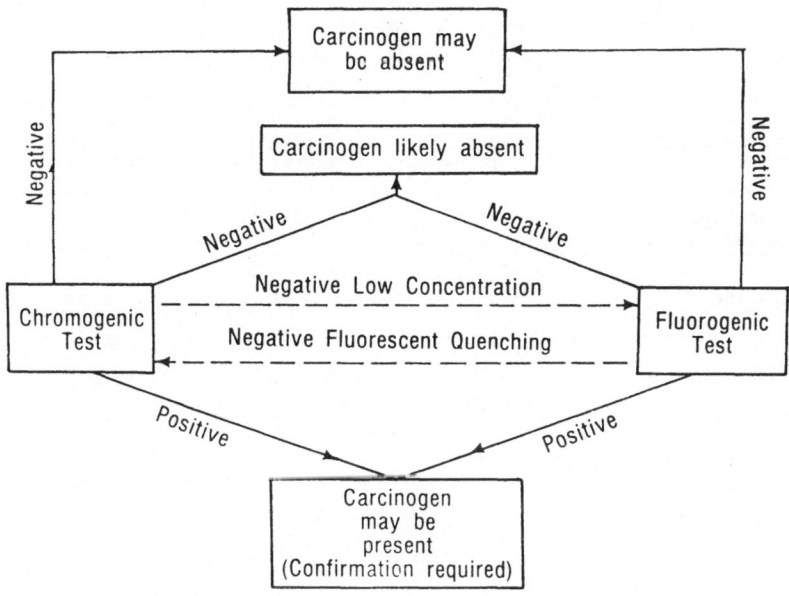

Figure 12. Flow chart depicting manner in which chromogenic and fluorogenic spot tests complement one another (42,43)

The most promising reagents employed by Weeks et al (42,43) were Ehrlich's reagent (p-dimethylaminobenzaldehyde), fluorescamine and o-phthalaldehyde. Table 2 lists the limits of detection utilising Ehrlich's reagent when utilised for the detection of benzidine, 3,3'-dichlorobenzidine, 1-naphthylamine, 2-naphthylamine, 4-aminobiphenyl and MOCA [4,4'-methylenebis (ortho-chloroaniline)]. For the painted and stainless steel surfaces, the limit of detection values for the 6 aromatic amines were all 150 nanograms. or less. Table 3 lists typical limit of detection values using fluorescamine as the visualization reagent for the 6 OSHA carcinogens shown. The detection limit for this reagent was of the order of nanograms or tens of nanograms of amine per cm^2 of surface. These levels are typically five-fold lower than those obtained using Ehrlich's reagent.

Table 2. Limit of detection (ng/cm^2).
          p-Dimethylaminobenzaldehyde

CANCER-SUSPECT AGENT	STAINLESS FILTER PAPER (WHATMAN 42) (DIRECT TECHNIQUE)	PAINT STEEL 316 0.5-3.5 inch (LEACHING TECHNIQUE)	MACHINE GRAY GLIDDEN (LEACHING TECHNIQUE)
4,4'-Methylenebis-(o-chloroaniline) (MOCA)	175	150	150
Benzidine	30	30	150
3,3'-Dichlorobenzidine	30	30	150
1-Naphthylamine	800	150	150
2-Naphthylamine	30	30	150
4-Aminobiphenyl	30	30	150

Ehrlich's Reagent Limit of Detection Values.

Table 3. Limit of detection (ng/cm^2)
          Fluorescamine visualization (42,43)

CANCER-SUSPECT AGENT	FILTER PAPER (WHATMAN 42) (DIRECT TECHNIQUE)	STAINLESS STEEL 316 0.5-3.5 inch (LEACHING TECHNIQUE)	PAINT MACHINE GRAY GLIDDEN (LEACHING TECHNIQUE)
4,4'-Methylenebis-(2-chloroaniline)	3	6	15
Benzidine	3	6	15
3,3'-Dichlorobenzidine	3	6	15
1-Naphthylamine	30	30	30
2-Naphthylamine	3	6	15
4-Aminobiphenyl	3	6	30

References

1. Parkes, H.G.   The Epidemiology of Aromatic Amine Cancers. In: Searle, C.E. ed., Chemical Carcinogens, American Chemical Society Monograph No. 173. Washington, D.C.: American Chemical Society, 1976:462-480.

2. International Agency for Research on Cancer. Monographs on the Evaluation of Carcinogenic Risk of Chemicals to Man.   Vol. 16, Some Aromatic Amines and Related Nitro Compounds - Hair Dyes, Colouring Agents and Miscellaneous Industrial Chemicals, Lyon: International Agency for Research in Cancer, 1978:43-142.

3. Kriek,   E. Aromatic Amines and Related Compounds as Carcinogenic Hazards to Man.   In: Emmelot, P., Kriek, E., eds.,   Environmental   Carcinogenesis.   Amsterdam: Elsevier/North Holland Biomedical Press, 1979:143-164.

4. Fishbein, L. Potential Industrial Carcinogens and Mutagens. Amsterdam: Elsevier; 1979:256-416.

5. Yashida, O., Miyakaga, M. Etiology of Bladder Cancer; Metabolic Aspects in Analytical and Experimental Epidemiology of Cancer. In: Nakahara, W., Hirayarna, T., Wishroka, K.,Sugans, A. eds., Baltimore University Park Press, 1973:31-39.

6. Jones, T.C. Preliminary Risk Assessment.   Phase I: Benzidine, Its Congeners, and Their Derivative Dyes and Pigments, Washington, D.C., Office of Pesticides and Toxic Substances, U.S. Environmental Protection Agency, 1980 (TSCA Chemical Assessment Services) (EPA publication no. 560/11-80-019)

7. Anonymous.   ITC Recommends Three Categories of Dyes, Two Chemicals for Priority Testing.   Toxic Materials News 1979:6:363.

8. U.S. Department of Labor. Occupational Safety and Health Standards, Part 1910 Carcinogens. Washington D.C.: Occupational Health and Safety Office, U.S. Department of Labor. Federal Register 1974:39:3756-3795.

9. Anonymous. Benzidine Dyes: Reduce Exposure, Use Substitutes,OSHA/NIOSH Hazard Alert Cautions. Chem. Reg. Repts. 1980:4:63.

10. U.S. Dept. Of Health Education and Welfare. NIOSH/NCI Joint Current Intelligence Bulletin No.24: Direct Black 38, Direct Blue 6, and Direct Brown 95; Benzidine Derived Dyes. Washington, D.C.: U.S. Department of Health, Education and Welfare, 1978 (NIOSH publication no. 78-148)

11. Shriver, C.R., Drury, J.S., Hammons, A.S., Tourll, L.E., Lewis, E.B., Opresko, K.M. Reviews on the Environmental Effects of Pollutants: II Benzidine. Washington D.C.: U.S. Environmental Protection Agency, 1978 (ORNL publication no. EIS-86; EPA Publication no. 600/1-78-024).

12. Radding, S.B., Holt, B.R., Jones, J.L., Liu, D.R.,
    Mill,T., Hendry, D.G. Review of the Environmental Fate
    of Selected Chemicals. Washington, D.C.: Office of Toxic
    Substances, U.S. Environmental Protection Agency, 1975.
    (EPA Publication no. 560/5-75-001).

13. Jenkins, R.L., Baird, R.B. The Determination of
    Benzidine in Wastewaters. Bull. Env. Contam. Toxicol.
    1975:13:436-442.

14. Bowman, M.C., King, J.R., Holder, L.C. Benzidine and
    Congeners: Analytical Chemical Properties and Trace
    Analysis in Fine Substrates. Int. J. Environ. Anal.
    Chem. 1976:4:205-233.

15. Bowman, M.C., King, J.R. Analysis of 2-Acetylamino-
    fluorene: Residues in Laboratory Chow and Microbiological
    Media. Biochem. Med. 1974:9:390-401.

16. Holder, C.L., King, J.R. Bowman, M.C. 4-Aminobiphenyl,
    2-Naphthylamine and Analogs: Analytical Properties and
    Trace Analysis in Fine Substrates. J. Toxicol. Env.
    Hlth. 1976:2:111-129.

17. Nony, C.R., Treglown, E.J., Bowman, M.C. Removal of
    Trace   Levels   of   2-Acetylaminofluorene (2-AAF) From
    Wastewater. Sci. Total Environ. 1975:4:155-163.

18. Bowman, M.C., Rushing, L.G.   Trace Analysis of 3,3'-
    Dichlorobenzidine in Animal Chow, Wastewater and Human
    Urine by Three Gas Chromatographic Procedures. Arch.
    Environ. Contam. Toxicol. 1977:6:471-482.

19. Bowman, M.C., Trace Analysis; A Requirement for Toxico-
    logical Research with Carcinogens and Hazardous Subs-
    tances. J. Assoc. Offic. Anal. Chem. 1977:61:1253-1262.

20. Nony, C.R. Bowman, M.C. Carcinogens and Analogs: Trace
    Analysis of Thirteen Compounds in Admixture in Waste
    Water and Human Urine. Int. J. Environ. Anal. Chem.
    1978:5:203-220.

21. Mancy, K.H. Elements of Instrumental Analysis. In:
    Mancy K.H. ed. Instrumental Analysis for Water Pollu-
    tion Control. Ann Arbor, Mich.: Ann Arbor Science,
    1971:70.

22. Gutman, H.R. Isolation and Identification of the
    Carcinogen N-hydroxy-2-fluorenylacetamide and Related
    Compounds by Liquid Chromatography. Anal. Biochem.
    1974:58:469-478.

23. Fullerton, F.R., Jackson, C.D. Determination of 2-
    Acetylaminofluorene and its Metabolites by High Pressure
    Liquid Chromatograph. Biochem. Med. 1976:16:95-103.

24. Thorgeirsson, S.S., Nelson, W.L. Separation and
    Quantitative Determination of 2-Acetylaminofluorene and

its Hydroxylated metabolites by High Pressure Liquid Chromatography. Anal. Biochem. 1976:75:122-128.

25. Mefford, I., Keller, R.W., Adams, R.N., Sternson, L.A. and Yllo, M.S. Liquid Chromatographic Determination of Picomole Quantities of Aromatic Amine Carcinogens. Anal. Chem. 1977:49:683-684.

26. Stanley, J.W., Newport, G.D., Weis, C.C., West R.W. An Analytical Approach to Metabolic Profiling of Aromatic Compounds Using Liquid Chromatography. J. Liquid Chromatog. 1978:1:305-325.

27. Riggin, A.M., Howard, C.C. Determination of Benzidine, Dichlorobenzidine and Diphenylhydrazine in Aqueous Media by High Performance Liquid Chromatography. Anal. Chem. 1979:51:210-214.

28. Morales, R., Rappaport, S.M., Hermes, R.E. Air Sampling and Analytical Procedures for Benzidine, 3,3'-dichloro-benzidine and Their Salts. Am. Ind. Hyg. Assoc. J.: 1979:40:970-978.

29. Yllo, M.S. Analytical Techniques for Ecological and Toxicological Monitoring. In: Venkataramank. ed., Analytical Chemistry of Synthetic Dyes. New York: Wiley and Sons, 1977:571-580.

30. Baker, R.K., Deighton, J.G. Metabolism of Benzidine in the Rat. Cancer Res. 1953:13:529-531.

31. Sciarini, L.J., Meigs, J.W. The Biotransformation of Benzidine. Arch. Ind. Hlth. 1953:18:521-530.

32. Elson, L.A., Goulden, F., Warren, F.L. The Metabolism of Aromatic Amines in Relation to Carcinogenesis. Brit. J. Cancer 1958:12:108-115.

33. El-Dib. M. A. Colormetric Determination of Aniline Derivatives in Natural Waters. J. Assoc. Offic. Anal. Chemists, 1971:54:1383-1387.

34. Meigs, J.W., Brown, R.M., Sciarini, L.J. A Study of exposure to Benzidine and Substituted Benzidines in a Chemical Plant. Arch. Ind. Hyg. 1951:4:519-533.

35. Butt, L.T., Stafford, N. Papilloma of the Bladder in the Chemical Industry: Analytical Methods for Determination of Benzidine. J. Appl. Chem. 1956:6:525-539.

36. Sciarini, L.J. Mahew, J.A. Rapid Technique for Estimating Benzidines in Industrial Exposure. Arch. Ind. Hlth. 1955:11:420-421.

37. Glassman, J., Meigs, J.W. Benzidine (4,4'-diaminobi-phenyl) and Substituted Benzidines, a Microchemical Screening Technique for Estimating Levels of Industrial Exposure from Urine and Air Samples. Arch. Ind. Hyg. Occup. Med. 1951:4:519-525.

38. Dangwal, S.K., Kadam, W.T., Jethani, B.M. Modified Method for Determination of Urinary Benzidine. Am. Ind. Hyg. Assoc. J. 1978:39:1019-1022.

39. Rice, J.R., Kissinger, P.T. Determination of Benzidine and its Acetylated Metabolites in Urine by Liquid Chromatography. J. Anal. Toxicol. 1979:3:64-66.

40. Nony, C.R., Bowman, M.C. Trace Analysis of Potentially Carcinogenic Metabolites by an Azo Dye and Pigment in Hamster and Human Urine as Determined by Two Chromato-graphic Procedures. J. Chromatog. Sci. 1980:18:64-74.

41. Nony, C.R., Bowman, M.C., Cairns, T., Lowry, L.K., Tolos, W.P. Metabolism Studies of an Azo Dye and Pigment in the Hamster Based on Analysis of the Urine for Potentially Carcinogenic Aromatic Amine Metabolites. J. Anal. Toxicol. 1980:4:132-140.

DISCUSSION ON CURRENT USES OF AMBIENT AND BIOLOGICAL
MONITORING

G. LEHNERT   It has generally been found that for toxicological studies it is useful to follow the system devised by
Rohmert, Wenzel and Rutenfranz (1966) for studying problems
of occupational physiology, whereby a distinction is made
between the external load, internal load, and response.
Information on the external load to which workers are exposed
when handling certain substances is obtained by ambient
monitoring, whereas information on the internal load and
response is obtained by biological monitoring. While ambient
monitoring is naturally geared to the health protection of
groups of employees, biological monitoring is primarily aimed
at preventive health care of the individual.

In his paper Goldstein quite rightly pointed out that haematological changes in the form either of cytopenia of some or
all factors of the peripheral blood picture, or in the form
of acute myeloblastic leukaemia, are the most serious hazards
of chronic exposure to benzene. He also drew attention to
the fact that early diagnosis of benzene-induced cytopenia is
made considerably more difficult by the wide fluctuation of
the normal peripheral blood picture in the same individual
and between different individuals, the relatively high
compensation capacity of bone marrow, and the non-specific
nature of the changes. It is still not clear whether acute
leukosis only follows cytopenia or whether it can also
develop out of normal blood status.

It was against this background that Goldstein recommended
that in cases of occupational exposure to benzene a complete
blood analysis should be made initially and followed up by a
series of further tests. The aim of this proposal is hardly
to establish an "individual norm range", but it would help
those responsible to identify trends in the results of later
routine examinations and establish causal links between changes in the blood picture. In this respect the basic examina-

tion recommended by Goldstein should also be considered as a routine part of subsequent check-ups. Incidentally one might also mention that in the Federal Republic of Germany compliance with the health insurance regulations would probably demand that such a procedure be followed.

Goldstein recommends that the blood status be checked periodically in subsequent routine examinations. This advice must needs be followed, partly because there has not yet been any scientific evidence for a threshold dose for benzene and partly because there are no alternative methods of diagnosing acute leukosis.

Nevertheless we are bound to ask whether blood analyses alone are sufficient for assessing the health hazards of benzene. It should be borne in mind that any change in the blood picture represents an undesirable response by the haemopoietic system. An obvious solution would be to carry out additional routine checks of internal benzene loads to keep the latter within certain boundaries. It is now thought that this can at least help to prevent the development of cytopenia. The internal load can be determined by measuring either benzene present in the blood or phenol present in the urine; the first method is preferable, as it is more specific. The "headspace" method provides a simple and reliable means of measuring blood benzene levels by gas chromatography. Given this situation, routine checks of the benzene concentration in the blood should be instituted without delay.

At least as important as the selection of a suitable preventive care programme, if not more so, is to decide on the level of external benzene load above which regular check-ups should be instituted. This is a universal problem when dealing with hazardous substances, but it is particularly urgent in the case of benzene, as with all carcinogens, because of its leukaemia-causing potential. It is not really possible to arrive at a scientifically-based decision in the present state of knowledge regarding carcinogens, but it would be

unrealistic not to endeavour to do so, if only because of the
limited personnel and material resources involved.

These comments on benzene apply equally to the second group
of organic compounds discussed here today, the aromatic
amines.

Foa pointed out that the category of aromatic includes a
large number of substances with widely differing toxicological properties. He stressed that for many of the substances
the skin is the main intake pathway and that for this reason
ambient monitoring of the substances in the atmosphere of the
workplace is usually no guide to the external load to which
workers are exposed. But in view of the carcinogenic potential of many aromatic amines, measurement of the external
load is of major practical interest. The situation is further complicated by the fact that many aromatic amines have
not yet received sufficient attention in toxicological
research.

Foa described the Technical Regulations of the Italian
Ministry of Labour for preventive care in cases of occupational exposure to aromatic amines. He himself asked whether it
was justifiable to include compounds whose toxicological
properties have not yet been researched in the same category
as substances which have been found to be non-carcinogenic in
various in vivo experiments. This problem will no doubt have
to be discussed in greater detail this afternoon.

In the second part of this talk Foa described the methods of
ambient monitoring for aromatic amines that he has used under
field conditions, although he pointed out that for lipotropic
amines ambient monitoring could never give a true indication
of the hazard because of the danger of absorption through the
skin. He therefore attaches great inportance to biological
monitoring as part of regular medical examinations. This
could be geared to parameters either of internal load or of
response. We will have to examine this subject again when we

come to discuss Fishbein's paper, but it is worth pointing out at this stage that as far as the carcinogenic potential of aromatic amines is concerned, any objective assessment of response is simply tantamount to an early diagnosis of cancer, as in the case of benzene-linked leukaemia. For preventive diagnosis, therefore, every possible effort must be made to measure the load, rather than the response, and to keep exposure to a minimum, since no biologically tolerable maximum concentrations can be specified for carcinogenic substances. Foa has already stressed that this will call for improvements in analysis techniques in many areas. We would also endorse his final plea that all research on aromatic amines sould be intensified in view of the gaps in our knowledge and the potential hazards. But in view of the urgency of the matter and the wide range of materials involved, interim measures will no doubt be unavoidable. Fishbein discussed the subject of aromatic amines from the point of view of analysis techniques, describing methods used for ambient monitoring and biological monitoring. Thanks to the clear account he has given, it should be possible to work out a general guideline, in the course of our discussion, for routine medical monitoring of persons at risk.

As Fishbein explained, the main analysis techniques for the purpose are gas chromatography, high pressure liquid chromatography and spectro fluorimetry. Bearing in mind Fishbein's comments on the sensitivity and specificity of these three methods for identifying amines, it is clear that gas chromatography is the most reliable for diagnostic purposes, and may therefore be regarded as the preferred method for assessment of external and internal loads.

We now have to decide which of the two forms of monitoring - ambient or biological - is of greater preventive value in cases of occupational exposure to aromatic amines. Two aspects have to be taken into account:

1. Practical experience shows that at many workplaces aromatic amines cannot be detected in the ambient air, even with the most sensitive analysis techniques, but that at the same time methaemoglobin formation is observed in the employees. This phenomenon can only be explained by assuming that fairly large amounts of aromatic amines are absorbed percutaneously, but that - owing to its low vapour pressure - the substance does not enter the ambient atmosphere.

2. Fishbein drew our attention to the fact that azo dyes can also be metabolic carcinogens.

Both these aspects oblige us to conclude that some quantification of internal load, i.e. biological monitoring, is of central importance in preventive check-ups. Tests would be based mainly on urine samples. In my opinion analysis should not be confined to the determination of free amines or their acetyl metabolites, but in view of the point made by Fishbein about the carcinogenicity of azo dyes, it would be better to measure the internal load in terms of total amines after urine hydrolysis. Independently of this, we should also discuss whether such routine checks should be supplemented by methaemoglobin tests, that is, by measurements of response to exposure.

E.G. HUGHES   I am particularly concerned with biological limit values being quoted for surveillance of cadmium workers. I do not believe that our present knowledge allows absolute numbers to be quoted. Analysis of blood for cadmium content and widely varying results are obtained. Similarly the use of neutron activation is still experimental and figures used by Lauwerys using this method are suspect for kidney values, due to variation in anatomical position of the kidney.

Further work must be carried out with the cooperation of Occupational Health physicians and academic departments.

G. KAZANTZIS There is no evidence at present that exposure to cadmium gives rise to hypertension in man, therefore no indication to modify the existing FAO/WHO Provisional Tolerable Weekly intake for cadmium established in 1972.

Workers in an environment where a cadmium process is carried out have all grades of exposure and body burden, from the low concentrations seen in the general population to the very high concentrations seen in chronic cadmium poisoning. However, there is no indication, from observations made on cadmium workers in Sweden, of an increased prevalence of hypertension in those workers with intermediate exposure; studies in Japanese populations with an increased cadmium intake have shown a decreased mortality from cerebrovascular disease; the small study from Shipham, England which purported to show an increased prevalence of hypertension disregarded epidemiological principles of investigation and cannot be interpreted. Rather than expend scarce resources on setting up further studies to elucidate the role of cadmium in hypertension the opportunity should be taken of investigating blood pressure in existing studies. The nationally based mortality study of cadmium workers in the UK should provide some data in this question, as should other existing morbidity studies.

L. MIKSCHE The approach of evaluating a permissible air level from the critical kidney cortex concentration of 200 μg Cd/g has several uncertain parameters involved. The critical concentration may be higher than stated due to technical problems such as kidney localisation. Furthermore there are no reliable data on pulmonary absorption rate of cadmium estimations running from 15% to 50% of retained cadmium.

As far as renal effects are concerned, no cases of severe
renal disease or kidney failure have been described in
cadmium workers. Proteinurea has been observed mainly in
workers exposed for more than 20 years and from earlier years
one may assume that exposure levels have ranged up to several
mg Cd/m^3 air. Thus workers showing proteinurea were
exposed for many years to high cadmium levels. (E. Adamsom
1979, G. Hughes 1980, R. Jeandot et al. 1980).

A. MUNN   Foa's paper on aromatic amines has demonstrated
the problem of "generic" regulations as opposed to regulations limiting specific compounds. The detailed health surveillance appropriate for benzidine or for aniline would be
quite inappropriate for the relatively harmless medicament
paracetemol (para acetylaminophenol), and for other aromatic
amines of which there is ample evidence, both experimental
and epidemiological, of low toxicity.

Fishbein's paper dealt with azo dyestuffs derived from benzidine and related intermediates; both benzidine and its acetylated derivatives had been demonstrated in the urine of
workers with such dyes. Neither benzidine nor its acetylated
derivatives are the ultimate urinary carcinogens - believed
to be the hydroxylated derivatives. It would have been more
convincing if somebody were to demonstrate the hydroxy-
derivatives as a hazard for workers with these dyes.
Ultimately it is likely that epidemiology will indicate
whether users of such dyes are really at risk.

A. BERLIN   On the basis of the proposed definition of
biological monitoring of Zielhuis, can one consider such an
approach?

Presentations of health effects, analytical techniques and
legislative provisions should not become the topic of
discussion.

J. LEWALTER Problems of cadmium analysis are due to errors occuring in atomic absorption analysis, as there are no biological standards for persons exposed to cadmium.

Has experience been gained in the analysis of cadmium transport protein complexes in correlation with cadmium in biological material? And why is collective examination of all persons exposed to cadmium (simultaneous urine sampling of all subjects) not taken into consideration?

V. FOA What experience has been gained in evaluating carbon monoxide absorption by determing COHb at the beginning and at the end of the workshift? A study of motorway toll workers carried out by us showed that the difference in COHb levels between the beginning and the end of the shift was super- imposable, both for smokers and nonsmokers, although the initial carboxyhaemoglobin levels were considerably different for both categories.

R. LAUWERYS The comments made on cadmium could be applied to all industrial toxins and to all methods of analysis, both biological and ambient; it is always possible to claim that the toxicological data available are limited; one can always show that conflicting findings call for improvements in the methods of analysis. This should not prevent objective anaylsis of data already available nor reasonable recommend- ations to protect worker health. Specifically, as regards cadmium, the scientific data gathered during the past few years enable us to propose critical levels in the biological environments; of course these levels would have to be reviewed at regular intervals but they are very reasonable health objectives at the present.

A.M. THIESS I have three questions referring to cadmium:

    i) Are there experiences on chromosome studies in human beings with long exposure to cadmium, and what are their results?

    ii) How sensitive and how specific are lung function tests performed on cadmium persons?

    iii) What should be done with persons with proteinuria? Sure, they should be removed from further exposure to cadmium but how should they treated? What would be their rate of compensation?

R. E. YODAIKEN What are the long term effects of CO exposure? Animal experiments particularly in primates have shown that CO exacerbates atheromatosis. In a personal survey of coal liquifaction workers who are exposed to CO I was struck by the apparent high incidence of myocardial infarction. Are there any current methods of assessing long term exposure to CO?

E.P. RADFORD In response to Foa's question, carbon monoxide exposure from ambient air should be additive to CO taken up from smoking, although not exactly so. His result differs from similar studies we have done, in which rise in COHb from start to end of a workshift was similar for smokers and nonsmokers. Perhaps his workers changed their smoking patterns during the workshift.

In response to Yodaiken's question, the experimental evidence is equivocal about chronic atherosclerotic effects of CO exposure but we have found that ex-smokers had larger infarcts from acute mycardial infarction than those who had never smoked.

Finally: because of the importance of smoking on blood COHb, no standard for CO exposure based on blood measurements has been proposed. We rely still on an air standard to protect workers.

B. GOLDSTEIN The relative role of ambient and biological monitoring will depend in part upon a safety factor. This is exemplified by benzene. If benzene only produced aplastic anaemia, one could use biological monitoring to detect the early reversible cytoprene phase. A platelet count of 120,000/cu mm is statistically abnormal, but not clinically abnormal. In aplastic anaemia one could rely relatively heavily on biological monitoring although not completely. No such safety margin exists for acute leukaemia where it is possible that minimal bone marrow damage may be associated with leukaemogenesis. Reliance must be on ambient monitoring with haematological tests as a back-up.

E. FOURNIER Measuring benzene in the blood is certainly still useful, particularly in view of the convenience of the "head space" technique but measuring concentrations in exhaled air is perhaps even more convenient since it is a non-invasive technique. The measurement of urinary phenol was useful for benzene concentrations in air of 25 and 50 ppm but would appear to be of little value where standards of 1 to 10 ppm are concerned.

V. FOA I agree with Munn's comments. A more pressing problem is what to do with the evidence of carcinogenic effects of certain aromatic amines on man. This has been so clearly established that all that remains to be done is to ban their production and use.

M. CORN I am disturbed by the emphasis on biological moni-toring as contrasted to ambient monitoring. The day-by-day, week-by-week techniques for engineering controls and ambient monitoring are highly effective, requiring only infrequent or periodic recourse to biological monitoring. In the case of excursions in exposure, biological monitoring is appropriate, but employees will not submit to routine, frequent biological monitoring, particularly if the techniques are invasive.

MULTIDISCIPLINARY APPROACH TO PREVENTION AND HEALTH
PROTECTION BY MONITORING: ROLE OF INDIVIDUAL DISCIPLINES, THE
HYGIENIST: AMBIENT MONITORING - WHERE WHEN AND HOW I

W. A. BURGESS (USA)

Summary

Monitoring the presence of toxic chemicals in the workplace
is a key element in any industrial hygiene programme. Al-
though the monitoring tasks are conducted by the industrial
hygiene group, other members of the occupational health team
join in the sponsorship of the work and the utilisation of
the data. This paper reviews typical workplace monitoring
activities in the United States and their value in occupatio-
nal health programmes.

Introduction

The principal monitoring tool available to the industrial hygienist to establish the identity of a chemical agent and its
concentration in the work-place is air sampling. Until the
1960s air samples were either taken at fixed locations at
each work area or the sampler was held at the workers'
breathing zone to establish the exposure during selected
industrial operations. If the time spent at each work location were known an approximate time-weighted average concentration for the shift could be calculated for each worker
from the results of the fixed location samples. Breathing
zone samples were normally taken to represent worst case
exposures; time weighted average concentrations were normally
not calculated from these data. In 1960 Sherwood and
Greenhalgh introduced the concept of personal air sampling
using battery powered pumps worn by the worker (1). Two
decades of industrial hygiene experience have demonstrated
that personal air sampling offers a more accurate definition
of exposure than fixed location sampling and today it is the
method of choice in the United States for monitoring worker
exposure to chemicals.

Personal air sampling utilises conventional collection methods -filters for particulates and sorbents for gases and vapours. The collected material is stripped or desorbed from the collector for analysis in the laboratory. Recent improvements in personal air sampling include lightweight, long duration pumps with flow regulation. The ease of conducting personal air sampling on large numbers of workers has been enhanced by the introduction of diffusion and permeation based passive samplers, self-contained colorimetric systems mounted on lapel badges and electro-chemical sensors. The rapid innovation in this area has been made possible by the close cooperation between the industrial hygienist and analytical chemist and the obvious market potential which sponsors the interest of manufacturers.

Routine monitoring

Routine monitoring of worker exposure by air sampling is one of the first steps in ensuring that workers are not placed at risk. Effective monitoring must, however, be coupled with critical evaluation of the exposure data based on exposure guidelines and standards. The protocol for conducting monitoring programmes varies widely in the United States depending on the goal of the programme and the individual style of the investigator. The National Institute for Occupational Safety and Health (NIOSH) has recommended the employee exposure determination and measurement strategy shown in Figure 1 for Occupational Safety and Health Administration (OSHA) regulatory requirements (2). The event that initiates repeat sampling in this plan is an exposure greater than the Action Level which is nominally one-half the OSHA Permissible Exposure Limit. The authors describe the action level concept as follows:

> The action level was set with the view that the employer should minimise the probability that even a very low percentage of actual daily employee exposure averages (8-hour time-weighted averages [TWA]) will exceed the standard. That is, the employer should

monitor employees in such a fashion that he
has a high degree of confidence that a very
high percentage of actual daily exposures are
below the standard. In statistical terms the
employer should try to attain 95% confidence
that no more than 5% of employee days are
over the standard.

This monitoring plan has a series of decision making steps
with adequate opportunity for feedback to modify the sampling
frequency based on changes in the work environment. Adequate
record keeping is required to make this approach effective.
A number of companies in the United States are using some
variation of this sampling strategy.

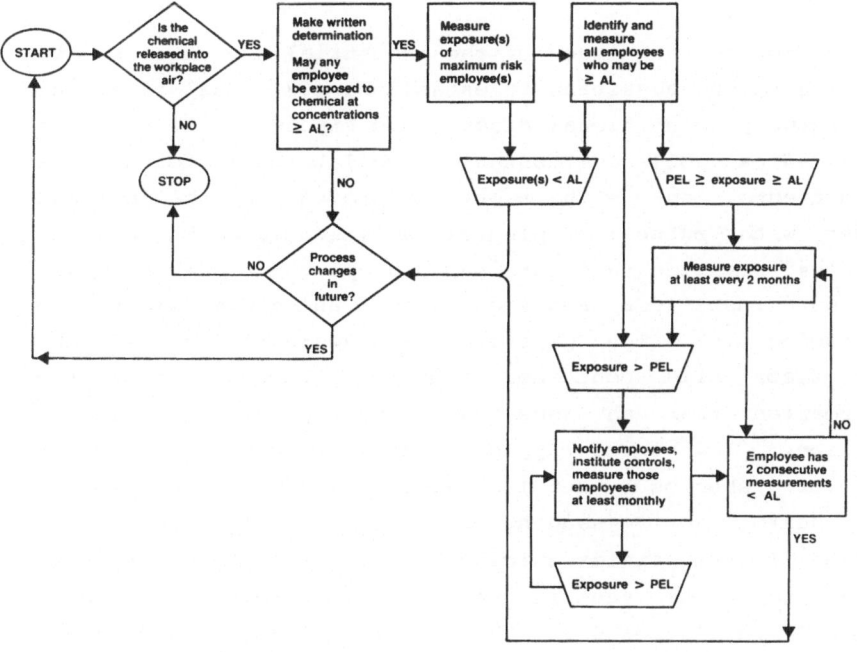

Figure 1. NIOSH recommended employee exposure determination and
measurement strategy. Each individual substance
health standard should be consulted for detailed
requirements. AL = action level; PEL = permissible
exposure limit

A monitoring plan of the type presented in Figure 1 can be the key to an effective prevention programme and becomes a resource for other members of the occupational health team. It targets the need for control action if air concentrations exceed the Permissible Exposure Limit and continuing periodic monitoring if concentrations exceed the Action Level. The physician is provided with data which are useful in establishing a biological monitoring programme, the epidemiologist may be able to use the limited monitoring data to establish exposure groups and the engineer is provided with data to monitor the effectiveness of installed controls.

Medical case studies

The monitoring techniques of the industrial hygienist may be of value to the physician in establishing a causal relationship between occupational disease and exposure. In one such case a medical colleague contacted our laboratory to describe two patients, one with a biopsy-proved mesothelioma and another with extensive pleural calcification. The medical histories revealed that both men had spent a number of years as floor installers and routinely sanded old tile before resurfacing it. The physician was aware that asphalt and vinyl floor tile contained asbestos, however, he wanted confirmation that an asbestos exposure could occur in the workplace. Industrial hygiene monitoring of air concentrations of asbestos by our laboratory revealed air concentrations during active sanding of greater than 1 fibre/ml. The membrane filter fields examined under phase microscopy were similar to those seen in other asbestos operations such as shipboard insulation work; the asbestos fibres were discrete and easily counted (3). The satisfactory conclusion to this case was due to the physician's knowledge of the monitoring capabilities of the industrial hygienist.

Epidemiological studies

The epidemiologist needs industrial hygiene monitoring data to develop dose information on populations under study. In

retrospective studies one is fortunate to study a work population in a plant where the materials and processes have not
changed in decades. In this unique situation it is possible
to monitor exposures under the operating conditions at the
time of the study and use these data as a valid basis for a
dose calculation. This situation did exist with a study
population exposed to asbestos at an insulation facility in a
small New England shipyard. The materials used and the
procedures employed in the work had not changed appreciably
over a twenty year period. Air sampling conducted during the
epidemiological survey was useful in establishing the
exposure occurring during the previous two decades (4).

A more normal situation was encountered in an epidemiological
study of silicosis in the granite monument industry of Barre,
Vermont. Under a NIOSH contract the Harvard School of Public
Health had agreed to determine dustiness at granite cutting
operations and relate, insofar as possible, work histories,
dust measurements and respiratory health. Limited historical
data of dust exposures were based on midget impinger sampling, the standard for dust counting in the United States
until the 1970s. To utilise the data it was necessary to
relate midget impinger data to the respirable mass sampling
data generated in our study. An early granite shed was reopened and four granite cutters were hired to work with old
tools and without local exhaust ventilation to simulate the
conditions existing in the 1920s and 1930s (5). Monitoring
of the dust exposure in the reconstructed shed operation was
useful in correlating the two sampling techniques and establishing a dose statement for the study population.

The design of an industrial hygiene monitoring programme to
complement a prospective epidemiological study would appear
to be a somewhat simpler matter. Such was not the case in a
five year study of the effects of automobile exhaust on
Boston traffic officers and toll booth operators. This monitoring programme involved sampling for contaminants associated with automobile exhaust, namely nitrogen dioxide,

carbon monoxide, total hydrocarbons, respirable particulates
and lead in addition to the general contaminant, sulphur dioxide (6). Ideally these contaminants should be sampled with
a personal monitoring unit, however, this was not feasible so
fixed location sampling was conducted where the officers were
stationed. This technique did provide the necessary exposure
data for the epidemiologist.

In many epidemiological studies it is not possible to identify a single chemical species or family of chemicals which
best correlate with the disease pattern observed in the work
population. One must frequently accept an index of exposure
which can be monitored by simple personal sampling techniques
and is useful in establishing gradations of exposure. In a
study of rubber workers there was concern about the exposure
of workers during tyre curing. Laboratory studies identified
a myriad of chemical compounds generated during the tyre
curing process (7, 8). In an epidemiological study of this
population the workplace exposure was established by monitoring respirable mass particulates, certainly a non specific
procedure but one felt to provide a reasonable index of exposure to the complex curing fume contaminant.

In many disease processes it may not be the average concentration of the toxic agent that produces morbidity but
rather repetitive instantaneous peak concentrations. This is
a difficult monitoring task for personal sampling since it
usually requires a continuous read-out instrument which has
considerable bulk and weight. Recent innovations in electro-
chemical sensors and miniature recorders may provide a solution to this problem in the near future.

Engineering studies

The general air monitoring data described earlier is of
obvious value to the plant engineer since it identifies those
operations that require additional engineering control. Once
installed the impact of the control can be assessed based on

this monitoring plan. Special industrial hygiene monitoring techniques can also be designed for engineering case studies.

Standard design plates on industrial processes include hood geometry, air flow rate, duct transport velocity, and entry loss (9). In general, these designs are empirically based and their performance has not been critically reviewed in plant settings. We have used a tracer particulate and a monitoring system to evaluate the collection efficiency of local exhaust hoods in tire plants. A contaminant is released at a given flow rate in the duct just downstream of the hood so that all of the contaminant is collected by the system. The duct concentration of the tracer particulate defines the 100% collection efficiency reference point. The contaminant is then released at the generation point in the process serviced by the exhaust hood under study. The concentration of the tracer in the duct is noted and the ratio of this concentration and the 100% concentration is an index of capture efficiency. This simple monitoring programme should be useful in assisting plant engineering in defining the efficiency of installed local exhaust ventilation facilities (10).

A second tracer monitoring procedure is of value to the plant engineer in defining reeentry of exhaust streams to the plant. To evaluate the extent of this problem a tracer can be released inside the exhaust hood while flow integrated air samples are collected at various work station locations inside the plant. Sulphur hexafluoride has found favour in this application due to its stability, low toxicity, and sensitivity for detection by an electron capture detector (11). We have used this tracer in cooperation with plant engineering to identify the problem and establish a control approach.

Analytical studies

The analytical chemist is the key to the success of any ambient monitoring programme. Few scientific analyses require the sensitivity, precision, and accuracy now routinely practised in industrial hygiene laboratories. Close cooperative effort must be developed between the industrial hygienist and the chemist to handle difficult sampling and analytical tasks. In a study of the exposure of municipal firefighters to eight air contaminants we tested the creativity of our analytical chemists. The result of a joint development project was a personal air sampling device which can be worn by the firefighter during his work (12).

Monitoring the exposure patterns of firefighters in over 200 structural fires in Boston, we noted life threatening concentrations of carbon monoxide and acrolein and less hazardous levels of benzene, hydrogen chloride, hydrogen cyanide, nitrogen dioxide, and carbon dioxide. As a result of the study the department introduced the mandatory use of breathing apparatus which reduced smoke inhalation cases by 40% in one year.

Conclusions

A number of ambient monitoring approaches are available to assist in the solution of complex occupational health problems presented by regulatory agencies, the medical clinician, the epidemiologist, and the plant engineer. The utilisation of current monitoring technology by the members of the occupational health team must be enhanced if worker health is to be protected. Future occupational health needs will require scientific and engineering advances if the potential value of ambient monitoring is to be achieved.

References

1. Sherwood R.J. and Greenhalgh D.M.S. A Personal Air Sampler. Ann Occup Hyg1960;2:127-132.

2. Leidel N.A., Busch K.A., and Lynch J.R. NIOSH Occupational Exposure Sampling Strategy Manual. NIOSH Technical Report No. 77-176, 1977.

3. Murphy R.L., Levine B.W., AlBazzaz F.J., Lynch J.L. and
    Burgess W.A. Floor Tile Installation as a Source of
    Asbestos Exposure. Amer Rev Resp Dis 1971;104:576-580.

4. Murphy R.L.H., Jr., Ferris B.G., Burgess W.A., Worcester
    J. and Gaensler E.A. Effects of Low Concentrations of
    Asbestos. Clinical, Environmental, Radiological, and
    Epidemiological Observations in Shipyard Pipe Coverers
    and Controls. New Eng J Med 1971;285:1271-1278.

5. Ayer H.E.,Dement J.M., Busch K.A., Ashe H.B., Levadie
    B.T.H., Burgess W.A. and DiBerardinis L. A Monumental
    Study - Reconstruction of a 1920 Granite Shed. Amer Ind
    Hyg Assoc J 1973;34:206-211.

6. Burgess W.A., DiBerardinis L. and Speizer F. Health
    Effects of Exposure to Automobile Exhaust, Part V.
    Exposure of Toll Booth Operators to Automobile Exhaust.
    Amer Ind Hyg Assoc J 1977;38:184-191.

7. Rappaport S. and Fraser D. Air Sampling and Analysis in a
    Rubber Vulcanisation Area. Amer Ind Hyg Assoc J 1977;38:
    205-210.

8. Burgess W.A., Peters J.M. and Monson R.R. The Rubber
    Workers Study at the Harvard School of Public Health.
    EPA Proc. Environmental Aspects of Chemical Use in Rubber
    Processing Operations Conference, Akron, Ohio, March
    1975.

9. Committee on Industrial Ventilation, American Conference
    of Governmental Industrial Hygienists, Industrial
    Ventilation: A Manual of Recommended Practice, 18th ed.,
    Lansing, Michigan, 1980.

10. Gempel R. and Burgess W.A. A Technique to Measure the
    Capture Efficiency of Local Exhaust Ventilation Hoods.

11. Drivas P.J., Simmands P.G. and Shair F.h. Experimental
    Characterization of Ventilation Systems in Buildings.
    Environ Sci & Tech 1972;6:609-612.

12..Treitman R., Burgess W.A. and Gold A. Air Contaminants
    Encountered by Firefighters. AIHAJ 1980;41(10):

MULTIDISCIPLINARY APPROACH TO PREVENTION AND HEALTH
PROTECTION BY MONITORING: ROLE OF INDIVIDUAL DISCIPLINES, THE
HYGIENIST: AMBIENT MONITORING - WHERE WHEN AND HOW II

A. HEUSE (BELGIUM)

Summary

The activities of an industrial hygienist cover two very important fields - monitoring of safety and health at work and collection of data for occupational health research. The paper discusses the roles that an industrial hygienist is required to fill and examines the appropriateness of where he should take samples, when he should take them and which sampling methods are to be used. It concludes by summarising a comparative survey carried out within the European Community.

Introduction

A brief survey of seven Community countries has shown that the profession of 'industrial hygienist' as such does not exist at all. There is no training officially leading to this title and the law does not require that such persons be employed. However, regulations often require various industrial hygiene measures which are performed by various other specialists: engineer/head of production, head of safety, occupational physician, toxicologist, chemist, production engineer, medical hygienist, etc.

What is the job of the industrial hygienist?

The industrial hygienist's job is to study the nature and to determine the importance of factors which may affect the health and well-being of people during their work. His activities cover two very important fields. They cover monitoring of safety and health at work and collection of data for occupational health research. They may take various forms.

i)   Detection of unhealthy working conditions. The indus-
     trial hygienist must:
     - identify places of work where harmful factors
       may be present and indicate where special
       supervision is necessary
     - define the techniques and organisation of such
       supervision
     - organise periodic or continuous monitoring and
       ensure that it meets health standards
     - investigate complaints about working condi-
       tions, determine their origin and analyse
       cases of excessive exposure.

ii) Improvement of working conditions.   The industrial
     hygienist must give aid and advice to improve working
     conditions and reduce harmful factors, etc.
     - when manufacturing processes are modified
     - by ensuring that certain contaminants have been
       eliminated
     - by verifying the effectiveness of protective
       measures on a general (ventilation, insulation,
       etc) or individual basis.

iii) Provision of aid to research and progress in occupation-
     al health and toxicology. The industrial hygienist must
     provide the data related to specific or non-specific
     health disorders and cooperate in the drafting of health
     standards.

These activities are impossible without an excellent knowledge of the industry concerned: the hygienist will therefore
spend most of his time at places of work in industry. He
will therefore base his findings on careful observation of
human and technical data in industry and on an inspection of
the quality of the environment (qualitative and quantitative
checks) involving the taking and analysis of representative
samples of various harmful agents to which workers are
exposed.

As regards human data he will note the number of workers normally employed, the absentee rate, sickness rate, accident
rate, etc; and as regards technical data the manufacturing
processes, raw materials used, by-products and impurities,
waste, frequency of maintenance, etc.

As regards inspection of the quality of the environment,
although analysis of these samples may sometimes be left to
specialist laboratories, the hygienist generally will play an
essential part in ensuring the statistical value of the
sampling. It is generally for him to decide where, when and
how the sampling is done.

Where should the samples be taken?
The site of sampling depends on the aims of monitoring. It
may be done:
- at the actual workplace, close to the workers, if the
  aim is to determine the degree of exposure to a
  specific pollutant
- in the general atmosphere of the place of work or
  workshop, often via a network of sampling points, if
  the aim is to determine the sources of atmospheric
  contamination or the quality of protective measures
  (ventilation, etc).
- at the location of the worker's respiratory tract
  (or of a sensory organ such as the eye or ear),
  possibly using a portable personal instrument; thus
  making it possible to check workers' exposure levels
  during their work, to determine exposure in nearby
  areas not directly affected by a given type of
  pollution and also to obtain objective data in
  connection with complaints.

When should samples be taken?
The frequency, duration and time of sampling depends on various considerations. Monitoring may have to cover a full
cycle of operations (for example in the study of non-routine
activities) or, depending on the job specifications, to

evaluate the effect of each stage in it. It will sometimes be necessary:

- to assess exposure over the whole working day (TLV monitoring), or to make comparative measurements;
- to cover each shift if shiftwork is involved, or different atmospheric conditions (seasonal variations).
- to carry out continuous monitoring in the case of highly toxic or irritant substances, or agents affecting the central nervous system (reduced vigilance etc), to detect any concentration peaks.

Apart from these factors which are connected with the type of work concerned, account must also be taken of the expected concentration, the amount of equipment necessary for accurate analysis (depending on the sensitivity of the analysis method), the degree of accuracy required (levels near the TLV), all of which must be discussed with the specialist who will make the analysis.

Which sampling method should be used?

The hygienist will have to choose between sampling methods with subsequent analysis or direct-reading methods (with or without recording), between 'spot' sampling (for short periods) and sampling spread over longer periods. This choice will depend upon the equipment available and the aim of the monitoring as shown in Table 1.

Table 1. Aims of Monitoring

	Type of Sampling	Aims	Equipment
Direct reading	instant measurement	to define the sources of contamination	Drager tubes[1]
	continuous recording	general monitoring (in connection with an alarm system)	direct reading dosimetry (cumulative or non-cumulative) dosimetry with continuous recording[2]
Sampling	spot	workplace analysis analysis of manufacturing processes	gas samplers (vacuum containers, plastic bags, etc.)
	spread over a long period	individual monitoring assessment of average exposure	film badges filters absorbent media (wash bottles) absorbent media (activated charcoal, silica gel)

[1] see Appendix 1
[2] see Appendix 2

By virtue of his training and experience, the hygienist must be able to select the method best suited to the problem in hand: Table 2 shows various possible circumstances.

Table 2. Selection of method of monitoring

Aims of monitoring	Where?	When?	How?
To identify and quantify new harmful agents, etc. (new manufacturing process)	at the workplaces concerned and at workplaces nearby	during a working cycle	direct instant reading before, during and after the work various types of sampling, spot sampling, sampling spread over the working period, continuous recording
To determine the extent of workers' exposure in the workplace environment	at the workplace or on the worker himself	during a working cycle or eight hours per day	sampling around the workplace, during work
In an individual case (complaint, suspected occupational disease, etc.)	at the location of the tract or a sensory organ (eye, ear, etc.)	eight hours per day	individual sampling, sampling throughout out working hours (activated charcoal, dosemeter etc.)
To monitor working conditions periodically	at the workplace	during a working cycle	sampling throughout working hours by means of a sampling network
continuously	throughout the premises	8 or 24 hours per day	continuous recording (coupled with an alarm) or sampling throughout working hours)
Epidemiological studies	combination of various data	data sometimes covering several years (long-term effects)	comparison with health statistics

An overall view of occupational health, however, can only be obtained by comparing data obtained simultaneously from the medical surveillance of workers, from biological tests made on them and from ambient monitoring. In Europe the initial trend was to give priority to medical and biological monitoring, which is generally performed only in large concerns or

under special or unusual conditions. Some legislation nevertheless does allow for situations where regular ambient monitoring could replace medical surveillance. Today, however,
the human being is still regarded as the absolute integrator
of the various harmful influences allowing for possible
synergistic effects, variations in individual sensitivity,
etc. Comparison of these different sets of data is none the
less essential to progress in epidemiological knowledge,
which is still fragmentary or non-existent in many fields.
In this respect, the medical hygienist is working at the
point where all this information converges and is especially
well-placed to integrate the data obtained.

The industrial hygienist in the European Community

A new concern of the hygienist moreover, is protection of
the environment outside the works: monitoring of the disposal
of solid and liquid waste, smoke emission, etc. In performing these different tasks, the industrial hygienist may act
at various levels and in various sectors of the industrial
organisation in his country. He may operate within central
or regional State structures: these duties involve inspecting
firms, preparing health standards, medical research, etc. He
may operate in the private sector, in industry, either
directly attached to a firm, or in a research unit or
laboratory in insurance companies which have an interest in
the prevention of occupational accidents and diseases.

In view of these considerations we felt it would be interesting to carry out a short survey in some countries of the
European Community. We have therefore summed up the opinions
of the appropriate authorities in these countries as regards:

i) The importance given to the various activities of the
hygienist. The emphasis is generally on the assessment of
harmful agents at the place of work. The procedures are in
rare cases standardised (Arbejdstilsynets - publikation No.
87/1979 in Denmark, Technische Regel fur gefahrliche

Arbeitstoffe - TRgA 401 Bl 1 in the Federal Republic of Germany, etc) or are concerned with particular pollutants or conditions (asbestos, chromium, confined spaces, vinyl chloride, etc). A very brief outline of this information is given in Table 3.

Table 3. Activities of the hygienist

Activity	EEC COUNTRIES					
	DK	I	IR	B	NL	UK
1. Assessment of harmful agents, etc. at the place of work	++	+	++	++	-	+++
2. Monitoring of health at the workplace	++	+	$+^2$ -	$+^2$ -	-	+
3. Technical surveillance	++	+	+	-	+	+
4. Obtaining objective data in connection with complaints	+ -	+	+	+ -	+	+
5. Education of personnel	+ -	+	+	+ -	-	+

1 regulations for asbestos, chromium and confined
2 regulations for asbestos and vinyl chloride

ii) The main aims of ambient monitoring. These depend on the industrial sectors involved and vary considerably from one country to another as shown in Table 4.

Table 4. Main aims of ambient monitoring

AIM / AIMS OF MONITORING	EEC COUNTRIES						SECTOR		
	DK	D	I	IR	B	NL	Government	UK Unions	Private
1. Government factory inspections	++	++	++	-	+	+++	+++	-	-
2. Periodic monitoring of harmful agents, etc.	++	+++	-	-	+ / -	-	-	-	+++
3. Occasional analyses	++	+	++	++	++	-	+	+	+
4. Investigation of complaints	-	-	-	-	+ / -	+	+ / -	+++	+ / -
5. Verification of protective measures	-	+	+	++++	-	++	-	-	+

iii)   The different structures within which the hygienist has to work in the public and the private sector. These are shown in Table 5. In some countries, like the United Kingdom, there is a trend towards regional structures (field consultant groups). In others, central bodies continue to supervise local organisations. In Europe there is an increasing tendency to supplement medical and biological surveillance with technical monitoring of workplaces. A good balance between these two approaches would indeed seem to be the ideal solution. It will not only permit a more careful study to be made of known situations but will make it possible, by the comparisons and research involved, to pinpoint new situations such as are perpetually occuring in today's industrial world. Such cases then become a matter for the epidemiologists.

Table 5. Position of the hygienist in various structures.

	EEC COUNTRIES						
STRUCTURE	DK	D	I	IR	B	NL	UK
Government - central	+	-	Instit Super	Labour Dept.	+ - Ministry of Labour	Social affairs	Headquarters consultant
- regional	-	Länder	Unita Sanit local.	-	-	Factory Inspect	Field consul- tant groups
Industry	?	Head of manu- facturing plant Medical dept.	Head of manu- facturing plant Medical dept.	Head of manu- facturing plant Engineering department	Safety and fire prevention	-	+ -
Insurance	?	Technical departments	I.N.A.I.L.	-	F.M.P.	-	-
Research units	-	+ - (recognised)	-	+ (not recognised)	+ (recognised)	-	-
Laboratories	-	Landes Inst.	-	-	+ (recognised)	-	-

We wish to express our gratitude to the authorities in the countries consulted for kindly answering our questions.

Appendix 1

ADVANTAGES AND DISADVANTAGES OF INDICATOR TUBES

ADVANTAGES
- rapid estimate
- permit large number of rapid measurements
- low cost (important for small firms)
- very easy to handle (often used at the workplace)

DISADVANTAGES
- adequate calibration often lacking
- estimates not very specific
- instant assessments, not spread over a period of time

Appendix 2

ADVANTAGES AND DISADVANTAGES OF DIRECT AND CONTINUOUS READING INSTRUMENTS

ADVANTAGES
- rapid and continuous estimates which can cover 24 hours per day (concentration peaks)
- possible to incorporate an alarm system
- no need for handling or laboratory analysis
- possible to keep documents as evidence
- reduce sampling costs

DISADVANTAGES
- expensive (suitable for large firms)
- assessment generally not very specific
- fixed equipment
- require frequent calibration

MULTIDISCIPLINARY APPROACH TO PREVENTION AND HEALTH
PROTECTION BY MONITORING: ROLE OF INDIVIDUAL DISCIPLINES.
THE NURSE: ROLE IN THE HEALTH TEAM I

D.M. RADWANSKI (UK)

Summary

*In addition to European Directives concerning qualifications
of nurses and their activities, there are statutory provisions in a number of Community countries concerning employment of nurses in workplaces. Although there are no statutory provisions in the United Kingdom concerning their
employment in workplaces, the training and qualification
governed by the Royal College of Nursing are increasingly
required by employers. The activities of the nurse at the
workplace may be wide-ranging and they change according to
the number of the specialists employed at the workplace.
This paper examines those activities and relates them to
those of other specialists.*

Introduction

The Directives relating to nursing were agreed by the Council
of Ministers of the European countries in 1977. They provide
for mutual recognition of the formal qualifications of nurses
responsible for general care, and the coordination of legal
and administrative provisions in respect of the activities of
general nurses. It seems likely that a considerable time may
elapse before specialist directives for Occupational Health
Nursing could be signed.

In a number of countries in the European Community, nurses
are required by statute to be employed in some workplaces.
We do not know the exact number, or what they all do, but it
seems that they are mainly involved in first-aid treatment
under the guidance of a physician. There are no statutory
provisions for the employment of nurses in workplaces in the
United Kingdom, but around 10,000 are employed in this field.

Occupational Health Nursing training in the United Kingdom has been established since 1934. The Occupational Health Nursing Course lasts six and a half months full-time, or eighteen months on a day-release basis. The training and qualification (Occupational Health Nursing Certificate) are governed by the Royal College of Nursing, and are not statutory but are increasingly required by employers. Courses are available in a number of centres throughout the country, and are strongly supported by the Health and Safety Executive, the body concerned with the health and safety of workers in the United Kingdom. Occupational Health Nursing training on this scale is not available in any of the other countries in the European Community. Without specialist training the nurse is unlikely to be able to fulfil the role discussed in this paper.

Although the title of the paper implies that the nurse works in a team of other health professionals, she is more likely to work in the United Kingdom in circumstances where she has very little medical or other support.

The role of the nurse

The role of the nurse changes according to the number of the other specialists employed in the workplace. Where the nurse is the only health care practitioner, she is likely to undertake a wider variety of duties from the one who works in a team composed of a number of specialists, such as physicians and hygienists. Every nurse in Occupational Health practice requires further training, but there is a special need for the nurse who is the only health care practitioner in the workplace to have this training. She is not a doctor, a hygienist or a safety officer or a substitute for any of these but a range of duties and procedures unlike those in general nursing must be undertaken if the nurse is to make a full contribution in the workplace. Without specialist training the nurse will simply try to use her hospital experience in the workplace, and will not even be able to assess when the advice of other specialists should be sought.

The aims of Occupational Health Nursing are the promotion of
health and the prevention of illness and injury occuring at
work, but in nearly all situations first-aid and treatment
are also undertaken by the nurse, within the limits of good
Occupational Health practice. It cannot be assumed that
every nurse is able to arrange, and carry out appropriate
first-aid in the workplace without further training which is
necessary if she is to be closely involved in the first-aid
provisions. The Occupational Health Nurse trains and
supervises first-aiders, so that when an accident occurs
there is no doubt that appropriate first-aid arrangements
have been made.

For ease of reading, the nurse is considered in this paper to
be female, but males are equally accepted in Occupational
Health Nursing.

Planning for disaster, in conjunction with the management and
other workers is also a part of the nurse's work.

Before the worker is employed, or when the worker changes
employment, the nurse may carry out a health interview or
examination. This is of little value unless she understands
the working environment and the requirements of all the jobs,
so that individuals can be placed in suitable work. Even
where a full-time occupational physician is employed, the
nurse is likely to carry out pre-placement health screening.
It is usual for the nurse to be able to advise management
that potential employees are fit, and to refer to a physician
in cases of doubt. This works simply where a physician is
employed, but where no occupational physician is available,
individuals can be referred back to their family physicians.
When the unsupported nurse in the United Kingdom requires
medical advice, pertaining to the workplace, she can apply to
the Employment Medical Advisory Service to be given
specialist medical advice.

As far as possible, each worker returning from absence attributed to illness or injury should be interviewed by the
nurse. This is not only to arrange job modifications or a
temporary shortening of working hours, but to observe changes
in known individuals, and provide the opportunity for advice
to be given.

A knowledge of current health and safety requirements affecting the workplace is essential. Known or potential hazards
may require biological monitoring of workers before they are
placed in a job, and at intervals throughout their working
life.

Routine screening procedures may be necessary, both at preplacement health examination and at regular intervals. Tests
involving the collection of urine and blood samples, measurement of respiratory function and audiometry are commonly
carried out by the nurse. These procedures can be carried
out by a technician, but when they are undertaken by a nurse
she takes the opportunity to discuss with workers the reasons
for biological monitoring, and to encourage them to participate in their own health care. She can recognise deviations
from normal and their importances relevant to the work situation. Arrangements are made for referral for further
specialist advice when necessary, or the removal of the
worker on a temporary basis.

The nurse visits the working areas regularly and frequently
to see all the workers not simply those who attend the health
department. She must begin by meeting foremen and supervisors and learning the details of the working process, and
what the jobs involve. It is easy also to check on such
matters as first-aid arrangements, barrier cream dispensers
and the hygience of canteens and toilets. On any walk
through the plant, the nurse will ntoice the general tidiness
and cleanliness of the plant, as well as obvious hazards to
health. With training she can carry out general environmental surveys, probably working to a check-list and instigate
investigations of possible health hazards.

It is recognised that investigation and advice related to the control of hazards new in any workplace should be carried out by specialist teams, of which the nurse may be a member. Where regular monitoring is required, the nurse can easily learn to use such hygiene tools as sound-level meters and gas detectors and interpret the results. The nurse who works as the sole health practitioner must be able to advise the management when further specialist help is needed. When faults are found during monitoring, reports must be made to the individual who can take remedial action. The value of the assessment made by the nurse is determined by her competence, but also by the recognition of other health and safety practitioners as well as the management, that the nurse must make a useful contribution.

Where safety officers and others concerned with safety are employed, the nurse coordinates her activities with theirs. Where the actual monitoring is the responsibility of others, the nurse is able to complete the picture from other parts of her work. She will use the records to help in health surveillance. The record of all attendances at the Health Department, and the reasons for attendance, together with individual records provide other tools for health supervision.

The nurse assists in the education and training of workers in hazardous occupations, supervisors, safety representatives and others, and has a responsibility to carry out health education related to the workplace. The well-informed nurse does much to allay anxiety, and encourage workers to use all the protective means available, not least by her own example.

The organisation and management of the health department is usually in the hands of the nurse, and where she is involved in planning she will make provision for the needs of the workforce including biological monitoring requirements. The nurse's role is not that of a Health Department attendant, who waits for clients to come to her. She makes her contribution through her knowledge of the workers, whom she must see at frequent intervals in their actual work situation.

Perhaps more than any other health care practitioner, the Occupational Health Nurse has the opportunity to observe a population closely over a period which may last for many years. If the care given by the nurse at work is well respected she can have considerable influence on the health and safety of the workers. She cultivates good relationships so that, exercising discretion and competence, she can contribute to the general wellbeing of the workforce.

Conclusions

The whole nursing process is concerned with assessment, planning, carrying out and evaluating care, and technical expertise is required of nurses in most situations nowadays. Some kind of Occupational Health Nursing has been going on for more than a hundred years. The Occupational Health Nurse of today has to be able to use all the tools available to her, to help the worker to maintain his health, and where necessary to interpret his needs to the management, offer excellent first-aid advice and support when necessary, and decide the priority order.

We have lately set up in the United Kingdom, a project to entrust the whole Occupational Health care of a group of small factories to an Occupational Health Nurse. We await with interest the experience we shall gain from this and intend to evaluate it after two years. We should be glad to share this experience with you.

References

1. Current Approaches to Occupational Medicine - Editor A. Ward-Gardner. Publisher J. Wright & Sons Ltd. 1979.

2. Nursing in the European Community - Editor Sheila Quinn CBE. Publishers Croome Helm. 1980.

3. Occupational Health Service - The Way Ahead - Health and Safety Commission. HMSO 1977.

4. Occupatinal Health Nursing - Editor Brenda Slaney. Publisher Croome Helm. 1980.

5. The Nurse's Contribution to the Health of the Worker. First Report of the Nursing Sub-Committee 1966-1969. Published by the Permanent Commission and International Association on Occupational Health. 1969.

6. Education of the Nurse. Second Report of the Nursing Sub-Committee 1971-1973. Published by the Permanent Commission International Association on Occupational Health 1973.

7. Occupational Health in Europe - 6 Comparisons by Ruth Alston from Occupational Health - Volume 27 No. 6. June 1975.

MULTIDISCIPLINARY APPROACH TO PREVENTION AND HEALTH
PROTECTION BY MONITORING: ROLE OF INDIVIDUAL DISCIPLINES.
THE NURSE: ROLE IN THE HEALTH TEAM II.

M.E. RAHJES (USA)

Summary

Development of comprehensive ambient and biological monitoring for worker populations is dependent on manpower, technology, administration, and support.

Occupational health nurses are potential manpower sources if they have the appropriate basic education and additional knowledge and skills to expand their roles into this area of prevention. The role of the nurse as part of the health team is dependent on team resources available in the industry or through consulation.

Many conferences, seminars, and symposiums are built around special topics in health care and sooner or later a panel of health professionals is called upon to relate what each specific discipline is doing in that area. Since many of the participants already have some idea of what is going on in the field, there are very few surprises in the presentations. Careful attention is given to avoiding any blatant infringements on territory or interpretations of what other disciplines should be doing. Consideration is usually given to the importance of the interdisciplinary or team approach. There seem to be no reasons for deviating from the pattern in this paper; there are no earth-shaking revelations to present, but perhaps there will be some insight into the present status of the role of the nurse in the health team, what factors are affecting the role, and an interpretation of what should and could be possible to achieve.

First of all may I present a definition of ambient and biological monitoring - the checking, testing, and observing of living beings, their life processes, and their surroundings.

For the occupational health team, the process involves worker populations. For monitoring processes the environment affecting the worker includes not only the industrial setting but also his home, community, and world as well. Practically speaking, we cannot possibly monitor this total environment, but we must constantly be aware of it.

For health professionals trained in treatment and who have practiced only in medical care settings, the environment has received only cursory attention. Many health professionals in occupational health have had a tendency to view workers as "vertical patients" in need of our services only when they are injured or sick. We need to realise that latent "horizontal patients" may be lurking in the wings.

Some progress has been made in recognising the influences of family, society, and culture on the health of people. This progress has been enhanced by a more recent realisation of the effects of emotional stress on health.

Occupational and public health practitioners are generally ahead of other medical specialisms in recognising the influence of the environment on the health of populations. Occupational and public health specialists realise that true primary prevention of disease is embodied in controlling the exposure of populations to hazards in the environment including the workplace. Until we reach the goal of safe and healthy working conditions for men and women, we must continue to monitor the worker for signs of impending or actual occupational disease.

The identification, monitoring, and control of health and safety hazards in the work environment constitutes primary prevention. Biological monitoring is a facet of secondary prevention and both are very important aspects of comprehensive programmes in disease and injury prevention in worker populations.

In order to conduct a comprehensive programme in ambient and biological monitoring for all working populations, we need the manpower, the technology, the administrative structure for the coordination of service delivery, and support for the effort from the public and private sectors.

In the United States, we are attempting to increase the manpower available through the development of occupational health and safety education resources. This effort is to provide for the training of new occupational health professionals and increasing the continuing education available to the health professionals already working in the field. Occupational health nurses are the largest group of health professionals in industry and with adequate education and training could help solve some of the immediate manpower problems.

I have been associated with occupational health and occupational health nursing since 1964 in various capacities: staff nurse in a multi-nurse health service; staff nurse in a one-nurse service; state health department industrial hygienist; student in masters' and doctoral-level programmes in public and occupational health; and faculty in a graduate occupational health nursing programme. With that background, I am sure that I would not be expected to say there is no place for nurses in ambient and biological monitoring. I hope that no one would expect me to say that all occupational health nurses should be engaged in all aspects of ambient and biological monitoring. What is left is the obvious. Some occupational health nurses should be performing some of the functions in ambient and biological monitoring.

Many occupational health nurses are the only full-time members of the health team in the plant. In small plants physician, industrial hygiene, and other specialty services are often limited to periodical visits from corporate level team members or consultation from outside sources. I will

speak to monitoring activities the nurse, if properly
educated, could perform based on having limited contact with
other team members. These activities can be modified and
integrated into team functions as the situation dictates.

Biological monitoring may be conducted to determine the
effects of known health hazard exposures on the health of
the worker, determine if engineering and administrative controls are effective, find hyper-susceptible workers who are
affected by lesser exposures, and find unexpected effects
on health due to synergistic or unexpected hazardous conditions. It is in the area of biological monitoring that the
occupational health nurse has assumed more responsibility.
The area of ambient monitoring is less well understood.

Appropriately trained nurses should be able to develop and
manage biological surveillance programmes; to perform health
and occupational histories and physical assessments including special examinations; and to relate untoward findings
to environmental factors. Nurses and nurse practitioners
trained in physical assessment, who do not have knowledge of
environmental health hazards and their related toxicology,
are not prepared to assist in comprehensive surveillance
programmes.

The expansion of their role into physical assessment has
been the most popular area for many occupational health
nurses. Physical assessment is an important part of the
occupational health nursing role, but it must not become the
major or only aspect. To continue to work only with individual employees can keep nurses locked in screening or secondary prevention.

Ambient monitoring is a team process and should involve the
worker and the supervisor; purchasing, engineering, maintenance, and production departments; and occupational safety
and health personnel. In the absence of in-plant industrial
hygiene and safety personnel the nurse could, if properly
trained and equipped, do surveys and limited monitoring.

Some activities of the nurse in ambient monitoring could
include:

initial plant survey done to locate health
and safety hazards and recommend further
evaluation by industrial hygiene and safety
specialists.

periodic inspection of known hazardous areas
and processes; inspection for correct functioning of environmental controls and consistent, safe operating procedures; proper
use and storage of materials; proper maintenance and housekeeping; employees adequately
trained in the use of production equipment
and personal protective equipment; number of
employees in the area and potential for
exposure; any changes in manufacturing
process or products; limited environmental
sampling including air sampling, noise
levels, checking ventilation systems, etc;

investigation of accidents or incidents and
documentation of findings for identification
of patterns and potential problems.

Ambient monitoring by the nurse must not be accomplished to
the exclusion of other nursing functions. The more comprehensive the nursing function, the greater the value to the
health of the worker.

In most of the accepted definitions of occupational health
nursing, there is reference to the worker, the work environment, and the relationship between both. Agreement on what
functions the nurse should perform in this role is difficult
to achieve even among occupational health nurses. The role
is quickly and constantly changing making new and increasingly complex demands on our practice. This has enabled

many who are willing to acquire additional knowledge and skills to move into new and exciting areas of practice.

Conversely, many nurses who are unable or unwilling to meet these new demands are frustrated and often become defensive regarding the changes.

There are many factors affecting the state-of-the-art and practice of occupational health nursing. The most important factor is educational preparation.

In the United States, there are several levels of basic nursing education. This causes fragmentation in the nursing profession and creates confusion among other health profes-sionals. It is extremely difficult for employers of occupa-tional health nurses to understand the different criteria for each level and what to expect from their nurse employees.

In the United States, any person who completes an accredited associate degree nursing programme (2 years average length), baccalaureate degree nursing programme (4 to 5 years average) or hospital-based diploma nursing programme (3 years average length) is eligible to take a state examina-tion to become a "registered nurse".

The basic education in the associate degree and diploma programmes is usually weak in science, public health, and mental health courses so important in occupational and public health practice. Very few of the basic nursing education programmes include any courses in the occupational health speciality, but most baccalaureate programmes require courses in public health and mental health.

A 1972 survey of registered occupational health nurses in the United States indicated that for 91 percent the highest educational credential obtained was the nursing diploma. Two per cent reported an associate degree and 7 per cent reported attaining a baccalaureate or higher degree. Five percent of

all nurses working in occupational health were licensed practical nurses with less than two years of education. Over 46
percent of the occupational health nurses were age 50 or
older and only 7 percent were under 30 years of age. The remaining 47 percent were between 30 and 50 years of age (1).

A 1964 survey of occupational health nurses noted that over
one-half had completed their basic nursing education before
1940 and 88 percent before 1950 (2).

What we have in the United States is a cadre of occupational
health nurses who are at least 30 years away from their
basic nursing education in hospital-based diploma schools.
Many of these nurses have upgraded their basic education
through continuing education courses and by completing
baccalaureate degree programmes. Some have done additional
study and coursework and have passed the test for certification in Occupational Health Nursing developed and given by
the American Board for Occupational Health Nurses.

There is a clear and pressing need to provide practising
occupational health nurses with opportunities to upgrade
and enhance their basic education at the baccalaureate level
and through appropriate continuing education courses.

An important contribution that practising occupational
health nurses can make to strengthen the future practice of
occupational health nursing is to lend their support to the
requirement of the baccalaureate degree in nursing for entry
into nursing practice.

In the past and now, there have been courses and master's
degree programmes in occupational health offered by schools
of public health. More recently, courses and master's
degree programmes in occupational health nursing are being
developed in graduate schools of nursing. Graduate programmes are hindered by:

- lack of qualified faculty with education and experience in occupational health nursing, and

- lack of occupational health nurses with baccalaureate degrees eligible to enter these programmes.

With the appropriate education, proper equipment, support and cooperation of management, and cooperation of the workers, occupational health nurses interested in expanding their role to include ambient and biological monitoring can do so.

In the United States, the nurse most adequately prepared for this expanded role would be the graduate of a master's programme in occupational health nursing whose programme included courses or entrance requirements in occupational health, industrial hygiene, toxicology, physiology, epidemiology (with special emphasis on worker populations), public health statistics, safety, physical assessment, research, clinical practice in industry, and public health administration.

This nurse should be expected to:

- survey and monitor the environment including basic air sampling and noise measurement;

- recognise potential health hazards and understand behavioural, physiological, and clinical symptoms associated with each hazard;

- understand threshold limit values, health and safety standards and regulations, occupational and public health laws, and related legislation;

- using the epidemiological method, identify
  high-risk individuals and populations;

- collect prevalence and incidence data for
  occupational diseases and injuries, demographic data, and data regarding environmental factors;

- plan and develop health surveillance and
  employee education programmes for special
  and high-risk individuals and groups;

- conduct biological monitoring including
  taking blood, urine, and tissue samples;
  vision and hearing testing; pulmonary
  function testing; and

- complete detailed health and occupational
  histories, perform physical assessments,
  interpret laboratory values, and appropriately refer any deviation from normal or
  suspicious findings.

This nurse should understand the importance of cooperation
and coordination of all health and safety related functions
and personnel. This nurse should be able to interpret
effectively the nurse's role to the health team and to
management.

Another factor affecting the function of the nurse is the
attitude of the peer group toward a particular or potential
function. These attitudes may be an endorsement or rejec-
tion of the behaviour by nursing leaders and educators as
reported in the literature. A review of the literature
indicates support for expanding the role of the occupational
health nurse into a worker and prevention centered practice
including biological monitoring. This concept is supported
by a great number of occupational health nursing leaders and
educators (3-7).

There is also support for the expansion of the nursing role in the work environment including hazards monitoring, industrial hygiene, and safety (8-15).

Also found in the literature is support for this expanded role by many management personnel in industry (16-18).

It is difficult to analyse the attitude of practising nurses without extensive surveys of attitudes and behaviours to determine perspectives and directions. These attitudes can be changed or strengthened by the influence of successful role models who have expanded their role into the desired function.

Technology is another major factor affecting the function of occupational health nursing. The scientific basis for predicting health consequences and the technology for control of health hazards has not kept pace with the overwhelming technological advances in industrial production and processes. However, the technologies needed for ambient and biological monitoring are becoming more advanced and there is growing emphasis on scientific measurement. Occupational health nurses should be constantly expanding their knowledge of the monitoring and control of hazards in their particular industry. They must also be aware of the advances in the technology for medical diagnosis and treatment.

An increase in technology in health care usually results in a decrease in direct personal service. In the future more time will be spent in monitoring and less in personal services including counselling, care and management of non-occupational illness and routine examinations for employees who are not considered to be in high-risk categories. Nurses will have to work diligently to offset the depersonalisation that can accompany increasing technology.

With the increase in technology we can expect increased specialisation including industrial hygiene, behavioural

science, genetics, occupational epidemiology, and specialists in specific diseases. We can then expect the continuing technological explosion to provide for the creation
of the "super specialist". It would not be surprising to
see specialisation in pleural and even connective tissue
disease.

Increased technology along with the accompanying specialisation is very expensive. Large population bases are needed
to support specialists. In the past, this dilemma has often
been solved by the regionalisation of technical and
speciality services and personnel. In order to tie into
these services, industry will have to look outside their
organisations. The occupational health nurse may continue
to be the major in-plant health professional having direct
and continuous contact with the employee and his work
environment.

The occupational health nurse and the other members of the
health team are an important source for the manpower needed
to develop comprehensive programmes in ambient and biological monitoring. All members of the team must work
together to increase their monitoring capabilities and to
develop worker and prevention-centered practices.

The technology for monitoring is improving but must be
constantly changing and expanding to meet the growing and
urgent need.

The organisational or administrative framework necessary for
conducting scientific measurements in the workplace is
inadequate in both government and private industry sectors
and is essentially non-existent in small industries.

The continued development of manpower, technology, and
administration for ambient and biological monitoring and
control technology is totally dependent on the support of
the private and public sector.

Support for this effort by industry is usually related to
enforcement of standards and regulations although some
enlightened managements are convinced of the potential for
maximization of production and profit through cost-effective
control of occupational injury and disease. The interest of
management in occupational health and safety is directly
affected by economic conditions. In the past, some of the
greatest advances in occupational health and safety have
occurred when there is a shortage of workers thereby creating a need to keep them well and functioning during periods
of increased production such as war. It is unfortunate that
the value of the worker is based on an inverse relationship
with the unemployment rate.

The performance and success of ambient and biological monitoring is totally dependent on the support of legislative
bodies. This support can be directly measured by the amount
of monies appropriated and the enactment and enforcement of
laws and regulations for occupational health and safety.

We must work in concert on all levels to bring together all
of the resources needed to protect our greatest resource -
the worker.

References

1. U.S. Department of Health, Education and Welfare,
    Division of Nursing. Surveys of public health nursing
    1968-1972. Bethesda, Md.: Department of Health,
    Education and Welfare, pp 75. (DHEW publication no.
    [HRA] 76-8).

2. U.S. Department of Health, Education and Welfare.
    Occupational health nurses: an initial survey.
    Washington, D.C.: Department of Health, Education and
    Welfare 1966. (PHS publication no. 1470).

3. Brown, M.L. Trends for the future of occupational
    health nursing. Occup. Health Nurs. 1973:21(8):7-11.

4. Ford, L.C. Opportunities and obstacles in occupational
    health nursing. Occup. Health Nurs. 1973:21(7):9-14.

5.   Tinkham, C.W.   Occcupational health nursing in the
     1980s.   Occup. Health Nurs. 1977:25(6):7-13.

6.   French, M.   The nurse's role in prevention and
     treatment.   Occup. Health Nurs. 1973:21(2):15-17.

7.   D'Ardenne, D.   The role of the occupational health
     nurse in industry.   Community Health 1973:6(6):326-
     329.

8.   Hayman, M.J.   The occupational health nurse in the work
     environment.   Can. J. Public Health 1976:67(supp 2):33-
     34.

9.   Onyett, H.P.   The nurse - valuable new resource in
     hazards monitoring.   Occup. Health and Safety 1976:
     46(6):18-22.

10. Raniere, T.M.   Chemical hazard indentification - our
     need to work together. Occup. Health Nurs. 1978:26(9):
     19-21.

11. Bodnar, E.M.   Management of toxic agents in the work-
     place: the role of the occupational health nurse.
     Occup. Health Nurs. 1979:27(3):7.12.

12. Kornbacher, G. The nurse's role in toxicology. Occup.
     Health Nurs. 1976:24(8):24-26.

13. Craley, E.W. New trends in occupational health nursing
     as they relate to industrial hygiene. Amer. Industrial
     Hygiene Assoc. J. 1977:38:230-232.

14. Burkeen, O.E.   The nurse and industrial hygiene.
     Occup. Health Nurs. 1976:24(4):7-10.

15. Simons, R.S.   The occupational health nurse: safety's
     over-looked resource. Occup. Health Nurs. 1980:28(5):
     7-12.

16. Stiens, W.L.   The expanded roles of the occupational
     health nurse. Occup. Health Nurs. 1975:23(4):18-21.

17. Krikorian, M. The occupational health nurse's emerging
     role in administering the plant employee protection
     program. Occup. Health Nurs. 1978:26(8):20-21.

18. Reznikoff, P.A.   Safety, management and nursing.
     Occup. Health Nurs. 1974:22(6):26-28.

MULTIDISCIPLINARY APPROACH TO PREVENTION AND HEALTH
PROTECTION BY MONITORING: ROLE OF INDIVIDUAL DISCIPLINES.
THE PHYSICIAN: ASSESSMENT OF WORKERS' EXPOSURE - ETHICS AND
RELIABILITY OF BIOLOGICAL MONITORING I

N.J. ROBERTS (USA)

Summary

*Viewed as periodic assessments to determine whether or not
workers have evidence of exposure to potential physical or
chemical hazards in their work environment, and even to
measure that exposure, biological monitoring is a valuable,
and in some circumstances necessary, tool for the physician
charged with protecting the health of workers.*

*Carried further, biological monitoring should include the
effort to detect adverse health effects which arise out of
the work environment, both by the direct search for such
effects and by providing a basis for epidemiological studies
to detect correlations between work exposures and subsequent
disease or disability experience.*

*The problems, complexities, and ethical considerations in
trying to accomplish such biological monitoring are
discussed.*

Biological monitoring can be thought of in narrow or broad
terms. To some, it refers only to the intermittent measurement of specific substances in the blood, urine, hair, nails
or expired air of workers to determine whether or not they
have been exposed, or even to quantitate their exposure, to
potential physical or chemical hazards in their work
environment. The potentially exposed workers thus serve as
a work environment sampling system to supplement other
measurements of that environment.

In this presentation, however, biological monitoring and
health surveillance are joined in a pragmatic way - just as
they usually are, and should be, in actual practice. Even
when we only measure a urinary metabolite of a toxin, we are
already looking at a health effect however harmless it may
be. Some portion of the worker's detoxification resources
has been utilised and to the extent that they are finite,
any spending of them can be thought of as a health effect.

In examining an individual worker in relation to a possible exposure to a hazard, we deal with a continuum starting with evidence of exposure, going to evidence of a health effect, and finally, though happily not often, to a significant or even fatal effect. As physicians, we must be sensitive to this whole continuum. We cannot look only for evidence of exposure to conform with an arbitary definition of biological monitoring. We must continue on to include the surveillance of the worker's health for evidence fo the effects of physical or chemical exposures related to work.

Thus biological monitoring should be redefined to include the surveillance of worker health for the detection of the effects of exposure to hazards. When workers are examined only for the purpose of helping to maintain or improve their health rather than because of possible exposure to hazards, or are examined to determine their fitness to work, or to measure disability, such examinations would not be classified as biological monitoring even though a semanticist might insist that the term remains appropriate. Interestingly, a worker motivated to discontinue cigarette smoking as a result of a health maintenance examination would obviously be doing something importantly related to the risks of some potential work hazards as well as diminishing risks not related to work.

For these reasons, our subject is here discussed broadly, and biological monitoring is assumed to encompass the initial thorough baseline examinations of employees, and then the intermittent thorough examinations performed to detect any evidence of exposure to work hazards, to measure such exposure, and to determine whether or not those examined have experienced any adverse effects of their work environment on their health. This expanded concept of biological monitoring would also include the collection of information about health and disabilities which might help us to recognise through epidemiological study any adverse health effects of their work exposures on them, on their spouses, or on their children.

It is the responsibility of the physician providing occupational medical service to recognise, alone or with assistance, the situations in which biological monitoring is indicated, to plan the type and frequency of such monitoring, to accomplish it or oversee its accomplishment, to have recorded and to interpret the findings, to communicate them to those examined, and to take, or to advise, and then monitor or have monitored, any actions that are indicated as a result of the findings.

There are situations in which laws or governmental regulations require the performance or offering of given examinations at prescribed intervals. In most areas, nothing precludes an employer from requiring employees to have periodic examinations for biological monitoring.

The proposal that employers should be enabled to require periodic health assessments of all employees potentially exposed to a chemical or physical hazard in relation to their work is a sound one. Undoubtedly, if any testing to be done poses significant risks or unacceptable discomforts, employees should be fully entitled to have adjudicated fairly and validly an unwillingness on their part to accept such portions of an examination.

The requirement of monitoring examinations is reasonable because they help assure the earlier recognition of adverse health effects resulting from work. Not only is it possible to detect or measure evidence of exposures, and to discover health effects, the potential for which we know, but good examinations also enable us to discover earlier, where they exist, other adverse effects of work exposures for which we would not be specifically searching upon the basis of our present knowledge.

It is self-evident that the findings from these examinations should not be used in an unscientific or improper way in relation to the welfare of those examined. Our counsel about an individual's fitness to continue specific work should not, for example, be based upon testing which has been done to expand our scientific capacities to protect worker health but the results of which we cannot yet interpret or apply with confidence.

To be realistic, however, we must consider some of the questions and complexities involved.

It is easy to say that physicians should "recognise the situations in which biological monitoring is indicated", but even this first step is an immense challenge. What can be accomplished is obviously limited by the extent of existing knowledge. The task requires that physicians be aware of the chemical and physical hazards to which employees might be potentially exposed, and it requires that they know or learn the possible evidence or effects of such exposure, and how best to detect them.

Our knowledge about potential work hazards is, and will remain, incomplete. Even in the case of such well-known and long-studied hazards as those posed by toxic lead compounds, controversy persists about the optimum testing to be done in biological monitoring, and about the interpretation of the results of such testing.

The need for biological monitoring varies from worker to worker, and varies greatly from work-site to work-site. For example, the employee with sickle cell anaemia is not able to tolerate a level of exposure to some lead compounds which might be acceptable for another employee. Even apparently healthy individuals with no known genetic defect may differ greatly in their sensitivity to certain insults. Successful control of the level of cotton dust in a textile mill will prevent byssinosis in almost all workers, but for a very few a level of dustiness low enough to prevent the disease is neither known nor presently achievable. A biological monitoring programme can, by enquiry about chest tightness and measuring pulmonary function, help assure the identification of these few workers before permanent harm is done to them.

Although biological monitoring is indicated however fine is the engineering control of potential exposure, or however certain is the use of good quality personal protection equipment, there is admittedly a greater need for this type of monitoring where we lack full confidence in the engineering controls, in the availability and use of satisfactory well-maintained personal protection equipment, or in the level of compliance with protective work practice arrangements.

Even when we have detected potential hazards in the workplace, it is often difficult to identify all of the workers who may be exposed to them, or may have been exposed to them. Furthermore, to compound our problems, few workers indeed are potentially exposed to one hazard, and one hazard only.

Beyond these difficulties, we know that many findings which could be adverse effects of work exposures can also be caused by something having no relationship to work. Additionally, a finding at the time of a monitoring examination may be demonstrated subsequently to have been a false positive finding, though sometimes only after further study which may have been anxiety-provoking, time-demanding, and resource-consuming in all senses.

We take it as a given, of course, that biological monitoring examinations should never be the primary or keystone means of protecting the health of workers. We know, however, that the best of environmental controls, or other exposure controls, are fallible, and that the human beings designing them, constructing them, using them, or being protected by them, are also fallible. Realising this, the proposal that potentially exposed employees have periodic health assessments appropriate to their potential exposures, and thorough enough to allow the detection of <u>any</u> adverse effects related to workplace exposures, is a most reasonable and responsible one.

While the use of the employee as his or her own exposure sampling device may seem objectionable to some, in certain situations biological exposure monitoring is better than other methods of exposure measurement, or may even provide the only really useful information about exposure. For example, individuals at risk of episodic contact with dimethyl formamide (DMF) in the chemical plant may receive the major portion of an exposure through the skin. Obviously in such cases measurement of the air concentration of DMF in the working area or even the breathing zone will tell only part of the story. In another example, a worker's blood carboxyhaemoglobin level is a more accurate measure of possible hazardous exposure than are ambient levels of carbon monoxide.

Deserving emphasis also is the observation that the detection of early changes resulting from workplace exposure can be a most effective means of impressing both an employer and the employees with the importance of a situation needing attention. The worker who needs but does not use ear protection may have second thoughts when confronted with the evidence of a measured loss of his or her own hearing.

In prospective terms, we naturally wish that we would never in the future have to learn about the ill effects of work exposures by discovering those effects at the time of biological monitoring. It would obviously be vastly preferable could they be known as potential hazards on the basis of study accomplished before they had to be experienced by human beings. In fact, however, there is no feasible way that we can fully achieve this goal. We must make a responsible effort to try to do so, but in view of our finite scientific resources, the limitations of our methodologies and our capacities to extrapolate their results to humans,

and the time required for the acquisition of knowledge, we
will continue to need biological monitoring.

For the ultimate welfare of workers everywhere, intermittent
health assessments of those potentially exposed to hazards
should be thorough, and thoroughly recorded. Data on potential exposures, or actual exposures, should also be well
recorded, as should all disabilities and the ultimate cause
of death. The possible relationship of any disability and
of the cause of death to work exposures should be considered
but this should be done with care, accuracy, and thorough
study and deliberation to allow the making of valid conclusions. As has already been said above, we know well that
innumerable disabilities which might be work-related are
also experienced by individuals who have had no work exposures that could cause them.

At the time of an examination performed for the purpose of
biological monitoring, we may encounter a) nothing abnormal,
or b) effects indicative of exposure but not necessarily of
harm, or we may find c) effects which we would have to
consider as harmful, sometimes reversible, at other times
not so, and lastly we may occasionally discover d) something
that we know will progress distressingly regardless of any
action taken.

In each of these cases, what we counsel and what is done has
to be custom-designed to the findings and to the situation.
In some cases temporary, in other cases permanent, avoidance
of further potential exposures to the harmful agent or
agents is indicated by the nature of the findings.

In all cases where there is evidence suggesting or demonstrating exposure to, or adverse effects from, environmental
hazards in the workplace, the environmental control programme that should have precluded such exposures must be
reviewed, reassessed, and improved where necessary. The
individual experiencing the evidence of exposure or ill

effects must be told clearly and fully about the findings, and advised appropriately. The employer must be notified of any need for attention to the engineering controls, to the adequacy and use of personal protective equipment, or to compliance with any work practice requirements that are in effect.

The identity of a worker having evidence only of undesirable exposure, and not of harm, should not be revealed to the employer. If, however, that worker alone, and not other workers, presents on repeated examinations comparable evidence of exposure, and cannot or does not successfully control or eliminate the exposure by the use of normal methods, professional judgement about the risk involved would be required to determine the proper course of action.

Where the findings in an individual worker justify temporary or permanent protection from specific potential exposures, the worker's identity must, of course, be revealed.

Some individuals propose that employees developing occupational disabilities should be free to keep this information from their employers if they wish to do so. It is hard to imagine logical, moral or legal justification for such a position. Employees wanting to continue in work which is known to be having an important adverse impact on their health should for their own sake be protected against what in at least some cases can only be viewed as the election of slow suicide. The employer who would be held liable for the preventable disability which an employee might elect to accept by continuing in work that is adversely effecting him or her could be expected to feel that this would be unjust if all feasible efforts have been made to prevent work hazards. Society, too, will feel some sense of injustice if it has passed on to it, as would inevitably happen, the costs of disability which could have been avoided.

In studying the possible work-relatedness of a health effect
or disability, the physician must, as stated above, be fully
aware of possible hazardous exposures. This is not easily
accomplished for a number of reasons. An accurate history
of past exposures is seldom attainable, though this does not
excuse a failure to make the best effort practical to obtain
it. Difficulties may be encountered in attempting to learn
the composition of substances to which a worker may have
been exposed, especially if these have been trade-named
products. Quantitation of exposures, which may be quite
critical to a decision, is often impossible. Knowledge of
the existence of comparable findings or disability in co-
workers of the employee is important, but sometimes difficult to elicit. An employee's nutritional habits or state,
avocation or second job, smoking history and habits, past
and present history of the use of alcoholic beverages or
other drugs, genetic endowment and resistance may one or all
be related to positive findings.

With respect to the reliability of biological monitoring,
the problems involved are well known. We must take all
steps available to us to try to avoid or overcome them.
However, even with the best equipment, frequently calibrated, and the most competent technicians, it can remain a
challenge, for example, to accomplish consistently good
spirometry, or audiometry. The margins of error in chemical
laboratory testing, and in haematologic studies, are familiar to all of us. Sincere and competent physicians differ
in the interpretation of the same findings even where there
are no doubts about their accuracy. The need for improving
our capacity to detect accurately, and at an earlier stage,
the potential ill effects of some work hazards is self-
evident. The ever-present conflict between sensitivity and
specificity plagues us when we want to be sure that we do
not miss anything significant but at the same time want to
avoid undesirable false positive results.

In spite of all the limitations referred to, it would seem that there is one clear and most responsible course for us to follow. To recapitulate, we should accomplish good biological monitoring of all employees potentially exposed to chemical or physical hazards in the workplace. We should have the findings of these examinations well-recorded, together with the best obtainable information about the past exposures of individual employees, and about pertinent health-related habits and activities.

We should at the same time be accomplishing the indicated monitoring of the workplace environment, and have the findings recorded in such a way as to study them in relation to the health of employees potentially exposed.

We should maintain disability records and cause-of-death records on all potentially exposed employees in such form as to allow their analysis for possible correlations with work exposures and work experience. We should share promptly with employees, employers, the scientific properly evaluated findings which constitute new knowledge relating to environmental hazards. And we should seek always to expand our knowledge and skills with respect to monitoring both the worker and the workplace, and our capacity to analyse the results and accomplish the actions indicated for the protection of the health of workers.

How feasible is this seemingly-idealistic proposal? In some situations and places it is not at all unrealistic, it is achievable. But if we face reality - our only option - overwhelming problems will long preclude its full accomplishment in even the most developed countries.

There are not many physicians in the entire world practising occupational medicine. Most physicians, already overworked caring for the ill, would neither be able nor inclined to do regular biological monitoring examinations of workers. Even were we to have sufficient properly-trained physicians able and anxious to do such work, the dedication and expenditure of the needed quantities of expensive resources in a "total effort" would probably prove socially unacceptable not only to those who now resent the proportion of all resources presently consumed in medical care, but to others as well. Even workers themselves would demur, for they too would ultimately share in paying the costs of these programmes. Because the productivity of biological monitoring would inevitably be called into question, we would have to measure that yield carefully, together with the costs of achieving it, and, where the monitoring is not done, the "costs" of not doing it.

We do not, however, require a physician to do good health assessments. His or her role need not extend beyond the planning of the programme, and then the analysis and communication, with the assistance of computers and other health professionals, of the findings. Nurses and technicians, or other types of assistants, could make the observations and measurements needed for high-quality biological monitoring. The most responsible course of action for us at this time is to stretch ourselves to do what can be done now, and to learn what must be done, and what can be safely left undone if society's resources are to be allocated optimally. We must design and implement imaginative pilot programmes using state-of-the-art knowledge and technology, perhaps even testing the value of positive incentives to employers who support such programmes. Whatever our course from here, however, our goal must remain the protection of those who work from being harmed by their work, and we must evaluate our performance in multiple ways, one of which is by searching for evidence of harm.

MULTIDISCIPLINARY APPROACH TO PREVENTION AND HEALTH
PROTECTION BY MONITORING: ROLE OF INDIVIDUAL DISCIPLINES.
THE PHYSICIAN: ASSESSMENT OF WORKERS' EXPOSURE - ETHICS AND
RELIABILITY OF BIOLOGICAL MONITORING II.

L. PARMEGGIANI (ILO)

Summary

This report covers the broad problem associated with the ethics and reliability of biological monitoring. This is seen mainly in the context of international labour standards and the problems likely to arise within the undertaking.

The legal status of biological monitoring

Reference is made to biological monitoring in Convention 136 on benzene adopted by the International Labour Conference in 1971, Recommendation 144 which supplements it, Convention 139 on occupational hazards caused by carcinogenic substances and agents (1974), Recommendation 147 which supplements it, Convention 148 on the working environment (air pollution, noise and vibration) (1977) and, in more detail, in Recommendation 156 which supplements it.

A general provision which appears in all these documents (e.g. Article 13 of Convention 136, Article 4 of Convention 139 and Article 13 of Convention 148) and which is also applicable to biological monitoring is the issuing of appropriate instructions to any worker exposed on the measures to safeguard health and prevent accidents.

The provisions of Recommendation 156 relevant to biological monitoring are as follows:
  - the supervision of the health of workers
    provided for in the Working Environment (Air
    Pollution, Noise and Vibration) (Convention
    1977) should include as determined by the
    competent authority biological or other tests
    or investigations after cessation of the
    assignment when medically indicated (Paragraph
    16.1);

- the competent authority should require that the results of any such examinations or tests be made available to the worker, and at his request to his personal physician (Paragraph 16.2);
- the supervision provided for in paragraph 16 of this Recommendation should normally be carried out in working hours and should be free of cost to the worker (Paragraph 17);
- the competent authority should develop a system of records of the medical information obtained in pursuance of Paragraph 16 of this Recommendation and should determine the manner in which it is to operate;
- provision should be made for the maintenance of such records for an appropriate period of time to assure their availability, in terms which will permit personal identification by the competent authority only, for epidemiological and other research (Paragraph 18.1);
- to the extent determined by the competent authority the records should include information on occupational exposure to air pollution in the working environment (Paragraph 18.2).

Recommendation 144 on benzene stipulates that medical examinations should be:
a) carried out under the responsibility of a qualified physician, approved by the competent authority, and with the assistance, as appropriate, of a competent laboratory
b) certified in an appropriate manner (Paragraph 17).

The recommendations are not ratifiable instruments; they nevertheless serve as a guide when the corresponding conventions are being implemented and national legislation drawn up. An important aspect of the recommendations referred to above is the idea of incorporating biological monitoring into any statutory preventive and routine medical examination of workers. Although biological monitoring cannot be regarded as an integral part of medical examinations, it does serve the same purpose-preventive medicine for persons exposed to risk. It can therefore be compared to biomedical research as described in the World Health Organisation's Helsinki Declaration (revised in 1975):

> "The purpose of biomedical research involving human subjects must be to improve diagnostic, therapeutic and prophylactic procedures and the understanding of the aetiology and pathogenesis of diseases."

Biological monitoring therefore appears to be quite ethical under the conditions laid down by the competent authority.

Where there are not legal provisions or regulations, biological monitoring is governed by the following clauses from the Helsinki Declaration:

> "3.2 The nature, the purpose and the risk of clinical research must be explained to the subject by the doctor.
> 3.3 (a) Clinical research on a human being cannot be undertaken without his free consent after he has been informed...
> 3.4 (a) The investigator must respect the right of each individual to safeguard his personal integrity, especially if the subject is in a dependent relationship to the investigator.
> (b) At any time during the course of clinical research the subject...should be free to withdraw permission for research to be continued."

In view of the ILO's recommendations for instructions for workers exposed to air pollution, provision should be made for those instructions to be given and for the workers' representatives in the undertaking to be consulted before a programme of biological monitoring is launched.

On the question of how to implement a programme of this sort, the ILO's practical guidelines on occupational exposure to airborne substances (4,3,5) recommend that wherever possible the examination methods used should not affect the physical wellbeing of the worker and should not themselves represent a risk. Priority will therefore have to be given to levels in urine and in expired air where these are as representative as blood levels.

Problems likely to arise within the undertaking

In practice, there may be a number of problems associated with biological monitoring in the undertaking and in this case the occupational physician should follow a line of conduct for which provision has already been made.

When a schedule for biological monitoring is worked out the following should be taken into account:

- biological monitoring can only serve as an adjunct to environmental monitoring whether this is already being done or has got to be instituted;
- taking biological samples means removing the worker from his workplace which represents a loss of production time the extent of which depends on local organisational factors - indeed sometimes all samples have to be taken at the same time which involves a break in the continuity of work;
- in some countries only doctors may take blood samples;
- if large numbers of workers are exposed, far more of biological analyses may be required than environmental analyses;

- biological analyses, particularly of blood,
  are usually more complicated and more delicate
  and therefore more expensive than air analyses;
- the study of controls may involve a considerable increase in the number of investigations
  and therefore in the cost.

With these points in mind, the occupational physician will be
able to assess whether the resources allocated to biological
monitoring would be better spent elsewhere - on preventive
measures with more immediate effects, for example.

To be efficient, biological monitoring depends not only on
the consent of the workers but also on their active cooperation. This cooperation is extremely important because the
sampling conditions have to be strictly observed. Workers
are sometimes against biological measures because of the physical discomfort it involves, because they feel like guinea
pigs and, still more important because they are afraid of the
results.

It is therefore essential to instruct the workers and their
representatives properly before instituting the system and to
agree on what is to be done about the results. Workers must
also be assured that the monitoring will be carried out under
the responsibility of a physician.

The management of the undertaking will not generally object
to environmental monitoring which is technical, collective
and covers an area (occupational exposure) which is entirely
under the control of the employer. They may be less in
favour of biological monitoring which involves loss of
production time and requires individual interpretation of
each case by physicians. The individual nature of biological
monitoring is more suited to a hospital than to an undertaking; however, as long as managerial staff are properly
informed in advance these problems should have been solved

before   monitoring starts.   It is essential for the employer
to   recognise   that biological monitoring is only part of the
overall   safety and health programme and must be followed up
by   every   technical   preventive   measure   which   proves
necessary.

Data management

Including   biological   monitoring   in   pre-employment and
routine   medical   examinations   of workers exposed to occupational hazards is important from the point of view of medical
ethics beccause it involves confidentiality.   One of the main
reasons   for   any   doubts workers   may   have about biological
monitoring   is   their   fear that the   results of the examinations will be passed on to the employer.   An abnormal result
may   simply   mean that the worker is using the wrong methods,
that his personal hygiene is not adequate, that he is sicken-
ing for a disease or that he is moonlighting, etc.   The occupational   physician   can,   with discretion, inform the health
and   safety committee or, where there is none, the management
of   the   undertaking   about   the   results   for the group as a
whole.   He must take these results into account in any advice
on health at the workplace which he is called upon to give in
his   capacity   as adviser to the employer and workers. Nevertheless, before giving details of a result which suggests bad
working   conditions or an increased risk, he must investigate
the   case   thoroughly,   find   the reasons for the anomaly and
discuss   it   with   the   worker   so that the latter can either
agree to the involvement of the management of the undertaking
or   be   informed when national legislation makes it necessary
to   notify   the   employer   of   the   worker's   unfitness.   The
physician   should   treat   the   results in the same way as the
abnormal   results   of   any   medical   examination   taking into
account   the fact that the results of biological examinations
provide   indications of a disorder much earlier than those of
clinical investigations.

It is important for the results of each examination to be given to the worker, even when the results are normal, and for the occupational physician to be ready to pass the information on to the worker's own doctor, if the worker so wishes; the relationship between the occupational physician and the worker's own GP will normally be defined in each country on the basis of local medical ethics.

Finally, the occupational physician should see biological monitoring not only as a way of protecting the health of the worker who is exposed now, but also as a way of ensuring better protection for the worker who will be exposed to occupational risks in the future. To achieve this objective, he must be in a position either to draw up biological monitoring and environmental monitoring data himself or to hand them over to the scientific authorities. In doing this, he must nevertheless respect medical confidentiality as described in the ILO's Recommendations 156.

The role of the competent authority

The international labour standards mentioned above clearly define the minimum the competent authority must do in this field.

The increasingly widespread use of workplace monitoring and biological monitoring has, in the more developed countries, led to the establishment of laboratories available to undertakings who do not have their own facilities for investigation and analysis. Some of these laboratories belong to universities and research institutes and others to the competent authority (labour, Public Health); some have been set up by employers' associations and others are private money-making concerns. Because of the importance of their activities in the field of health surveillance, the public authorities should quite clearly give the subject all the necessary attention.

The methods the authority uses to this end vary according to national convention. In Belgium the administrative practice is to have authorised laboratories; in France the laboratories are authorised to carry out specific analyses such as the measurement of asbestos fibres or certain industrial poisons; in Denmark laboratories recognised by the competent authority are recommended by it to the undertakings. A special system has been adopted in France whereby the INRS has statutory recognition as the national reference institute for the choice and standardisation of methods to be applied by laboratories working for undertakings. In other countries official laboratories may carry out spot checks on private laboratories; laboratories belonging to public institutions may be asked by workers' representatives to carry out analyses and, where necessary, biological workplace measurements.

To ensure that the results are reliable it is essential for:
- regular checks to be made at national level for comparison of the results of examinations of the same samples by different laboratories;
- standardised methods not only for analysis but also for sampling to be recommended at national level and then at international level because perfect analysis techniques are not much use if optimum sampling conditions are not achieved;
- technical standards and biological limit values to be set for each method used to obtain results;
- biological monitoring to be based, wherever possible, on a dose indicator and an effect indicator.

Programmes of comparison have not actually been very satisfactory for atmospheric monitoring at workplaces but biological tests and quality controls have been more successful.

Ultimately comparisons of this sort could be made at international level following the example of the Commission of the
European Communities.

Good monitoring depends on the cooperation of the workers,
the time the samples are taken, their freedom from contamination and strict adherence to the technical sampling
conditions.

It would be desirable for the competent authority to
encourage:
- the use of biological monitoring in conjunction with routine medical examinations wherever this is possible;
- the measurement of biological reference data
  at the medical examination preceding exposure
  to risk;
- systematic comparison of biological data with
  the atmospheric workplace concentrations.

I should like to thank Drs Denonne, Eustace, Notten, Rossi,
O'Callaghan, Svane, Wagner and Woodcock for their valuable
advice and the documents they provided for this report.

MULTIDISCIPLINARY APPROACH TO PREVENTION AND HEALTH
PROTECTION BY MONITORING: ROLE OF INDIVIDUAL DISCIPLINES.
THE EPIDEMIOLOGIST: VALUE OF MONITORING.

J.M. PETERS (USA)

Summary

Monitoring of exposure and monitoring of effects deserve equal attention. In the past most studies have not paid attention to both the careful assessment of exposure and the careful assessment of disease outcome. Rarely have the two been put together in a coordinated fashion. Until this is done routinely we shall continue to have fragmented information and results of limited use. The number of people interested in occupational health research is small enough that we cannot afford to make these same mistakes again. Epidemiologists must work with industrial hygienists. Industrial hygienists must work with epidemiologists. Toxicologists, medical directors, chemists, etc., must all put their best efforts into the determination of the relationship between exposures and effects in the occupational health setting.

Introduction

The epidemiologist interested in occupational disease has traditionally been interested primarily in health effects, either as morbidity or mortality. This relates to the fact that most epidemiologists have medical training by background. This preoccupation with health outcome or response has frequently led to a neglect for the exposure part of the dose-response equation. Attention to better ways of measuring outcome is commendable but not when exposure does not receive equal attention.

Those studies which provide the most useful information for occupational health purposes are those in which the same attention is paid to the dose or exposure as to the response or outcome element. Obviously, monitoring of the health is required on the one hand and monitoring of the exposure is required on the other. The principal thrust of this presentation is to emphasise that both deserve equal energy and effort if the resultant data are to have the most meaning with respect to understanding the disease and to controlling the occupational health problem. This point may be emphasised by presentation of examples of how things can be done and how they should not be done. For the most part it is easier to find bad examples than good ones. It also should be emphasised that generally one individual is not capable of conducting a useful study by himself or by herself. Multiple disciplines are required and the input of both expertise in environmental assessment and disease response is required. In almost every case it requires two or more individuals.

The value of monitoring for epidemiological purposes considering both health outcome and exposure has relevance from two major standpoints; the first being medical surveillance, the second being research studies with applicable results.

As far as medical surveillance goes, there are two principal reasons for its conduct. One is to detect disease which might not have been previously suspected and the other is to be sure that disease which might result from an exposure is not occurring at the existing exposure level. Frequently, multiphasic health testing is conducted on work populations without paying attention to the exposures of the individuals in question - in my view a sin. More and more companies are now attempting to link the exposures with the health effects information, although to date successful linkages have not been frequent. Linkage obviously requires the input of both the epidemiologist or physician interested in the health effect and the industrial hygienist who is interested in the exposures. Joint planning can lead to meaningful screening. Two examples of this approach that have yielded useful information come from the studies of the rubber industry. The first example involves mortality, the second morbidity.

The mortality experience of approximately 25,000 past and current employees from one plant in Ohio going back to 1925, has been reviewed by Monson and Nakano. (1,2) Ascertainment of vital status was made and death certificates on those deceased were located. A comparison was made between numbers of deaths observed among rubber workers as compared to the number of deaths expected on the basis of death rates in the USA. In this comparison, race, sex, age, and time of death were taken into account. Comparisons were made for all rubber workers as well as for groups of rubber workers who had worked together in specific areas of the plant. This latter analysis was crucial. When reviewing the overall mortality, the results showed mortality between 62% and 82% of that expected based on the death rates in the USA. One could have stopped here and said that there is no problem in the rubber industry. However, further analysis of death experience by department revealed some very interesting associations. Excess gastrointestinal cancer was seen in workers from the processing area. Excess lung cancer was demonstrated in tyre-curing areas and excess bladder cancer was seen in men who worked at least 35 years and who died at age 75 or above. While exposures in this study were not quantified and no estimates of dose were derived, it was possible to relate certain cancer excesses to certain departments on the basis of mortality and departmental categorisation.

In another plant 744 workers were examined by multiphasic health testing. (3,4) In addition, estimates were made of their exposure to respirable particulates, solvents, and noise. By employing these indices of exposure it was possible to demonstrate excess respiratory morbidity in those individuals working in areas in which exposures to dusts and fumes were high. This was despite the fact that no standards were being exceeded and no obvious over-exposures were occurring. That is, it is likely that the Occupational Safety and Health Administration would not have found any violations based on specific exposures to toxic materials. In addition to the excess respiratory morbidity associated with respirable particulates, certain other findings of interest occurred which deserve further attention.

For example, workers exposed to emissions from heated uncured rubber reported chest tightness on return to work; workers in the cutting department exposed to oil mist reported more gastrointestinal symptoms (nausea and abdominal pain); and elevated levels of serum creatinine were seen more often in mill workers who also reported both more difficulty while urinating and red or brown urine.

The previously cited examples simply illustrate the advantage of considering exposure on a very crude basis, namely by departments in which the worker spent the majority of his time. There are obviously many examples of studies in which specific hypotheses have been tested, taking advantage of careful environmental assessment and careful ascertainment of health effects.

In considering the relationships between exposures and effects one can think about acute exposures vs acute effects, acute exposures vs chronic effects, chronic exposures vs chronic effects or chronic exposures and acute effects. The principal problem involved in those four possibilities centres around chronic exposures. Said another way it is a great deal easier to measure either acute or chronic effects and acute exposures than it is to measure chronic exposures. The only element that does not require a cross-sectional measurement is the ascertainment of lifetime dose or the best estimate of chronic exposure. A crucial need then is to find better ways of collecting these data.

Acute exposure, acute effect

The simplest kind of epidemiological study involves acute exposure and acute effects. (Some researchers might not refer to these studies as epidemiological in future, but I

am using the term epidemiology as a broad term considering
any study of groups of individuals.) It is obviously possible and quite simple to put an individual in an exposure
chamber and expose them to "X" parts per million of a toxic
agent and measure the effect of such after a period of a few
minutes to a few hours. The occupational health literature
is replete with studies of this kind. These studies provide
much of the "hard" evidence of toxic effects of many materials. Examples include exposure to carbon monoxide, sulphur dioxide, ozone, etc. In most instances these studies
consider only the ambient environment of the individual and
do not attempt to measure actual delivered dose. The closer
one comes to the true ascertainment of delivered dose, the
higher the value of the information will be. In the case of
carbon monoxide, this is obviously possible as carboxyhaemoglobin can be measured.

It is interesting that at least for three substances -
sulphur dioxide, cotton dust and toluene diisocyanate (TDI) -
the level of exposure at which acute effects are seen is
approximately the same level at which chronic effects can be
detected. It is important to determine whether this is true
for other substances. If it is, the implications for
standard setting are obvious.

Acute exposure, chronic effects

Most acute exposures which result in chronic effects involve
accidental over-exposures to materials. It is frequently
difficult, therefore, to assess the magnitude of the exposure, except in some instances by re-enactment of the
accident. Examples which come most easily to mind involve
respiratory damage from acute over-exposures, for example
from nitrogen dioxide or other toxic agents that can produce
severe respiratory effects which may be permanent. Acute
over-exposures to radiation can likewise produce long-term
sequellae (viz the atomic blasts in Japan and cancer).

It is possible, of course, to follow up individuals who have had acute exposures to ascertain the health effects. Examples of this include individuals who might have been over-exposed to benzene, or individuals who suffered chloracne from exposure to chlorinated compounds.(5) Opportunities to follow cohorts of workers acutely exposed to substances that can produce chronic effects are not common but obviously when they do occur advantage of this circumstance should be taken.

Chronic exposures, acute effects

Examples demonstrating acute morbidity from chronic exposures are not frequent and generally involve "allergic", hypersensitive or idiosyncratic reactions. For example, an individual could work with a solvent for many years before the development of an acute severe contact dermatitis. Individuals can also work with respiratory irritants on a chronic basis and suddenly develop a respiratory sensitivity to these materials. Examples would be formaldahyde and TDI. Fatal anaphylaxis has been known to occur from the latter. The acute onset of aplastic anaemia can also occur following a chronic exposure to a material such as benzene. It is probable, however, that premonitory signs of the acute disease manifestations would be detectable if monitoring of the exposed individuals had been conducted. That is, certain subtle changes in the red blood cells, white blood cells, or platelets would likely have been possible to observe before the full disease.

Chronic exposures, chronic effects

This is by far and away the most important of the four possibilities being described in this paper. Most of the important occupational health questions involve relating chronic exposure to chronic effect and this is the challenge for the epidemiologist. At this point almost no quantitative information exists on exposures of interest in the

past.   If a cohort is studied today and certain disease is
found,   relating that disease to past exposure becomes
extremely difficult.   Frequently, the best that can be done
is   to   know the number of years the individuals worked in a
specific work setting. Sometimes weightings can be established   that   allow dividing people into exposure categories
by qualitative estimates, for example, low, medium and high.
A word of caution must be added however. One must be absolutely sure that an estimate of past exposure is valid.
Otherwise the results can be misleading. A common approach
is to ask a company industrial hygienist or other individual
familiar with the company work processes to estimate the
extent of exposure.   In these cases the professional judgement of the industrial hygienist is relied upon and in some
cases (but not all) it is valid. A recent example involved
a mortality study of pesticide workers in which the company
had provided information on the extent of the pesticide
exposure.   The study involved two plants, one in which
exposures were allegedly high, and one in which exposures
were allegedly low.   However, in the plant in which exposures were high there was a respirator programme to control
the exposure.   When the question was asked, are the people
in the high exposure area really being exposed to more
pesticide than the people in the low exposure area, the
answer was no.   Because those individuals working in the
high exposure area were wearing respirators their overall
exposure was lower than those working in the low exposure
area without respirators.   This was proven by biological
measurements of pesticide body burdens in the individuals.

Deriving estimates of lifetime exposure is not always a
losing battle, and efforts should be made to make this
important determination.   There are many cohorts with
interesting past exposures that need to be studied. We
cannot afford to conduct studies beginning today that will
take 30 or 40 years to complete. There is however a particular study in which serious efforts were made to derive a
lifetime estimate of dose.   While one must make certain

assumptions in order to derive such an assessment of exposure, the crudeness with which these estimates must be made
still do not invalidate the effort to do such. The example
involves Vermont granite workers exposed to silica. These
individuals work in a variety of work settings and a variety
of jobs. Many mass respirable samples for dust and silica
were taken representing most jobs and most work settings.
On the basis of these measurements and on the basis of a
knowledge of the time and occupations of each individual in
the study, and on the basis of making dust measurements in
sheds which were reopened for the purpose of assessing "old"
exposures, it was possible to accumulate a lifetime dose of
exposure to silica and to relate these findings to the
disease outcome measures of X-ray abnormality and pulmonary
function test abnormality. (6) The dose estimate clearly
refined the relationship between the exposure and effect,
and revealed a clear-cut relationship between exposure and
the development of X-ray abnormalities, (7) and exposure and
the development of abnormalities of pulmonary function. (8)
These studies provided information relevant to both standard
setting for silica and to the best approach for medical surveillance. That is, when the effects on pulmonary function
were compared to the effects on chest X-ray, the effects on
pulmonary function are found earlier than those in the X-ray,
thus suggesting that pulmonary function testing may be a more
relevant medical monitoring procedure than chest X-rays.

Certain new approaches can be followed that provide a tremendous amount of promise at the present time; for example the
determination of change in function related to exposure during the period in which the change is measured. Any organ
which has an easily measured functional capacity is susceptible to such an approach. Ageing usually results in decrement of function of most organs. If the magnitude of this
ageing decrement can be determined, then the opportunity is
provided to compare the change in functional capacity of an
organ with that expected from ageing. An organ which clearly
provides that opportunity is the lung. However, consideration

should be given to conducting similar studies of the kidney, brain, heart and liver.

At the present time we know enough about the lung to realise that ventilatory capacity changes at a predictable rate. If a group of individuals is being exposed to a material which can affect the lung, one expects that this rate of decrement will increase. Depending on the change in the rate of decrement and the size of the study population, effects of chronic exposures can be revealed in periods as short as one year. The examples of workers exposed to TDI, (9) Boston fire-fighters, (10) and copper smelter workers (11) are relevant. One simply needs then, to monitor a group of workers over a relatively short period of time, namely one or more years while determining the rate of decrement. If the rate of decrement is normal, one can assume that the exposure is not immediately harmful. I believe this kind of information is better than relying on the acute exposure, acute effect, information for standard setting. Few studies have involved other organs. It would appear that this approach has great value and will serve to provide much information relevant to monitoring in epidemiological studies and obviates the two big problems in dealing with chronic exposures: guessing at past exposures or studying populations prospectively for long periods of time.

The line between medical surveillance and research relevant to occupational health is not a clear one. The level of our ignorance is such that medical surveillance conducted well, that is, with careful measurements of exposure and careful measurements of disease outcome, is likely to be of direct use for standard setting, for medical monitoring and will likely yield information of research value.

References

1. Monson, R.R., and Nakano, K.K. Mortality among rubber workers. I. White male union employees in Akron, Ohio. Am. J. Epidemiol. 103:284 (1976).

2. Monson, R.R., and Nakano, K.K. Mortality among rubber workers. II. Other Akron employees. Am. J. Epidemiol. 103:297 (1976).

3. Weeks, J.L., Peters, J.M., Monson, R.R. Screening for occupational hazards in the rubber industry. Am. J. Ind. Med. 2 (2) 125-41 (1981).

4. Weeks, J.L., Peters, J.M., Monson, R.R. Health hazards in the curing department. Am. J. Ind. Med. 2 (2) 143-51 (1981).

5. Zack, J.A., Suskind, R.R. The mortality experience of workers exposed to tetrachlorodibenzodioxin in a trichlorophenol process accident. J. Occup. Med. 22 (1):11-14 (1980).

6. Theriault, G.P., Burgess, W.A., DiBerardinis, L., Peters, J.M. Dust exposure in the Vermont granite sheds. Arch. Environ. Health 28:12-17 (1974).

7. Theriault, G.P., Peters, J.M., Fine, L.J. Pulmonary function in granite shed workers of Vermont. Arch. Environ, Health 20:18-22 (1974).

8. Theriault, G.P., Peters, J.M., Johnson, W.M. Pulmonary function and X-ray changes in granite dust exposure. Arch. Environ. Health 20:23-27 (1974).

9. Peters, J.M. Cumulative pulmonary effects in workers exposed to toluene diisocyanate (TDI). Proceedings Royal Society of Medicine 63:372-375 (1970).

10. Peters, J.M., Theriault, G.P., Fine, L.J., Wegman, D.H. Chronic effect of fire fighting on pulmonary function. New Eng. J. Med. 291:1320-1322 (1974).

11. Smith, T.J., Peters, J.M., Reading, J.C., Castle, C.H. Pulmonary impairment from chronic exposure to SO_2. Am. Rev. Resp. Dis. 116:31-41 (1977).

MULTIDISCIPLINARY APPROACH TO PREVENTION AND HEALTH
PROTECTION BY MONITORING: ROLE OF INDIVIDUAL DISCIPLINES.
THE ENGINEER: EQUIPMENT, PLANT MODIFICATIONS, AND DESIGN I.

J.M. EVANS (USA)

Summary

This paper shows that the chemical engineer's role in
occupational health extends from the laboratory, where the
fundamental elements of a process are developed; to the
pilot plant, where questions of unit operation and equipment
design can impact heavily on elements of occupational health
and safety; and then to the commercial operation, where
monitoring and improved equipment design are intertwined to
lower fugitive emissions and reduce worker exposure to
potentially toxic products.

This paper illustrates how the chemical engineer's involvement in occupational health can extend beyond these normal
uses of his skills to the development of data for use in
defining safety measures and in the development of regulations themselves.

Examples are drawn from experiences in the conversion of
coal to gas and oil.

Introduction

The role of the chemical engineer in health protection
extends from the laboratory, where the fundamental elements
of a process are developed; to the pilot plant, where
questions of unit operation and equipment design can impact
heavily on elements of occupational health and safety; and
then to the commercial operation where monitoring and
improved equipment design are intertwined to lower fugitive
emissions and reduce worker exposure to potentially toxic
products. The involvement of the chemical engineer in
occupational health can extend beyond these normal uses of
his skills to the development of data for use in defining
safety measures and in the development of regulations.
Examples are used from experiences in the conversion of coal
to gas and oil.

Training of the chemical engineer

In the past in the United States, a chemical engineer's training did not include people, and little or no mention was made of occupational or community health. Rather, the chemical engineer was trained in the engineering sciences. He was taught to be pragmatic; he learned that it was his job to develop, design and/or operate chemically-related processes in a cost-effective manner.

Despite this lack of people or health-related training, it did not take the chemical engineer long once on the job to comprehend from either a humane or mechanistic viewpoint that to design, develop, or operate a plant in a cost-effective manner he had to be aware of the adverse health and safety effects of the chemicals and the process with which he and the plant workers were dealing. An unhealthy or injured worker decreased productivity and increased the cost of doing business. The chemical engineer had to design and operate the facility in such a way as to protect the worker within the plant and the community outside the plant.

We are speaking here of an educational system that is several decades out of date - or we hope it is. Today, the chemical engineer is part of a multidisciplinary team of engineers, industrial hygienists, toxicologists, medical doctors, etc., whose complementary skills are used to see that the plant operation is efficiently attuned to the safety and occupational health of its employees.

The chemical engineer's place in the occupational health team

Any one or combination of the following steps may be instituted by such a multidisciplinary team to achieve the following objectives:

- changing the process to eliminate a toxic product
  or by-product;
- developing and implementing the use of proper
  emission control technology;
- monitoring both the process and the workers to
  detect potentially harmful substances before they
  reach hazardous concentrations; and
- instituting work practices or using protective
  equipment to protect the worker when there is a
  potential that he may be exposed.

The chemical engineer has a key role to play in each of
these methods of achieving a safe, healthy work environment.
Although each individual case is different, the engineering
approach is sufficiently similar that examples of what can
be done are worth describing.

Process modifications

In general, coal gasification and liquefaction processes do
not readily lend themselves to modifications which reduce or
eliminate toxic by-products. However, there are two notable
exceptions; one is the Synthane coal gasification process
and the other is the solid-liquid separation unit operation.
The first involved a fundamental change in chemistry,
though only a simple design change, while the second was
almost the opposite.

For the Synthane process the problem was twofold - operating
problems and the generation of a toxic by-product. The
potential for operator exposure was intensified by operating
problems. The Synthane process is a fluidised-bed process
designed to operate at approximately 1550 F (843 C) and 1000
psig (69 atmospheres). The pilot plant would not operate
when the first attempts were made to start it up in 1977.
During these startup attempts, tar and solids plugged the
recycle quench-liquor heat exchangers, caused emulsions in
the gas-liquor separation vessels and finally plugged up the
internal cyclones.(1-3) Each time this happened the equip-

ment had to be opened and cleaned. Analyses of process
tars, which were similar to those removed from the Synthane
pilot plant equipment, indicated that they contained carcinogenic compounds. These analyses were substantiated by
highly positive in-vitro (Ames) tests.(4) In the laboratory
engineering experiments to define fundamental properties of
the fluidised-bed gasification process indicated that if the
process were altered by moving a pipe so that the coal was
fed into the bottom of the fluidised-bed rather than above
it, the tar by-products could be almost eliminated.(5) When
this alteration was made to the pilot plant, tar production
dropped drastically and operating and maintenance problems,
with their consequent potential for worker exposure,
decreased significantly.

The second example is that of solid-liquid separation. One
of the primary reasons for liquefying coal is to separate it
from the mineral matter. The German practice through World
War II, and American practice until the late 1970s, was to
filter the liquefied coal to accomplish the separation.
The high-temperature, high-pressure equipment used for filtration leaked incessantly and required constant maintenance
to keep it in operation.(6) Operators and maintenance
personnel were exposed to the toxic solvent vapours and/or
carcinogenic tars. Today a number of these liquefaction
processes - e.g., Solvent Refined Coal-II, H-Coal and Exxon
Donor Solvent - have eliminated the filtration step. Rather,
these processes are now being designed with a distillation
operation as the solid-liquid separation step, using a
minimum of moving mechanical equipment. The distillation
equipment is subject to far less mechanical breakdown than
was the filtration equipment and consequently its use is far
less likely to result in worker exposure.(7-9).

Thus, alteration in the Synthane process affected the process
chemistry while the changes to the liquefaction unit operation involved physical chemistry and mechanical alterations.
In both instances, these alterations, defined and designed by

chemical engineers, resulted in a profound improvement in the emission control technology as well as the operational parameters of the processes.

Equipment design

Equipment design modification is probably the most fruitful approach to reducing or controlling fugitive emissions and for reducing exposure to maintenance workers as exemplified by a National Institute for Occupational Safety and Health (NIOSH) programme and from a more common industrial experience for examples of this approach to improving occupational health.

The chemical engineer has a key role to play in the design of emission control technology, especially as defined by NIOSH. This definition may be paraphrased by defining emission control technology as improvements to process or equipment that result in fewer emissions in the workplace and, subsequently, that result in a substantial decrease in equipment maintenance with a consequent decrease in the potential exposure of operators or maintenance personnel.

During the past several years NIOSH has made a number of fugitive emission control technology studies that used this concept as the basic philosophy. The team approach was found best suited to implement these studies - a team consisting of chemical engineers, industrial hygienists, and toxicologists. It might be assumed that it was the contention of NIOSH in designing the fugitive emission control studies that the engineer who was familiar with the specific processes and with the equipment could both recognise the problems and identify solutions or partial solutions to these problems through the expanded opportunity to observe operators and question personnel at a wide variety of installations.

The objective of NIOSH's control technology study for coal liquefaction and gasification facilities was to examine a

number of coal gasification and liquefaction projects to
determine where occupational hazards might exist. Of more
importance, the study was to define problem areas, whether
they were in the process, in instrumentation, in mechanical
equipment, or if they were metallurgical in nature. The
second part of the study was to determine what, if anything,
was being done to correct the problems identified, then to
correlate the information gathered from the various coal
conversion facilities that had been visited and make the
information available to the public. Two of these problem
areas are chosen as examples.

i) In the coal liquefaction plant the first unit
where a potential for occupational exposure exists
is at the mixing vessel where the solid coal is
mixed with the coal-derived hydrocarbon solvent.
The coal slurry is warm [100 F (177 C)] and is
continually agitated; consequently, vapours are
given off which condense in the fine-coal feed
chute, causing it to plug. Once plugged, the
chute has to be cleared, so that the operator of
this particular unit is frequently exposed to
hydrocarbon vapours and condensed liquids.(10)

ii) The hot slurry letdown valves, control valves and
centrifugal pumps are also recognised as potential
fugitive emission or maintenance problem areas.
The hot high-pressure slurry erodes the valve
internals after only hours of operation. Likewise,
centrifugal pump casings and impellers erode after
less than 100 hours of service. Pump seals fail
even more rapidly. All such failures result in
potential operator or maintenance personnel exposure.(10,11)

A satisfactory engineering solution to the coal solvent-
mixing vapour emission problem was found at one plant the
control technology team visited - this was to operate the
coal-solvent mixing tank under a slight negative pressure.

The vapours were discharged to a flare system.(12) At other
plants, the chemical engineers identified approaches to the
valve and to the pump problem while the industrial hygienist
devised techniques for cleaning equipment which required
frequent maintenance in such a manner as to reduce worker
exposure.   However, it would seem that pump seal solutions
will involve a combination of process chemistry, equipment
design, and lubricating oil specifications.

My final example of the engineer's role in equipment design
to reduce the potential for occurrence of occupational
exposure is of a type which is more commonly encountered by
commercial plant chemical engineers. At Sasol-I, the engineering department early recognised that the most dangerous
devices on a vessel - to the maintenance men - were the
purge connections.   While purge valves at Sasol-I are normally locked shut or blanked off before maintenance personnel are permitted to enter a vessel, such precautions can be
circumvented either accidentally or by vibration, releasing
inert gas (purging is usually done with an inert gas) into
the vessel and endangering the maintenance worker. Sasol
engineers eliminated this potential problem by eliminating
inert gas purging. Instead, steam purging was used wherever
possible.   Steam not only displaces the toxic atmospheres,
but in addition air is drawn into the vessel as the steam
condenses.   Should a purge connection containing steam be
inadvertently opened, the worker can see the leak (or, if it
is large, perhaps can feel it).(13)

Monitoring

Monitoring for fugitive emissions has generally been regarded as the province of the industrial hygienist. He uses
area and personnel monitoring to determine whether a potential for exposure to toxic materials in the workplace has
become an actuality, as well as to determine the degree of
this exposure.

The chemical engineer, with his knowledge of process chemistry and equipment design, is an important adjunct to the industrial hygienist in any monitoring programme. A typical example of teamwork between the chemical engineer and the industrial hygienist to establish a monitoring programme occurred during the inception of an occupational health programme at the low-Btu gasifier located on the campus of the University of Minnesota at Duluth. A team of several industrial hygienists, several instrumentation specialists, and a chemical engineer was given the task of setting up a three-year industrial hygiene monitoring programme. In this situation, the engineer defined the potential leak points in the process and helped to define the most likely paths that leaking gases would follow within the equipment. Despite a low operating pressure of approximately 20 to 30 inches of water at the top of the gasifier, coal feed lockhopper valves and all flanges were identified as potential leak points. Because the original design was based on handling non-toxic, non-carcinogenic materials, it was expected that leakage would be extensive. Based on the engineering evaluation of gasifier products, and the industrial hygienists' evaluation of the relative toxicity of the materials involved, carbon monoxide was chosen as the indicator compound. In addition, a large [120 lb (254 kg)] mercury seal at the base of the gasifier was identified as a potential source of problems.

Based on engineering advice, no formal monitoring programme was to be established until the gasifier had been through a three-month shakedown run, but monitoring of all potential leak-points was to begin immediately, as both a precautionary and a training measure.

One year later the same team returned to the University to reevaluate the industrial hygiene programme. They found that the monitoring programme had identified high carbon monoxide (over 500 ppm) concentrations in the building on several occasions and that a number of design changes had

been made, including boxing in all piping flanges. The
mercury seal, which had blown out twice, had been replaced
with a mechanical seal.

This is a prime example of an instance where a monitoring
programme set up by a team including both chemical engineers
and industrial hygienists not only protected an operating
crew from excessive exposure but, in fact, saved their lives
several times when leaks occurred which the operators had
not anticipated.(14)

There is still another example of the involvement of the
chemical engineer in occupational health monitoring programmes at the Sasol-I plant. The Sasol engineers knew that
many of the toxic gases generated in the process or used for
pre-maintenance purging of vessels were similar to and just
as deadly as those found in gassy coal mines. So, not having
any industrial hygienists at the time, and having become experts at technology transfer, they adapted the same monitoring instrumentation which was used in coal mines for use in
purged vessels which have to be entered for maintenance.
Even then (in 1977) Sasol maintenance people would not enter
a vessel if the canary wasn't there.(13)

Workplace characterisation studies

Workplace characterisation is considered a special category
of the industrial hygienist's monitoring duties. However,
pilot plants are not staid, industrial operations and
require new approaches. NIOSH, in its twin characterisation
programmes for coal gasification and liquefaction pilot
plants, used a team consisting of both chemical engineers
and industrial hygienists. In this programme, the lead
roles could shift rapidly. Chemical engineers, leaning
heavily on the emission control technology study discussed
previously, defined areas, locations, plant operating
conditions and potential emission points for a representative sampling programme. The industrial hygienists then

took charge of the personnel and area sampling and, together with the engineers, directed the complex chemical analyses of the samples obtained, then reported the data.(6,10)

It was anticipated that the engineers could then take the data from the various plants characterised in both the liquefaction and gasification studies and extrapolate it to obtain a first approximation of the potential workplace exposure in the larger demonstration or commercial plants. Such an effort would help identify potential sources of excessive emissions where further emission control techno- logy studies are required for larger plants. Although the study has not been completed, at least one engineering and construction firm has used a portion of these data from NIOSH demonstration plant design studies.

Criteria documents

An area not normally thought of as being of interest to chemical engineers is that of criteria document development. However, when NIOSH became interested in the development of process-oriented documents several years ago, chemical engineers were key members of the document-development team, along with the industrial hygienist, toxicologist, medical doctor, and other health or biological science-related specialists. The first of these efforts was managed by a chemical engineer.(15,16) Here, it was the chemical engi- neer's task to describe the process chemistry, to define how the product and by-product composition altered as it passed from one part of the operation to another, to describe the design of the process equipment, and to identify the mechanism by which emissions were most likely to occur. Working on a broader scope, the engineer categorised the process based on variations in process chemistry so that different technologies would be regulated according to individual merit.

Once this effort was accomplished the other specialists involved in the task - the industrial hygienist, the toxicologist, and the medical doctor - could efficiently apply their own speciality to the criteria document development. Without very close teamwork by all of the specialists, this type of document could not be developed accurately or efficiently.

Conclusions

The chemical engineer has a definite and important role in the development of a healthy and safe workplace. This role extends from the laboratory where the chemistry and the fundamental developments of a process occur, to the pilot plant where questions of process configuration and equipment design take place, to the commercial plant where the process and individual should be monitored and where continuing efforts should be made to improve health and safety measures. Further, the chemical engineer should and must take a significant role in the regulatory process. His services should be made available to those agencies developing data on pilot or industrial processes. He can and should contribute significantly to the regulatory development process itself by applying his process background. He may thus aid the development of practical regulations that can be implemented and which will enhance the occupational health and safety of the worker.

Acknowledgments
I would acknowlege and thank Dr. Ralph E. Yodaiken, M.D., M.P.H., NIOSH, Division of Extramural Coordination and Special Projects; Mr. James A. Gideon, Research Chemical Engineer, NIOSH, Division of Physical Sciences and Engineering; and Mr. Lynne R. Harris, Chemical Engineer, NIOSH, Division of Extramural Coordination and Special Projects, for the encouragement which they gave me before and during the development of this paper. I would also like to thank Cherryl M. Crouch for her assistance in typing and editing this paper.

Bibliography

1. Report of visits to Synthane Pilot Plant, Pittsburgh, Pennsylvania. Rockville, Md, Enviro Control, Inc. September 1976, February 1977, and April 1979 (submitted to NIOSH under contracts 210-76-0171 and 210-78-0084).

2. Lewis, R., Santore, R.R., Dubis, D. Coal pressurisation and feeding: use of a lockhopper system. Pasadena: California Institute of Technology, 1977.

3. Lewis, R., Strakey, J.P., Haynes, W.P., et al. Update of Synthane Pilot Plant status. Presented at the Tenth Synthetic Pipeline Gas Symposium, Chicago, Illinois, October 30-November 1, 1978.

4. Epler, J.L., Young, J.A., Hardigree, A.A., et al. Analytical and biological analyses of test materials from the synthetic fuel technologies - I, mutagenicity of crude oils determined by the Salmonella typhimurium/microsomal activation system. Mutat. Res. 1976; 57:265-76.

5. Nakles D.V., Massey, M.J., Forney, A.J. Influence of Synthane gasifier conditions of effluent and product gas production. Pittsburgh: Pittsburgh Energy Research Centre, 1975-76; [PERC/RI-75/6].

6. Report of the industrial hygiene comprehensive survey for the Cresap Test Facility. Rockville, Md, Enviro Control, Inc. (submitted to NIOSH under contract 210-78-0101), 1980.

7. Committee on Processing and Utilisation of Fossil Fuels. Assessment of technology for the liquefaction of coal. Washington: National Research Council for the National Academy of Sciences, 1977.

8. Friedman, S., Akhtar, S., Yavorsky, P.M. An overview of coal liquefaction projects. Presented at the Technology and Use of Lignite Symposium, Grand Forks, N.D., May 14-15, 1975.

9. Stotler, H.H., Schutter R.T. H-Coal Pilot Plant status and operating plans. Presented at the AIChE meeting, Philadelphia, Pa, June 5-7, 1978.

10. Report of the industrial hygiene comprehensive survey for the Solvent Refined Coal Pilot Plant. Rockville, Md, Enviro Control, Inc. (submitted to NIOSH under contract 210-78-0101), 1980.

11. Report of visit to HYGAS Pilot Plant, Chicago, Illinois. Rockville, Md, Enviro Control, Inc., November 8-11, 1976 (submitted to NIOSH under contract 210-76-0171).

12   Report of visit to the Solvent Refined Coal Pilot
      Plant, Fort Lewis, Washington. Rockville, Md, Enviro
      Control, Inc. February 1979 (submitted to NIOSH under
      contract 210-78-0084), 1980

13.   Report of visit to South African Coal, Oil and Gas
      Corporation, Ltd (SASOL), Sasolburg, South Africa.
      Rockville, Md, Enviro Control, Inc., Dec 5-8, 1977
      (submitted to NIOSH under contract 210-76-0171).

14.   Industrial Hygiene Review Panel of the Oak Ridge
      National Laboratory's Life Sciences Synthetic Fuels
      Program. University of Minnesota, Duluth gasifier,
      industrial hygiene review. Oak Ridge: Oak Ridge
      National Laboratory, 1980.

15.   National Institute for Occupational Safety and Health.
      Criteria for a recommended standard...occupational
      exposures in coal gasification plants. Rockville, Md:
      US Department of Health, Education and Welfare, 1978.
      (DHEW [NIOSH] publication No. 78-191).

16.   National Institute for Occupational Safety and Health.
      Recommended health and safety guidelines for coal
      gasification pilot plants. Rockville, MD: US Depart-
      ment of Health, Education and Welfare, 1978 (DHEW
      [NIOSH] publication No. 78-120).

MULTIDISCIPLINARY APPROACH TO PREVENTION AND HEALTH
PROTECTION BY MONITORING: ROLE OF INDIVIDUAL DISCIPLINES.
THE ENGINEER: EQUIPMENT, PLANT MODIFICATIONS AND DESIGN II.

P. LARDEUX (FRANCE)

Summary

*Broadly speaking an engineer is one employed to apply his
knowledge, according to his training, in the production of
awide variety of goods. ᵀn France it has been recognised
that an engineer's training needs to be improved in the area
of industrial safety. In this paper specific training
requirements are highlighted and ways are discussed in which
preventive planning can be initiated and acted upon.*

Introduction

A dictionary definition of an engineer is someone who has
received scientific and technical training equipping him to
direct certain projects or engage in research. Nothing pre-
disposes him to concern himself with safety, which, again
according to the dictionary, may be either the feeling of
confidence and calmness of one who believes himself sheltered
from danger or the situation or untroubled state which
results from a real absence of danger. Depending on his
natural inclinations, the engineer may adopt an approach
corresponding to the first definition or act so as to achieve
the second.

Broadly speaking, an engineer is someone employed in industry
to apply his knowledge in the production of a wide variety of
goods according to his training. At any time, therefore, he
may have to cope with occupational hazards threatening himself or his associates.

The ability to take precautions against industrial accidents
or diseases obviously depends on one's awareness of the risks
involved and of the ways of preventing them. But this is not
enough, since all existing risks are not known and are far
from being immediately apparent to the untrained eye.

It is impossible to foresee all the new hazards brought about by new technologies, products, organisations and structures. In industry there are always special cases which call for a high degree of vigilance both at the design stage and in operating conditions. If prevention is to be effective, all the available skill and know-how must be applied at all levels and stages of the manufacturing process, as they are in the pursuit of productivity and profitability.

Improvement in safety

It might be assumed that a substantial part of an engineer's scientific and technical training is concerned with safety at work, or even that special training is available for safety specialists. The situation is, in fact, quite different, even though there are "safety engineers", a minority of whom have been given special training and who are concerned exclusively with industrial safety. it is not very desirable to develop this specialisation on a large scale; it would be much better for engineers working in production, design or any other departments to consider health and safety at each stage of their plans. To do this they must, if not specially trained, at least be informed of safety factors and made sensitive to them.

Although the idea of improving safety by training is not new, training in safety was for a long time confined to instruction given in various forms by official organisations to specialists in accident prevention. There are many engineering colleges in France, but only a few offer training in industial safety.

Mindful of these problems, the French committee concerned with engineers' qualifications drafted a report in 1979 on the improvement of training in industrial safety. This states that there is at present a lack of courses in industrial safety for engineers and that they should be given special training geared towards their responsibilities both inside and outside the working environment. There should be two aspects to such training -a general aspect designed to ensure that all action and planning are considered from the standpoint of safety, and a specific aspect concerned with the hazards encountered at work, how to train their associates and make them sensitive to safety problems and to the environmental hazards entailed by their work.

Training and planning for safety

This specific training should be given as part of special courses of instruction. Training courses on the use of sub-stances, the operation of equipment or the design of new products should include a safety aspect. Supervised work could provide a practical illustration of industrial hazards and of the precautions taken by designers and users. In-service training should provide an opportunity for trainees to include safety aspects in their reports. Visits to companies and organisations involved in health and safety research should also be included in training programmes to give an idea of the type of work being carried out in this field.

Some educational establishments have already introduced specialised courses of instruction in health and safety. In France, these are the university institutes of technology at Bordeaux, Lorient, Paris XI and Aix-Marseille. Elsewhere in Europe there is the school of safety technology of Wuppertal University in Germany and the University of Aston in Birmingham in the United Kingdom. Similar projects are being prepared in Belgium.

As far as the problems under discussion here are concerned, namely safety in the use of toxic agents, it is true to say that chemical engineers are at an advantage, even though they too have not been specially trained. Nevertheless, they are taught about the chemical and physical properties of sub-stances and their interactions, and sometimes a few rudiments of toxicology, so they are the first to be consulted in industry whenever a problem arises concerning the use of a product. They are often consulted for their knowledge as analysts, but again, without special training, they may overlook certain little known effects. We therefore urgently need, as an initial measure, to explore all possibilities for creating an awareness of safety problems among those in middle management and elsewhere, as well as top management, because it is ultimately their decisions which count.

When new installations are used, preventive planning and action should begin in the design office, which should be given all useful information by the research and experimental departments on the properties of the substances being used. But the point raised by Mr J. Evans elsewhere in this publication applies only to the future and to certain major undertakings which have been aware of this phenomenon for some years. Engineers, who are responsible for safeguarding production equipment, cannot shirk their responsibilities towards people.

In most cases engineers are faced with existing situations calling for immediate solutions. They should therefore:
- find out whether the substances being used or manufactured are intrinsically dangerous (toxic, inflammable, irritant, etc.);
- study the manufacturing process to discover possible associated factors obtained deliberately or otherwise (fumes, degradation products, etc.) which are also intrinsically dangerous;
- recognise hazards at work (the possibility of man/product, machine/product or product/product contact);
- assess the risk involved (measurement and analysis);
- devise safeguards by modifying the process or products, or by providing protection.

Engineers cannot do this work alone. In the first step they have to be assisted by occupational physicians and toxicologists, in the third by management and workers, and in the fourth by analysts. In the final step, on the other hand, they should help preventive specialists by providing justification for requirements imposed on the manufacturing process.

The engineer should deal directly with the occupational physician in determining the hazards of a particular process, since the latter cannot perform his tasks as medical supervisor unless he is familiar with the products and processes to which staff are exposed, and the engineer cannot accurately ascertain the effects of working conditions without consulting the doctor.

The engineer should also be in direct contact with the organisations concerned with technical control and the observance of regulations. In particular, he should be conversant with the regulations in force on the shop floor. This is particularly true since company heads tend increasingly to delegate their responsibilities for health and safety at work to middle management personnel in direct touch with the workers.

In preliminary research the charts showing the various stages in the manufacturing process could have superimposed on them a chart indicating not only the physical state of the substances used (solid, liquid, temperature and pressure) but also the nature of the hazards (burns, poisoning, inflammation, etc.). This would be supplemented by a test using a model or equipment of actual size to identify the danger zones and the interaction between zones (e.g. the risks of an inflammable substance being released into a zone where there are sources of heat and flames, etc.).

In such tests the production engineer, who must be very familiar with his own working unit, plays a particularly vital part in pinpointing these trouble-spots. He must have a

particularly critical eye and be able to foresee the unfore-
seeable. What would happen if a reactor, designed so as to
be perfectly adequate for the tasks it is required to perform, should burst or spring a leak? What product would be
released, and in what amount and at what temperature? What
would be the area affected? Would personnel be exposed?
What can be done to minimise the effects of such an accident,
and what emergency measures should be considered? Such
questions should be asked at all stages of production. A set
of priorities should be established in order of seriousness
to permit a more thorough examination of possible counter-
measures. All these questions should be discussed by the
health and safety committees, since this is their job, and
everyone will be able to contribute towards accident prevention through the use of appropriate equipment and processes.

This brings us quite naturally to the question of the preventive maintenance of plant and equipment; this should be based
on careful analysis, with the maintenance procedure having
been scrupulously studied and explained to the operators, who
should be informed of the reasons for the procedure. However, emergency measures by maintenance services, which sadly
tend to be ill informed about what they can come up against,
should also be discussed with the engineers responsible for
the equipment in question.

In the case of certain highly sensitive materials, emergency
measures could even be prepared in advance.

The engineer also has a part to play with the other members
of the production team in applying his technical knowledge of
the processes and installations to the analysis of accidents
and incidents. An accident is considered to have occurred
when a person has been the victim of an incident. When there
is no victim, there is only an incident.

The methods of analysing accidents have already been discussed on numerous occasions, and all that needs to be said

here is that the analysis of an accident should not be regarded as complete as long as a solution has not been found
ensuring that it does not happen again.

It could almost be argued that accidents or incidents occur
because insufficient preventive measures are taken, although
this does not raise any question of personal responsibility.
It simply means that the scientific community lacked the
information which would have made it possible to carry out
the preliminary analysis in sufficient depth.

The engineer should ensure that safety is never sacrificed
for the sake of routine. Everyone must be aware of the
problems and honestly informed of the hazards facing him.
The engineer's role is therefore to pass this information on
to the personnel and to top management so that the necessary
measures can be taken to improve safety.

The engineer should take time to think about safety, without
allowing it to become an obsession. All operations should be
considered in this spirit, and everyone involved in production and profit-making has a part to play.

Conclusions

In conclusion, safety cannot be regarded as a separate discipline like, for example, electronics or chemistry. It
implies rather an attitude towards one's behaviour in one's
private life and at the workplace. It would be impossible to
assign a safety specialist to every individual to think for
him. But every individual must be made sensitive to and
informed of the risks he is likely to encounter at work and
be prepared to adopt the attitudes needed to safeguard his
own health and that of other people. Because of their
function as coordinators and organisers, engineers provide a
particularly useful means of conveying information and of
organising safety measures. They should also be trained to
be receptive to these attitudes. Happily, there now appears

to be a greater awareness of safety problems, and training in industrial safety, which will one day no longer be optional, is now available in the engineers' training schools.

MULTIDISCIPLINARY APPROACH TO PREVENTION AND HEALTH
PROTECTION BY MONITORING: ROLE OF INDIVIDUAL DISCIPLINES.
THE ANALYTICAL CHEMIST: SAMPLE COLLECTION, METHODS AND
LIMITATIONS I

B. FALLENTIN (DENMARK)

Summary

Determination of pollutants in ambient air includes sampling, sample processing and analysis. The whole process may be carried out at the workplace, a sample of the ambient air may be transferred to the laboratory or a sample may be retained in solution or on absorbents. Relevant procedures and techniques are examined and discussed within this paper. Trends and needs are reviewed from the standpoints of the science and from practice in Member States of the European Community.

Introduction

The determination of pollutants in ambient air includes as other analytical procedures sampling, sample processing and analysis. No analytical procedure can give a true description of the composition of the material to be analysed unless the sample taken for analysis is representative of the material.

With ambient air as the material there is an inhomogeneous mixture with gaseous and particulate contaminants; there is a dynamic system with variable composition in time and space. This of course makes sampling very delicate. The variability with respect to time and space necessitates a well elaborated sampling strategy.

The questions where and when to sample have to be answered by the hygienist. But the questions how and even what to sample must involve the analytical chemist. Naturally, sampling strategy and sampling methods have to be coordinated.

In practice the sampling (or monitoring) of ambient air could be performed by three methods:

i) <u>Sampling and analysis at the workplace</u> The sampling and analysis are performed in one operation at the workplace by using the same direct reading field instruments which have to be calibrated at the laboratory.

ii) <u>Samples of ambient air transferred as such to the laboratory</u> A sample of the ambient air as such is collected in some suitable container and transferred to the laboratory for analysis.

iii) <u>Sampling through liquid or solid sorbents or filters</u> A measured volume of ambient air is sucked through a filtering or sorbing device, which retains the air contaminants. The contaminants thus collected are transferred to the laboratory for analysis. This type of sampling involves concentrating the contaminants.

Sampling and analysis at the workplace

In the early days very primitive methods were used for analysis "on the spot". For instance porcelain dishes containing a solution of palladium chloride were placed in work rooms for qualitative detection of carbon monoxide by reduction of palladious chloride to a finely devided block precipitate of metallic palladium. The same reagent was even used to prepare test papers for detection of carbon monoxide.

Test papers were developed for several gases. When used in adequate equipment the test paper method even allowed a semi quantitative determination in many cases.

Detector tubes

Much wider perspectives were however found in the use of reagents deposited on granules of silica gel or other suitable material.

Likewise this method is used for the determination of carbon monoxide in the hoolamite indicator. Hoolamite is a mixture of iodine pentoxide and fuming sulphuric acid on granular pumice stone (Patented by Hoover and Lamb 1919). The original white colour of the reagent changes by contact with carbon monoxide into bluish green to violet brown to black depending on the concentration of carbon monoxide.

The colour produced is compared with a standard colour scale and the indicator evaluated. Such evaluation is of course dependent upon the colour vision of the observer and the lighting conditions.

Today a great many detector tubes have been developed for the detection of numerous gases and vapours. Of the detector tubes used today the majority are based on the length colorimetric principle which should reduce the subjective factors in the evaluation. In these tubes a stain of variable length is produced according to gas concentration when a fixed volume of air is passed through the tube.

In the development of detector tubes there has been rather ingenious application of several chemical reactions. In some tubes preclensing layers are used for removing interfering substances. In other tubes two-step-reactions are involved which necessitate a special conversion layer before the indicating layer. The method has however its limitations. Detector tubes are very simple to use and they may be used by unskilled personnel. However many potential errors and pitfalls are inherent in the method. Therefore the sampling procedure has to be supervised and the results interpreted by an experienced hygienist.

Of course there will be many substances for which no detector tubes are available and mixtures where the use of detector tubes is not applicable. There may be limitations in the technique due to lack in sensitivity, specificity or precision. Another limiting factor is that the tubes normally are used in connection with a hand pump, which means a short sampling period. To overcome this problem special long term tubes have been developed for use with a battery driven pump which operates for up to 8 hours.

Direct reading physical instruments

Another type of sampling and analysis combined in one opera-tion and performed at the workplace is found in the direct reading instruments based on different physical principles.

One may assume that this type of analysis is not a matter of concern for the analytical chemist. Yet on the one hand analytical chemistry of today has for many years depended on physical methods; on the other hand the direct reading instruments need a careful calibration which may involve standardisation against other analytical methods.

It is not intended here to give a detailed description of instrumentation in this field but just to give a survey of different principles on which detection is based with some typical examples on instruments.

The thermal properties of a gas may be used for detection in a thermal conductivity cell or a thermal combustion cell as in the combustible gas detectors and explosimeters. The method is non-specific and generally of low sensitivity. More sensitive but even non-specific detectors are the photo-ionization detector and the flame ionization detector as used in total hydrocarbon analysers.

Photometry in the ultraviolet range is used for the detection of mercury vapour and ozone. Infrared analysers for carbon monoxide provide a selective detection by using gas filters. Likewise infrared spectrophotometry is used for determination of solvent vapours, and a high degree of selectivity is achieved by proper wavelength selection. Instruments based on chemiluminescence are available for determination of

nitrogen oxides based on their reaction with ozone. Similar
instruments for the determination of ozone are based on the
chemiluminescent reaction between ozone and ethylene.

Several other detecting principles are found in the variety
of direct reading instruments for determination of gases and
vapours; in addition there are the direct reading instruments
for the determination of particulate matters.

A special variety of air monitoring may be categorised as "on
the spot" analysis - the transfer of "the laboratory" to the
workplace as exemplified by the use of portable gas chromato-
graphs.

Samples of ambient air transferred as such to the laboratory

Under certain circumstances one could to advantage collect a
whole-air sample in a suitable container and transfer it to
the laboratory for analysis. In some cases this can provide
a useful opportunity for an orientating analysis of the air
contaminants present in an "untreated" sample. The method
could even be applied for the quantitative analysis of peak
concentrations. Containers used for collecting such "grab"
samples are gas sample tubes, bottles or bags. The sampling
is performed either by using evacuated containers which are
opened on the spot or by using displacement containers, e.g.
gas sample tubes provided with stopcocks in which the original air is displaced by drawing 10-15 times container volume
of ambient air through the container.

For the analyst the question is does the air sample in the
container have exactly the same composition as the ambient
air from which it is sampled, and if so for how long a time?

Deviations in composition may be due to container leak or
there may be losses of air contaminants due to adsorption on
container walls, or due to diffusion through container
material. Positive errors may arise from impurities given
off from the material of the container.

It is generally recognised that there is adsorption of constituents in air samples on the surface of glass walls. When we started to use gas sample tubes for sampling solvent vapours more than 20 years ago we observed losses immediately after filling. The remedy we used then was to heat the tube for desorption before transfer of a sample for gas chromatographic analysis.

When bags are used for sampling special care should be taken in respect of the choice of material. A variety of materials have been used for air sampling bags. Typical examples are PVC, polyester, different fluoroplastics, laminated plastics on aluminium foil etc. In each case the material has to be evaluated for the specific gas for which it is to be used. While rigid containers are normally used for grab samples, bags are preferred for integrated sampling over longer periods. For long term sampling in bags the ambient air is pumped into the bag by, for example, a battery driven pump. It is important to be aware of the possible contamination or losses due to the passage of the air sample through the pump.

Finally, mention should be made of a recently developed new type of whole-air sampler. It is a small evacuated container of 100 ml provided with a flow-limiting orifice at the air inlet. By regulation of the orifice a sampling time of 8 hours or more may be achieved.

Sampling through liquid or solid sorbents or filters

The most widespread methods used for accurate ambient air monitoring are those based on retention of the air pollutants. They are characterised by integrated sampling over longer periods and concentrating up the sampled pollutants.

Liquid absorbents

Sampling in liquid absorbents, with rather bulky and heavy
equipment, has been in use since the days of the early
industrial hygienists. Absorption of the air contaminants in
the liquid may be based on pure solution. Since gas or
vapour will never dissolve 100% in a liquid and to increase
retention efficiency a train of 2 or more liquid absorbers
in series, is often used.

Sampling efficiency may be increased dramatically by cooling
the absorbing liquid, e.g. by placing the absorbers in dry
ice. In other cases the absorption may be based on the use
of a reactive liquid, which retains the air contaminants by a
chemical reaction.

Some drawbacks in the use of liquid absorbers may be summarised:
- although spillproof absorbers exist the
  method is not well suited for personal sampling;
- the use of liquid may induce practical problems during sampling and shipping;
- there may be limitations in sampling capacity
  and sampling time due to evaporation of
  absorbent liquid;
- the dilution means that the method may not be
  sufficiently sensitive for determination of
  low concentrations.

On the other hand liquid samples are convenient for transfer
to analytical laboratory instruments.

Solid adsorbents

These days sampling in solid adsorbents is very often performed with the adsorbent placed in small tubes; this makes
the method very suited for personal sampling.

The most widely used adsorbent in air sampling is activated charcoal but a number of other materials are used including silica gel, alumina, molecular sieves, porous polymers and loaded gas chromatographic column fillings. It should be noted that gases and vapours tend to some degree to adhere on any solid surface; such adsorption is especially seen on porous solids.

Collection efficiency and break-through capacity are deciding factors for the choice of adsorbent. The break-through capacity for a given substance on a specific adsorbent is dependent on sampling rate, air concentration and relative humidity. The sample tubes often contain two sections of adsorbent, one primary section followed by a back-up section to indicate break-through.

Another factor of importance for the suitability of an adsorbent is the desorption efficiency. Normally the desorption may be achieved by solvent extraction or heat desorption although other methods have been used. Solvent extraction by carbon disulphide as solvent is most widely used for desorption from charcoal. By this method desorption efficiencies are reported from less than 50% up to 100% for different substances. Other solvents or solvent mixtures have been used for extraction; we are, for instance, using dimethylformamide in our laboratory.

In heat desorption the sample tube is placed in a flash heater and the desorbed compounds are swept directly into the analytical column of a gas chromatograph by the carrier gas. The advantage of this method is that no foreign substance is introduced and dilution of the trapped compound is thus avoided; this leads to higher sensitivity. A drawback is that only one analysis may be performed per sample.

As previously mentioned the use of small sample tubes with solid adsorbents makes the method extremely suited for personal sampling. A small portable battery driven pump draws

ambient air through the sample tube which is placed close to
the nose of the exposed worker. Typical sampling rates are
less than 1 l/min.

A recently developed personal sampler for organic vapours
does not use any pump at all but allows the vapours to
diffuse passively on to the adsorbent. The desorption is
then performed by solvent extraction.

Particulates

Particles may be collected by thermal precipitation, electro-
static precipitation or impaction. Sampling of particulates
on filters represents however the most versatile method.

Generally speaking the particulate sampling presents more
problems than gas or vapour sampling. The aerodynamic
conditions in the surrounding of the sampling head depending
on geometry and flow-rate play a deciding role in sampling
efficiency towards different particle sizes. For sampling
"total dust", i.e. all air borne particulates, an air velocity of 1.25 m/sec. at the inlet of the filter holder is
recommended.

For sampling respirable particles a preseparator e.g. a
cyclone is placed in front of the filter holder. Different
filter media are available: commonly used are membrane
(cellulose) filters and glass fibre filters. Small filters
(25 or 37 mm diameter) placed in light-weight filter holders
are convenient for personal sampling.

Analysis of samples

Any analytical procedure may include sample collection,
transport, storage, extraction, concentration, isolation,
identification and quantitation although there is not always
a clear-cut separation between all the steps.

When only the sample collection is located to the workplace then the next steps (transport and storage) may cause problems when volatile materials or reactive compounds are involved. Losses and contamination must be avoided, or at any rate minimised during sample processing. The processing of adsorbent tubes includes extraction - or heat desorption. Filter samples often require a destruction of organic matter with the risk of loss of products through volatilisation. This risk has to be reduced by suitable wet ashing or low temperature ashing (oxygen plasma).

For the final analytical determination of the components in the samples a multitude of analytical techniques are available but two methods dominate the field: gas chromatography and atomic absorption spectrophotometry.

Gas chromatography achieves in one operation separation, quantitation and to a large extent identification of the single components in a mixture and is applicable for a majority of organic air pollutants. For further identification if necessary gas chromatography may be combined with mass spectrometry or spectrophotometry of different kinds (IR, UV and fluorescence). Other chromatography techniques, especially high pressure liquid chromatography (HPLC), have been applied for analysis of organic pollutants e.g. polycyclic aromatic hydrocarbons (PAH). For determination of inorganic constituents (metals) atomic absorption spectrophotometry (AAS) has found general application.

Other methods used though not so wide-spread may be mentioned in this connection. They include anodic stripping voltametry, ion specific electrodes and X-ray fluorescence. For examination of the crystal structure of particles (e.g. quartz) X-ray diffraction is the main method. Particle geometry is examined by microscopy, and by combination of scanning electron microscopy and energy dispersive X-ray analysis it is possible to determine elements in single particles. In spite of a great variety of new analytical techniques classical procedures such as colorimetric methods are still in use and of application.

Trends and needs

The development of analytical techniques during the last decades has led to methods of high selectivity and sensitivities up to more orders of magnitude higher than previously known. Parallel to the development of analytical techniques there have been developments in sampling equipment and methods.

Looking into the future some promising analytical techniques applicable for ambient air monitoring come into view.

In the first place there is Inductively Coupled Plasma - Optical Emission Spectroscopy (ICP-OES) which permits multi-element determinations with low detection limits and very little matrix effect and in the second place, Ion Chromatography (IC) which is especially suited for the determination of anions.

Commonly, only elemental analyses have been performed on inorganic pollutants. It might be desirable with improving analytical procedures to obtain a more detailed chemical description including information on molecular structure, although the toxicological significance is not always clear. It must however be expected that there will be an interaction between analytical procedures and toxicology. As for analysis of particulate matter there might even be a need for information about the chemical composition of different particle size fractions.

Turning to sampling equipment the trend is clearly a development from bulky and heavy equipment to light-weight and small devices suitable for personal sampling.

Up to the late sixties, in Denmark, ambient air monitoring
practically always was performed as stationary sampling.
Since then personal sampling has taken over, and today
monitoring of workers' exposure whenever possible is performed by personal sampling.

It seems that the situation in the United Kingdom is very
much the same, whereas stationary sampling seems to be the
dominant method in France and in the Federal Republic of Germany. In the other member states of the European Community
personal sampling seems to be used to a varying extent.

By the selection of a method for environmental monitoring
including sampling and analysis the criteria are as for any
analytical procedure: specificity, sensitivity, precision and
accuracy. Efforts to achieve standardisation in this field
have been carried out. However, a problem with standardisation is that the procedure often leads to a standardisation
of the methods of yesterday. Perhaps it would be preferable,
in order not to restrain the development of new methods, to
make reference to recommended or validated methods.

In Denmark we have published guidelines for air monitoring
with reference to recognised sampling methods published by
the National Institute for Occupational Safety and Health
(NIOSH), D. Henschler ("Analytische Methoden zur Prufung
gesundheitschadliche Arbeitstoffe") and National Board of
Occupational Safety and Health, Sweden. (1-4) We intend to
elaborate these guidelines further in future.

In the Federal Republic of Germany a collection of approved
air sampling methods - as mentioned above - is published by a
working group under the MAK-commission. In France likewise
authorised methods are elaborated by the Institut National de
la Recherche sur la Securite (INRS). In the United Kingdom
the Health and Safety Executive is publishing recommended
methods for monitoring ambient air. In Belgium a standard
has to be followed when stationary air sampling is performed.

In spite of differences in methodology and in the legal
status of air monitoring in the member states there should be
a general interest in keeping a reasonable high quality of
such monitoring. With this in mind establishment of inter-
calibration of comparable methods at national and international level is strongly recommended.

References

1. Arbejdstilsynets vejledning om udforelse af arbejds-
   hygiejniske luftforureningsmalinger.
   Publikation nr. 87/1979.

2. NIOSH Manual of Analytical Methods, DHEW Publication,
   Cincinnati 1977 -.

3. Analytische Methoden zur Prufung gesundheitsschäd-
   licher Arbeitsstoffe. Bd. 1. Luftanalysen.
   D. Henschler: Deutsche Forschungsgemeinschaft/
   Arbeitsgruppe Analytisch Chemie.
   Verlag Chemie, Weinheim 1976.

4. Metodserien. Rapporter om bestämning av luftföro-
   reningar. Arbetarskyddsstyrelsen.
   Stockholm 1977.

MULTIDISCIPLINARY APPROACH TO PREVENTION AND HEALTH
PROTECTION BY MONITORING: ROLE OF INDIVIDUAL DISCIPLINES.
THE ANALYTICAL CHEMIST: SAMPLE COLLECTION, METHODS AND
LIMITATIONS II

R.H. BELL, G.R. SCHULTZ AND L.F. SEFTON (USA - OSHA)

Summary

*Most OSHA standards require the monitoring of worker chemical
exposure levels through the measurement of chemicals in the
ambient air of the worker's breathing zone. Biological monitoring is expected to become increasingly important as a tool
for evaluating worker exposure to chemicals.*

*Frequently, the OSHA chemist is involved in adapting chemical
methods or sampling techniques to OSHA's enforcement needs. A
sample storage stability problem for 2-butanone (MEK) was
solved to meet OSHA's needs by substituting silica gel for
charcoal as the adsorbent. A second sample storage stability
problem for hydrazine was solved by using Gas Chrom R coated
with sulphuric acid in place of silica gel coated with sulphuric acid as the adsorbent. A third problem was the development of analytical techniques specific to three benzidine-
based dyes. "Stop gap" analytical methods were developed
utilising paired-ion chromatography and separation by high
performance liquid chromatography for C.I. Direct Blue 6, C.I.
Direct Black 38, and C.I. Direct Brown 95. These examples
show the value of a close working relationship between the
analytical chemist and the industrial hygienist in solving
workplace sampling and analytical problems.*

Introduction

There are approximately 42,000 chemicals in the work environment; production exceeds one million pounds per year for
about 5,000 of these chemicals. According to Section 5(a)(1)
of the Occupational Safety Health Act (OSH Act) of 1970, the
employer is charged with the responsibility to "...furnish to
each of his employees employment and a place of employment
which are free from recognised hazards that are causing or
are likely to cause death or serious physical harm to his
employees." Enforcement of this charge is assigned to the
Occupational Safety and Health Administration (OSHA), an
Agency located in the United States Department of Labor.

OSHA Standards for chemicals

The OSH Act of 1970 was signed into law on December 29, 1970, and became effective on April 28, 1971. OSHA was permitted, for two years after the effective date of the OSH Act, to accept consensus standards and guidelines as regulations. These were produced by nationally recognised groups such as the American National Standards Institute (ANSI), the American National Fire Protection Association (NFPA), and the American Conference of Governmental Industrial Hygienists (ACGIH). Some 400 Threshold Limit Values (TLVs) for toxic chemicals were taken from ACGIH as OSHA Permissible Exposure Levels (PELs).

These PELs are listed in Tables Z-1 and Z-2 of the General Industry Standards, 29 CFR 1910.1000. The law requires that all new OSHA standards go through a public rule making procedure which is long and time consuming. It can take three or four years to promulgate a standard.

There is a provision of the OSH Act that permits the Agency to issue an Emergency Temporary Standard (ETS) when a hazard is so great that worker health is best served through immediate action. An ETS expires after six months and a permanent standard still must be produced. The ETS is valuable because it goes into effect immediately and worker exposure to a hazardous substance is minimised while a permanent standard is developed. It must be emphasisd that issuance of an ETS requires a major commitment of resources by the Agency because it still is necessary to proceed with the formal permanent standards setting process.

OSHA cannot set PELs for all of the chemicals in the workplace and for all of the new chemicals that will be introduced to the work environment. Regulations will be developed for some of these chemicals as hazards are identified. Others can be controlled by enforcement of the General Duty Clause of the OSH Act and will require support on a case-by-case basis.

Most standards for chemicals regulated by OSHA refer to air levels for monitoring worker exposure. Specific reference to biological monitoring of chemicals is made only in the more recent standards. For example, OSHA's new Lead Standard calls for medical removal protection for the worker based on blood lead levels. Biological monitoring will be incorporated where applicable, in future standards; however, it is unlikely that major revisions will be made to the existing standards because of the complexity of the required regulatory process.

OSHA's analytical laboratory

OSHA's Analytical Laboratory is located in Salt Lake City, Utah. Approximately 70,000 chemical samples are analysed in this laboratory each year. These samples are submitted to the laboratory as a result of OSHA compliance inspections throughout the United States. OSHA does not have specific responsibility under the OSH Act to develop methods for chemical sampling and analytical procedures. For the most part, methods for chemical analysis are developed by the National Institute for Occupational Safety and Health (NIOSH) - OSHA's sister agency for research established in Section 22 of the OSH Act. Although methods for chemical analysis are developed by NIOSH, the Salt Lake City Analytical Laboratory (SLCAL) of OSHA often adapts these methods to fit OSHA's field compliance needs and activities. If NIOSH has not developed a method for a given chemical then OSHA chemists generate "stop-gap" analytical methods. A "stop-gap" method is one that is developed by SLCAL to meet a given compliance activity and the method remains in effect for OSHA until NIOSH issues a replacement or a superior method becomes available. In 1979, OSHA revised methods for 30 chemicals and generated "stop gap" methods for another 50.

Discussion

An analytical chemist is often stereotyped as a person in a white laboratory coat, pipette in hand, working laboriously over seve-

ral test tubes filled with chemicals. The modern OSHA analytical chemist has many and varied responsibilities beyond
those of the stereotype. The analysis of chemical sample is
just one phase of work for an OSHA chemist. Participation in
court hearings, lecturing at the OSHA Training Institute, and
serving on various intra and interagency committees fill the
professional's busy schedule. The chemist plays an integral
part in the collection of ambient air samples by the industrial hygienist. In many cases, the sample collection method
used by the industrial hygienist has been adapted by the
laboratory chemist specifically for the requirements of a
given field problem. It is essential that the chemist and
industrial hygienist understand and appreciate each other's
problems. Because the industrial hygienist depends on the
chemist for providing the most convenient and proper sample
collection methods, there must be close communication between
the two. Only through this effective working relationship
can the chemist properly assist the industrial hygienist.

A sample collection method must meet two basic requirements:
it must satisfy the needs of the industrial hygienist and it
must be compatible with the method of analysis used in the
laboratory. These two requirements are best met by a chemist
who considers such things as collection efficiency, capacity
of the adsorbent, recovery efficiency, and storage stability.

The chemist has many alternatives for the development of a
sample collection method because of the wide variety of
adsorbents, filters, and bubbler solutions available.
Adsorbents may be considered for gases and vapours while
filters may be more adaptable to the collection of aerosols.
A combination of an adsorbent tube and a filter may achieve
the desired results for an analyte with both vapour and
aerosol components. Passive monitors are available that
utilise adsorbents and do not require sampling pumps.

Chemists at the OSHA laboratory are constantly confronted
with developing and improving sample collection methods.

The following three examples represent recent method modifications by OSHA chemists:

2-Butanone (Methyl ethyl ketone)

A storage stability problem was identified with the well established method for collecting methyl ethyl ketone (MEK) on charcoal adsorbent followed by desorption with carbon disulphide for analysis of MEK by gas chromatography. The breakthrough of MEK on charcoal was studied. It was found that 5 percent breakthrough occurred at 60.2 minute when the concentration was 1176 mg/m^3 at 80 percent relative humidity with a sample flow rate of 0.1 l per minute. A study of storage stability revealed that the percent recovery of MEK on charcoal dropped from about 85 percent to about 52 percent over 16 days at room temperature. Similar sample storage results were obtained with either coconut shell or petroleum based charcoal.

A number of adsorbents were evaluated and silica gel was found to provide adequate capacity (5 percent breakthrough at 29.5 minute with a sample concentration of 1174 mg/m^3 at 80 percent relative humidity and at a sample flow rate of 0.1 l per minute.); good storage stability was demonstrated by a constant 98 percent recovery of MEK through 16 days when dimethylsulphoxide was used for desorption. The storage stability test was carried out at an MEK concentration of 531 mg/m^3 at 80 percent relative humidity. All samples were stored at room temperature. These factors are summarised in Table 1.

```
┌─────────────────────────────────────────────────────────────────┐
│ Table 1:   Comparison of MEK Sampling Procedures                │
│                                                                  │
│                         Charcoal - CS₂        Silica Gel-DMSO   │
│ Breakthrough capacity    7.1 mg               3.5 mg            │
│ Desorption efficiency    85%                  96%               │
│ Storage stability        85% (day 1)          98%               │
│                          to 52% (day 16)                        │
│                                                                  │
└─────────────────────────────────────────────────────────────────┘
```

Table 1: Comparison of MEK Sampling Procedures

	Charcoal - CS_2	Silica Gel-DMSO
Breakthrough capacity	7.1 mg	3.5 mg
Desorption efficiency	85%	96%
Storage stability	85% (day 1) to 52% (day 16)	98%

All chemical samples collected by OSHA's industrial hygienists are sent to SLCAL for analysis. Thus, storage stability
of the collected samples was considered to be the critical
factor in adopting the silica gel collection method for MEK
by OSHA. Although the capacity of the silica gel to adsorb
MEK is much less than that of charcoal, it is adequate to
give a sufficiently low detection limit. This work illustrates the factors to be balanced by the chemist to arrive at
the most suitable sampling procedure.

Hydrazine

A storage stability problem was reported (1) with the proposed NIOSH method for collection and analysis of hydrazine.
(2) Sample collection involved the use of sulphuric acid
coated silica gel as the adsorbent. As much as 89 percent of
a sample was reported to be lost by the third day of storage.
A temporary solution to the problem was to have the industrial hygienist desorb the acid coated silica gel immediately
after sample collection since the desorbed solution was
reported to be stable. (1) Our industrial hygienists found
this procedure to be inconvenient. A new sample collection
method was adapted from a procedure developed by U.S. Air
Force (USAF) personnel ("Hydrazine in Air," USAF Method by
USAF School of Aerospace Medicine, Brooks Air Force Base, San
Antonio, Texas) which uses Gas Chrom R, a gas chromatography
support, coated with sulphuric acid as the adsorbent. The
storage stability of hydrazine on acid coated Gas Chrom R was

found to be very good; recovery remained above 90 percent for a period of 14 days. These efforts resulted in a new and improved "stop gap" sampling method for hydrazine.

Benzidine and benzidine-based dyes

OSHA issued an ETS on benzidine in 1973 followed by a permanent standard in 1974. Benzidine-based dyes are defined as those that contain benzidine attached to other substituents by diazo linkages. No mention of benzidine-based dyes was made in the standard. In 1978, the National Cancer Institute (NCI) published the results of a 13-week subchronic feeding study of C.I. (Colour Index) Direct Blue 6, C.I. Direct Black 38, and C.I. Direct Brown 95. (3,4) Two of these benzidine-based dyes induced both hepatic neoplastic nodules and hepatocellular carcinomas in male and female rats. The NCI bioassay for these dyes included analyses of urine samples for benzidine. Benzidine was detected in the urine of all the rats monitored. Analyses of the dyes prior to administration demonstrated no residual or contaminating benzidine. Studies with other benzidine-based dyes in a variety of animals (5,6,7) and tissues (8,9) revealed that biological conversion of the dyes to benzidine had occurred. NIOSH and NCI published a Current Intelligence Bulletin in 1978 as a result of the NCI bioassay results on C.I. Direct Blue 6, C.I. Direct Black 38, and C.I. Direct Brown 95.(4) NIOSH published a "Special Occupational Hazard Review for Benzidine-Based Dyes" in 1980. (10) OSHA issued an enforcement instruction to its field staff in 1980 with guidelines to follow when issuing citations under section 5(a)(1) of the OSH Act, and pertinent standards of a general nature, for employee exposure to Direct Black 38, Direct Brown 95, and Direct Blue 6 benzidine-based dyes. (11) NIOSH and OSHA are in the process of jointly issuing a Health Hazard Alert on "Benzidine-, o-Tolidine-, and o-Dianisidine-Based Dyes." The alert is informational and contains recommendations and several actions that should be taken by employers, employees, and their physicians in order to protect workers from exposure to the dyes.

The process as described is a typical one for the development
and reporting of toxicity data for a chemical or set of
chemicals. In this case the basic chemical, benzidine, was
covered by an OSHA standard, but dyes derived from the basic
material were not. Thus, these dyes became part of the some
40,000 chemicals in the workplace not covered by specific
standards. OSHA determined that the data base for three of
the benzidine-derived dyes (C.I. Direct Black 38, C.I. Direct
Brown 95, and C.I. Direct Blue 6) was sufficient to recommend
guidelines for the issuance of citations to employers who did
not provide a safe and healthy workplace for employees. This
action created immediate responsibilities for the OSHA
chemists. The existing NIOSH analytical method was for dia-
zonium salts and azo dyes in air. (12) It was not specific
to the three benzidine-based dyes in question. OSHA chemists
were requested to devise sampling methods for air and wipe
samples, to develop analytical methods specific to each of
the three dyes, and to verify the reliability of a test for
benzidine in urine since benzidine was reported as a metabolite of the dyes.

Paper, glass fibre, and polytetrafluoroethylene filters were
used to collect wipe samples. Desorption of the benzidine-
based dyes from the Whatman paper filters was found to be
inadequate. Glass fibre filters and polytetrafluoroethylene
were found to have better desorption characteristics than
paper with the glass fibre filters the better of the two.
Glass fibre filters were recommended for collection of both
wipe and air samples. An air flow rate of 1 l/minute with an
air volume of 100 l to 300 l was recommended for collection
of air samples.

High performance liquid chromatography was chosen as the
vehicle for the "stop-gap" method. C.I. Direct Blue 6, C.I.
Direct Black 38, and C.I. Direct Brown 95 are ionic in character; they are all sodium salts. The technique of paired-
ion chromatography was used for analysis of these dyes.
Paired-ion chromatography incorporates the use of a large

organic ion of opposite charge to the ionic ultraviolet or visible absorbing species so that the resulting "ion-pair" can be retained on a reverse-phase liquid chromatographic column. The ion is incorporated into the mobile phase of the liquid chromatograph. Tetraethylammonium phosphate was the ion of choice. The dyes were separated with high performance liquid chromatography through the use of solvent programming. Detection was at 546 nm and 436 nm using a dual wavelength detector. Different retention times were observed for each of the dyes.

An analysis for benzidine in urine was developed using a literature method for another aromatic amine as a starting point. (13) The method consisted of ether extraction of urine followed by high performance liquid chromatogrpahy analysis with fluorescence detection for benzidine.

Acknowledgement

The authors thank Ronald J. Freking, David C. Armitage, John M. Linkletter, and Carl J. Elskamp of the OSHA Salt Lake City, Utah Analytical Laboratory for their assistance and support in preparing this paper.

Mention of company names, or products does not constitute endorsement by the Occupational Safety and Health Administration.

References

1. National Institute for Occupational Safety and Health, NIOSH Manual of Analytical Methods, Vol.1, 2nd ed., Method No. P & CAM 248 Hydrazine Compounds in Air, April 1977 (DHEW Publication No. 77-157-A).

2. Cook, L.R., Glenn, R.E., and Podolak, G.E. Monitoring and analysis of personnel exposure to hydrazine at a rocket propellant plant. Am. Ind. Hyg. Assoc. J. 1979: 40: 69-74.

3. Joint NIOSH/NCI Current Intelligence Bulletin 24, Direct
    Blue 6, Direct Black 38, Direct Brown 95 Benzidine-
    derived Dyes. DHEW (NIOSH) Publication No. 78-148.
    1978.

4. 13-Week Subchronic Toxicity Studies of Direct Blue 6,
    Direct Black 38, and Direct Brown 95 Dyes.
    Carcinogenesis Technical Report. NCI DHEW Publication
    No. (NIH) 78-1358. 1978.

5. Rind, E. and Troll, W. Metabolic Reduction of Benzidine
    Azo Dyes to Benzidine in the Rhesus Monkey. J. Nat'l.
    Cancer Inst. 1975:55:181-182.

6. Lynn, R.K., Danielson, D.W., Ilias, A.M., Wong, K.,
    Kennish, J.M. and Matthews H.B. (1980). Metabolism of
    bis azobiophenyl dyes derived from benzidine, 3,3'-
    dimethylbenzidine or 3,3'-dimethoxybenzidine to carcino-
    genic aromatic amines in dog and rat. Toxicol. Appl.
    Pharmacol. 56 2 248-58 (1980).

7. Genin, V. Formation of Blastomogenic Diphenyl Amine
    Derivatives as a Result of Direct Azo Dye Metabolism.
    Vopr. Onkol: 1977: 23: 50-52.

8. Yoshida, O. and Miyakawa, M. Etiology of Bladder
    Cancer: "Metabolic" Aspects. In: Analytical and
    Experimental Epidemiology of Cancer (Nakahara, W. and
    Hirayoma, T. eds.) Baltimore, University Park Press,
    1973: 31-39.

9. Korosteleva, T., Skachkov, A., Scvaydestskiy, I.
    Detection of carcinogen-protein Antigens in serum from
    workers exposed to aniline dyes. Gig. Tr. Prof. Zabol.
    1974: 5: 21-24.

10. Special Hazard Review of Benzidine-Based Dyes. NIOSH
    Report. DHEW (NIOSH) Publication No. 80-109. 1980.

11. OSHA Instruction CPL 2-2.27, Benzidine-Based Dyes:
    Direct Black 38, Direct Brown 95, Direct Blue 6 Dyes,
    February 22, 1980.

12. National Institute for Occupational Safety and Health,
    NIOSH Manual for Analytical Methods, Vol. 1, 2nd ed.,
    Method No. P & CAM 234 Diazonium Salts and Azo Dyes
    in Air, April 1977 (DHEW Publication No. 77-157-A).

13. Linch, A.L., O'Connor, G.B., Barnes, J.R., Killian,
    A.S., Neeld, W.E. Methylene-bis-
    orthochloroaniline (MOCA): Evaluation of hazards and
    exposure control. Am. Ind. Hyg. Assoc. J. 1971: 12:
    802-819.

MULTIDISCIPLINARY APPROACH TO PREVENTION AND HEALTH PROTECTION
BY MONITORING: ROLE OF INDIVIDUAL DISCIPLINES. THE ECONOMIST:
ECONOMIC ANAYLSIS OF PREVENTION AND PROTECTION I.

L.B. LAVE AND E. CALLISON (USA)

Summary

*It is recognised that the elimination of all risk is imposs-
ible; the goal has to be optimum safety. This can be defined
by classical economics from the standpoint of determination
of risk being left to the market place. Several objections
to this concept are discussed. The role of biological
monitoring is examined as a bargaining, decision-making and
litigation tool for employees, employers and unions;
monitoring of benzene is used as an example.*

Optimizing worker health

"..... no employee will suffer material impairment of health or functional capacity even if
such employee has regular exposure to the
hazard dealt with by such standard for the
period of his working life (1)."

This is an ideal to inspire the public and win elections, but
it is a pernicious guide to action. The point of debunking
this rhetoric is not to chastise politicians or force us to
change our moral principles; we all suffer loss whenever a
worker is hurt or made ill. Rather, this is a plea for a
more helpful guide to action. With a proper statement of the
social goal, much of the current confusion concerning
occupational safety in the United States would disappear and
a clearer plan for action would emerge.

The Supreme Court recently stated the obvious: The
elimination of all risk, even of all risk in the workplace,
is impossible; zero risk is not a relevant goal (2). All
human activity involves risk. The individual, and society,
can reject some risks, but must be prepared to accept others.

The goal is not absolute safety, but rather "optimum safety".
Two principles can be used to elaborate this concept. The
first principle is that, from society's standpoint, an activity should be undertaken only if its output good or service
outweighs the health and other risks. For example, some old
coal mines around Pittsburgh recently were being reworked by
taking the coal used in pillars to support the roof; clearly,
the risk exceeds the social value of this output, at least
under normal circumstances. The second principle is that
resources ought to be directed to lowering risk until they
are no longer productive, i.e., until diminishing productivity of safety resources has fallen to the level where the
social value of a reduction in occupational disease is just
equal to the cost of achieving it.

The above paragraph used a number of loaded phrases, such as
the "social value of reduction in occupational disease" and
the "social value of output". Defining these concepts requires valuing risk (which risks are acceptable?) and equity
(do those who must bear a risk benefit from it?). Individuals disagree about these values and society must decide on
the mechanisms for resolving these conflicts. Resolving
value conflicts is one of the most important political
tasks.

One major proposal for defining optimum risk comes from
classical economics (3,4). Assuming that people can be
informed and are capable of making decisions for themselves,
economics emphasises presenting each worker with information
on the implications of various decisions, but then leaving
the determination of risk to the market place. Employers and
workers, through millions of small decisions, would determine
the risk-wage trade-offs to be offered and individual workers
would select their preferred trade-offs. This framework
emphasises efficiency of resource allocation and, under a set
of standard assumptions, can be shown to lead to a solution
which maximizes efficiency while giving workers their
preferred choice (within their available choice set).

The economic solution is regarded sceptically for a number of reasons. The first is that legislation would be required prohibiting risks above some level, just as in some countries suicide is illegal.

A second objection is that workers are not capable of making decisions involving risk (5). Such an objection is in direct conflict with the vast freedom of choice given individuals to behave in ways that society considers dubious. Society is curiously inconsistent: We allow alcohol, but not drugs. In the USA we allow individuals to subject themselves to risk by riding motorcycles without helmets and by smoking ciga-rettes, but we prohibit employers from offering jobs that have a similar level of risk. Economists search for consist-ency and object that, since we cannot and do not want to stop individuals from taking high risks in some activities, we ought to allow them to determine their own risk level in all activities. This plea to rationality and consistency is often lost on practitioners.

The third objection is that individuals with different back-grounds and levels of talent face different choices. Risky, dirty jobs generally fall to the poorest persons, whose alternatives are most limited. We who earn comfortable incomes in non-risky jobs can neither assume that the poor who take risky jobs are happy to do so, nor that their acceptance of the jobs is socially equitable. We must also be careful not to assume our preferences for risk apply to others, which is clearly contradicted by the recreational activities of many of these workers.

In some cases there are no opportunities for low risk employ-ment within a community, for example in a coal mining community, and the worker must leave if he rejects the risk. However, for most cases in the developed countries, there are many opportunities for non-hazardous employment within the community. As a rule, jobs with higher risks have higher pay and are taken by those who are less afraid and more influenc-

ed by income. This would be true, even if income levels were
ten times as high as today, although it is doubtful that jobs
as risky as those with the highest risks today would still be
accepted.

Even if one rejects this never-never-land of economic theory,
it is important to understand that people desire social goals
to be achieved efficiently and at low cost; they desire
safety and high consumption. Thus, analysis is needed to
clarify the implications of alternative approaches and to
find ways to accomplish our goals more efficiently. This
requires quantification and estimation of social benefits and
costs of each proposal. Analysis can be used to set
priorities, standards, and to allocate resources for
enforcement, but there are many areas requiring further
thinking, including the treatment of uncertainty.

The role of biological monitoring

The current system of regulating and managing occupational
risk is unsatisfactory in dealing with a number of problems.
Can an acceptable protective device be made? How good should
maintenance be? Should production be shut down when the
protective equipment breaks down? What should be done about
"hot spots" and periodic excursions? Whatever the rules of
the Occupational Safety and Health Administration (OSHA), or
even of the parent company, answers to most of these questions are currently worked out at a plant or subplant level
with little or no knowledge about the health implications.
Biological monitoring would provide decisions, presumably
with sufficient speed that health effects could be avoided.
The reason for using a toxic substance in the workplace is
that it lowers costs in producing a particular good or
enhances satisfaction from producing a more desirable good.
However, using it increases the risk or actual incidence of
disease. In order to retain the advantages of the former
while lowering the costs of the latter, we attempt to lower
worker exposure. The current methods are either to formulate

a standard which is believed to be protective or to select the most stringent standard which doesn't threaten the existence of the industry.

Uncertainty arises both in environmental monitoring and in the selection of a level believed to be harmless. Current safety standards are usually stated in terms of concentrations in air (or water, etc.); uncertainties in monitoring concentrations lead to the building in of a substantial safety factor to account for variations over time and location. Biological monitoring could eliminate this safety factor by measuring exposure directly, thus lowering uncertainty about variations in time and space.

A second large safety factor is encountered in setting an exposure level deemed to be safe. Little evidence is available that would provide confident estimates of what constitutes a safe level of exposure, or even of the level of damage that might be expected at each level. This safety factor could be eliminated by biological monitoring in cases where there is a precursor of serious disease that is a strong indication of future trouble, but is itself reversible or at least not a significant health problem. As long as a worker manifests no sign of ill-health or of the precursors to disease, exposure would be considered satisfactory. If no precursor exists and the first noticeable condition is serious and non-reversible, biological monitoring might still be used to stop the disease from progressing, but this stage is too late to be able to ignore other indicators, such as biological indications of dose.

These two types of biological monitoring, obtaining better indications of exposure and discovering precursors of disease, could do much to lower the cost of controlling the toxic substance and to lower the incidence of occupational disease. Biological monitoring might be more or less expensive than current ambient monitoring, although comprehensive monitoring of each employee at risk would presumably be more expensive.

The major point about both types of biological monitoring is that they are more direct measurements of the point of concern: the actual exposure of each worker and the precursors of disease. Not only is it more intellectually satisfying to measure the issues of interest, but there is the possibility of lower costs and better health. If we had confidence in biological monitoring, we could rescind emissions or ambient standards, except possibly for standards designed to prevent acute effects. Ambient standards would be redundant and less satisfactory than the standards for biological monitoring. More importantly, setting the biological standards would provide the maximum incentives for industry to find ways of lowering occupational disease at least cost. If satisfactory personal protection devices could be developed, they would prove their merit through the biological monitoring. If workers refused to wear the device, or the device wasn't reliable, it would become evident in the monitoring. Industry would be free to find the cheapest way of lowering the incidence of disease be that by substituting a compound or lowering emissions.

Currently, there is a debate as to whether a company can meet exposure standards by removing workers after they have reached the permitted level of exposure. Biological monitoring provides a more satisfactory way of dealing with this question. Work rules are suspected of giving insufficient protection; however, biological monitoring would give a better indication of whether they were protective of worker health.

An important advantage of biological monitoring is the direct information it would give about dose and biological changes indicative of disease. Armed with this information, the individual worker and his union could make more intelligent decisions. If workers desired lower exposure, they could negotiate this at collective bargaining. If individuals found the resulting biological changes intolerable, they could insist on changing jobs, even at the cost of quitting their jobs. This biological information would be invaluable in civil suits, both to establish an employee's claim and to protect the employer from false claims.

There is a fundamental difficulty in determining how much of the dose and change in physiology is due to the occupational exposure. For example, a worker being tested for benzene exposure might have received a substantial dose while filling his automobile on the way to work. Biological monitoring for chronic respiratory disease could not discern what part of the effect was due to smoking habits and other non-occupational causes. Statistical analysis could attempt to discern the contribution of other factors (by contrasting workers who smoked with those who did not for example, but uncertainty would remain. If the employer were deemed to be responsible for all adverse effects, employers would insist on excluding workers who smoked or were at higher risk for whatever reason (5). Present standards are enforced via fines, civil suit, or eventually forcing plant closure (3,5,7). Current fines are small and are not an effective deterrent (3,5); higher fines have been proposed, some of which have been upheld by the courts, and could prove effective (1). Litigation is cumbersome, expensive, and filled with difficulties and uncertainty. Plant closure is such an extreme measure that it is not an effective deterrent. To these enforcement devices for biological monitoring might be added the forced removal of a worker to less risky sites. Such forced changes in work rules might serve as the most effective deterrent, since a plant could run out of workers to perform crucial jobs.

Alternative enforcement procedure would levy a series of fines depending on the dose that each worker had received. For example, in monitoring for benzene by testing phenol in urine, the level of fines could be related to phenol concentration as shown in Figure 1, where the fine gets prohibitive at higher concentrations.

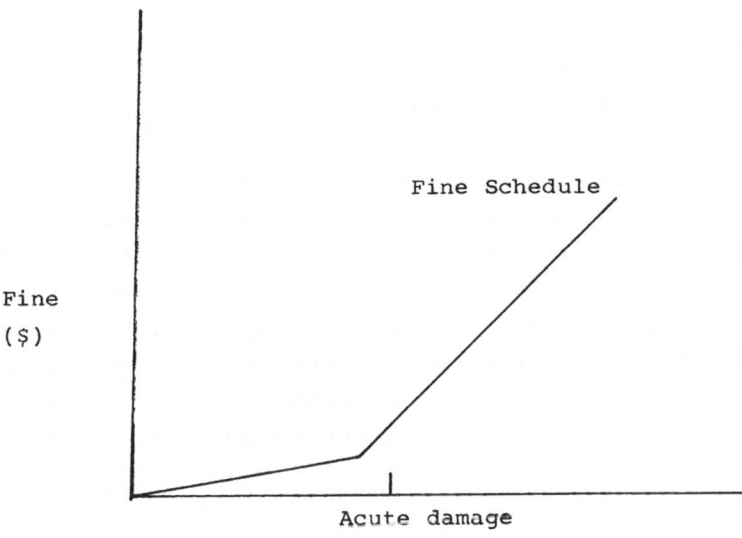

Figure 1.   Sample fines for phenol in urine

Benzene case study

Benzene is a clear, aromatic liquid used widely in industry
and commercial products (2,8). Chronic exposure to several
hundred parts per million of benzene in air has been fouond
to cause haematological disorders, including pancytopenia and
mylogenous leukaemia; there is some indication of effects at
exposures down to perhaps 10 ppm. Occupational exposure is
regulated, and there are proposed regulations for the general
population in the United States (9,10).

Ambient air concentration, currently used to measure exposure, is not a good indication of the dose received by individual workers; concentrations vary markedly depending on the
precise location of the air being sampled. A personal dosimeter might capture the relevant concentration during a short
time period, but can account for neither variations over time
nor the volume of air breathed (which varies with exertion
level). A continuous monitoring device corrects for the
first problem but not the second. More important is the
tenuous link between ambient concentration and haematological
disorders, since susceptibility differs among individuals.

Two methods of biological monitoring, measurement of benzene in exhaled air and of phenol in urine, provide better indications of individual dose (11,12,13). Monitoring exhaled air is easy and cheap, with few risks of laboratory or subject error. However, the physiological mechanisms which eliminate benzene through exhalation make the time of sampling crucial. Immediately after exposure, exhaled benzene comes largely from resevoirs in the air sacs in the lung and then from benzene in the blood. After perhaps ten hours, benzene stored in fatty tissue (which is more likely to indicate harmful exposure) becomes the predominant source of that being exhaled.

Benzene is metabolised by the liver, with phenol as the major oxidative product (13). This phenol is conjugated as phenyl-sulphate and excreted in the urine within 24 hours. Phenol concentration in urine is linearly related to benzene exposure. A fairly easy, reproducible method of measuring phenol exists, but its accuracy has been challenged (12,14, 15). Unfortunately, varying amounts of phenol are present in the urine due to other sources such as foods and drugs (13, 16).

While neither monitoring exhaled air nor urine involves invasive procedures, both require worker compliance and are likely to be resented as invasions of privacy. These methods are improvements over ambient air sampling in estimating total dose, although neither focuses on the adverse effects of benzene. Since health is the concern, it should be measured directly by counting blood cells and searching for irregularities. Several methods focused on blood disorders have been proposed. However, a major drawback is the necessity for taking frequent blood samples. Unfortunately, by the time blood disorders are observed, substantial harm has already been inflicted. A complication is that benzene's effects cannot be distinguished from those due to other causes.

Biological monitoring of the harm caused by benzene is not practical at present. Monitoring urine or exhaled air can be an improvement over ambient air monitoring for estimating total dose. The measurement of phenol in urine appears to be the best method for biological monitoring at present.

Information and costs are the primary considerations in deciding among monitoring techniques. Where one technique gives the same information at lower cost or more information at the same cost, decision is easy. Where techniques differ both with respect to information and cost, an examination of the value of the information is necessary. A useful comparison between the costs of ambient and biological monitoring can only be made if the methods yield comparable information, i.e., both yield information on exposure. When the biological monitoring technique measures health effects, as blood monitoring does for benzene exposure, a comparison of its cost with that of ambient monitoring means little.

In estimating the total cost of a monitoring programme, there are a number of costs which must be considered. For ambient monitoring, the estimate must include the capital cost of the equipment, technician labour, equipment maintenance, and materials costs. The cost estimate for biological monitoring must include the costs of technician labour and record-keeping as well as laboratory costs.

Since ambient monitoring and urinary phenol analysis yield the same type of information, i.e., the exposure level, their costs can be compared. The firm's cost of owning and operating a continuous benzene sampler is in the range of $20,000 - $30,000 per year (17). Assuming 35 employees per plant are routinely exposed to benzene (18), the cost per year of urine analysis is approximately $40,000 for one sample per week and $200,000 for five samples per week (18). These costs may be high as they use a laboratory fee which is not based on techniques mass analysis. However, continuous ambient monitoring would probably remain the least costly method for measuring exposure to benzene.

The cost estimates for blood monitoring, the only technique to measure the health of benzene, are based on a sampling frequency of one per week. This may be too frequent depending on how much blood is taken and from where. Also people vary in their ability to have blood taken on a frequent basis; for some it may not be possible to take blood nearly that frequently. Based on 35 employees routinely exposed and blood sampling once a week, the cost of blood monitoring is approximately $30,000 per year.

For benzene, ambient monitoring provides comparable data at lower cost than testing phenol in urine. Monitoring blood provides additional data that might spot disease at a stage where it could be reversed, or at least arrested. The greater cost of monitoring blood is justified only if the information on irregularities would have a large effect in lowering disease incidence, given high quality ambient monitoring.

The best route to take in monitoring occupational exposure to benzene may well be the use of continuous ambient monitoring in conjunction with a less frequent routine blood monitoring.

References

1. The Occupational Safety and Health Act of 1970. Public Law 91-596. Passed on December 19, 1970.

2. Supreme Court of the United States. Industrial Union Department, AFL-CIO v. American Petroleum Institute et al. No. 78-911. Argued October 10, 1979. Decided July 2, 1980.

3. Smith RS. The Occupational Safety and Health Act. Washington,D.C. : American Enterprise Institute for Public Policy Research, 1976.

4. Thaler, R., Rosen S. The Value of Saving a Life: Evidence from the Labor Market. In: Terleckyj NE ed, Household production and consumption, Washington, D.C. : National Bureau of Economic Research, 1976: 25-98.

5. Ashford, N.A. Crisis in the workplace: occupational disease and injury. Cambridge, M.A. : The MIT Press, 1976.

6. For example, see the Johns Mansfield rule regarding employment of smokers in their asbestos plant.

7. Economic report of the President, 1976. Washington, D.C. : Government Printing Office, 1976.

8. Bartman, T. Benzene. Working paper, Carnegie-Mellon University.

9. 43, Federal Register 5918 (February 10, 1978).

10. 43, Federal Register 29332 (June 9, 1977).

11. Sherwood, R.J. Benzene: The Interpretation of Monitoring Results. Ann. Occup. Hyg., 1972; 15:409-21.

12. Sherwood, R.J., Carter, F.W.G. The measurement of occupational exposure to benzene vapor. Ann. Occup. Hyg. 1970; 13: 125-46.

13. Walkley, J.E., Pagnotto, L.D., Elkins, H.B. The measurement of phenol in urine as an index of benzene exposure. Ind. Hyg. J. 1961; 22: 362-7.

14 Rusch, G.M., Leong, B.K.J., Laskin, S. Benzene metabolism. J. Toxicol. and Environ. Health 1977; supp. 2: 23-26.

15. Docter, H.J., Zielhuis, R.L. Phenol excretion as a measure of benzene exposure. Ann. Occup. Hyg. 1967; 10: 317.

16. Volterra, M. Urinary phenols II. Their significance in normal and pathological conditions. Amer. J. Clin. Path. 1942; 12: 580-7.

17. Personal communication with Bendix Corporation.

18. Occupational Safety and Health Administration. Economic impact statement: Benzene vol. II. Washington, D.C. : U.S. Department of Labor, 1977.

MULTIDISCIPLINARY APPROACH TO PREVENTION AND HEALTH PROTECTION
BY MONITORING: ROLE OF INDIVIDUAL DISCIPLINES. THE ECONOMIST:
ECONOMIC ANALYSIS OF PREVENTION AND PROTECTION II.

P.B. MEYER (THE NETHERLANDS)

Summary

*Economics has often been defined as the science which stu-
dies the problems connected with the distribution of scarce
resources. The potential to perform measurements in occupational hygiene is such a scarce resource. In a number of
examples based on problems of air pollution at the workplace
- which can be generalised easily to other problems in occupational hygiene - it is shown how cost calculations can be
used to formulate measuring strategies which from the point
of view of available resources try to attain an optimum.*

Introduction

"The philosophical significance of money is that
it represents within the practical world the most
certain image and the clearest embodiment of the
formula of all being, according to which things
receive their meaning through each other and
having their being determined by their mutual
relations.
G. Simmel The Philosophy of Money (1900)

During the last decades increasingly sophisticated measuring
instruments have been developed which can provide us with
detailed information on agents in our environment, which
might be a potential risk to health and wellbeing. Some of
these instruments are used to monitor the environment of the
working place. Before going into the cost aspects of these
measuring systems, it might be useful to mention a number of
criteria which have an important impact on this magnitude.
These criteria are:

- what has to be measured;
- what should be the sensitivity, the repeatability, the reproducibility, the accuracy and the
  dynamic properties of the instrument (band
  width) (see Appendix I);
- how often (frequency), how long and where (at
  how many locations) should measurements be
  carried out.

More trivial factors in this connection are: the money which
has to be invested in a measuring system, reliability of the
system, personnel cost and interest rates. They all will
influence the choice of measurement techniques and overall
costs of a monitoring programme.

Discussion

Assuming that the yearly costs of such a system can be presented
in the following way.

$$c_j = a_j \left(I - \sum_{j=1}^{j-1} I_j \right) + I_j + M + V$$

yearly costs due to amortisation
in year j + loss of interest due
to the investment in the year j

c_j = yearly costs in year j;
a_j = rate of interest in year j;
I = investment;
I_j = amortisation of investment in year j;
M = costs of yearly maintenance;
V = variable costs.

Variable costs are often at first approximation a linear function of production which in this case are the number of
measurements, e.g. this might stand for human effort if the
system is not automated.

The parameters affecting the cost equation can vary widely. As an example the costs of determining gravimetric concentrations of particles in air by an operator and by an automatic system are compared (figure 1).

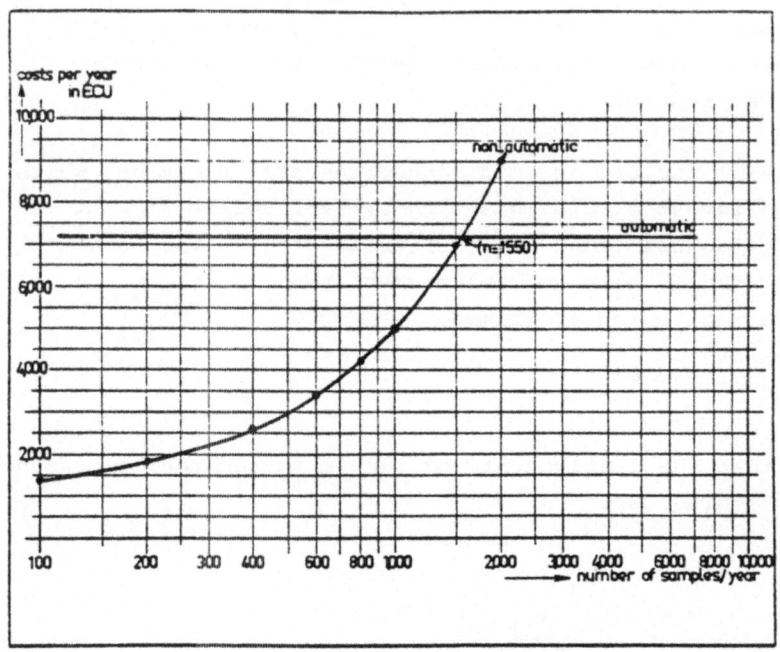

Figure 1. Costs of the determination of particle concentrations in air as a function of the number of samples taken per year.

Figure 1 is based on the following assumptions (see data Appendix II):

	A Non-automatic determination	B Automatic determination
Investment	high volume sampler	automatic instrument (β-ray attenuation) plus electronics to store results on magnetic tape
	ECU 4000	ECU 16000
Amortisation	10 years	5 years
Interest rate	10 %	10 %
Maintenance costs per year	10 % of investment costs	20 % of investment costs
Fixed costs per year		
Amortisation	ECU 400	ECU 3200
Average loss of interest interest	ECU 200	ECU 800
Maintenance	ECU 400	ECU 3200
Variable costs		
Material + personnel	ECU 1 + ECU 3/sample	negligible

It should be mentioned that in the first place this example
is meant to show how such a problem can be approached instead
of giving a definite answer. The answer would anyway strongly depend on local conditions, e.g. the still prevailing
tendency in most industrial countries for personnel costs to
rise more steeply than costs of instruments, while maintenance costs have a tendency to decrease, due to the higher
reliability of the newer versions of instruments. Although
there might be considerable local differences in the rate of
change of these costs.

It should be noticed that cases A and B are not quite comparable due to the difference in reproducibility of the two
methods (see Appendix II). It should also be remarked here
that the relation between costs and reproducibility is complex and highly non-linear. Costs have a tendency to rise
very steeply beyond a certain value of the reproducibility.
This point depends strongly on the "present state of the
art", e.g. increasing reproducibility demands, generally
speaking, increasing control of external factors such as
airflow, temperature of this flow, etc.

A simple example is derived from the determination of the
asbestos concentration in air, which in its final step comprises the counting of fibres in a sample using an optical
or electron microscope. In practice only part of the sample
can be investigated in this way. Assuming that the distribution of the fibres on the sample is governed by a poison distribution, the reproducibility of this part of the analysis
of the sample is inversely proportional to the square root of
fibres counted $\left(\dfrac{1}{\text{fibres counted}} \right)$. Using this rather
crude model, figure 2 shows costs as a function of
reproducibility.

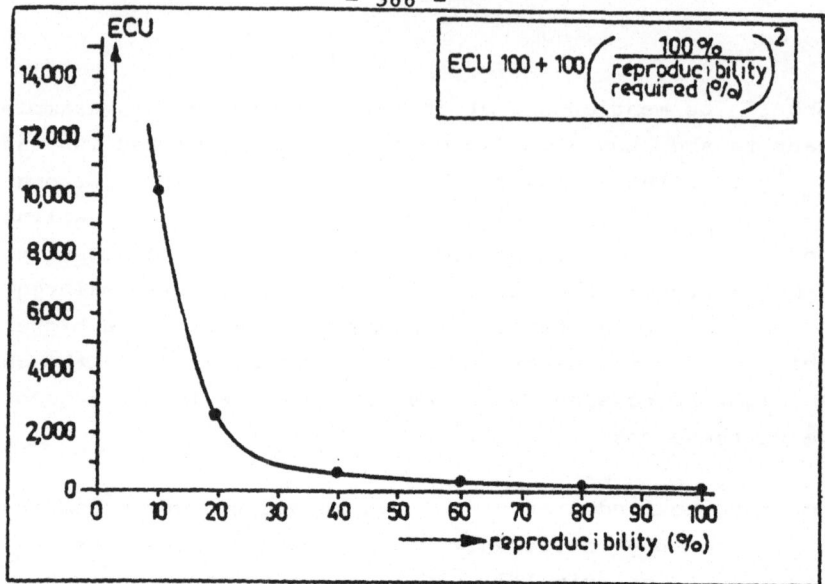

Figure 2. Approximate costs of electron microscope analysis of a sample as a function of reproducibility.

On the basis of theoretical and empirical considerations reproducibility accuracy (see Appendix I) for submicroscopic particles, as there is no sampling bias.

After the comparison of the costs of relatively simple measuring systems and the demonstration of a strong depen-dence of the costs on the required reproducibility a more complex system will finally be analysed. As an example the comparison of a system for the determination and identifi-cations of fibre concentrations in air will be taken.

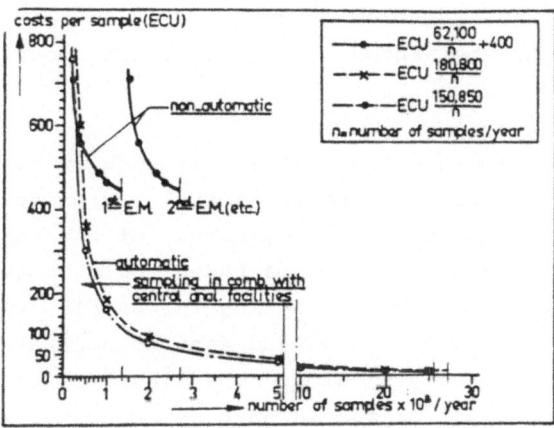

Figure 3. Costs of the determination of the fibre concentration in air as a function of the number of samples investigated per year.

Figure 3 is based on the following, still hypothetic, factilities:

	Non-automatic	Sampling in combination with central automatic analysing facility*	Automatic*
Investment			
High volume air sampler	ECU 10 000	ECU 10 000	ECU 10 000
Sample preparation	ECU 15 000	ECU 30 000	ECU 30 000
Electron microscope	ECU 150 000	ECU 150 000	ECU 150 000
Analyser with auxiliary equipment	--	ECU 200 000	ECU 200 000
Buildings	ECU 30 000	ECU 30 000	ECU 150 000
Amortisation of instruments	5 years	5 years	5 years
Building	30 years	30 years	30 years
Interest rate	10 %	10 %	10 %
Maintenance of instruments	8 %	10 %	12 %
Maintenance building	2 %	2 %	2 %
Fixed costs per year			
Amortisation	ECU 36 000	ECU 79 000	ECU 83 000
Average interest	ECU 11 500	ECU 22 250	ECU 32 000
Maintenance	ECU 14 600	ECU 39 600	ECU 49 800
Fixed personnel costs	negligible	ECU 10 000	ECU 16 000
Variable costs			
Material + personnel	ECU 400/sample	negligible	negligible
Cost equation	ECU $\frac{62\ 100}{n}$ + 400	ECU $\frac{150\ 850}{n}$	ECU $\frac{180\ 800}{n}$
Estimated maximum number of determinations per year	1350	25 000	27 000
Reproducibility $\approx$ repeatability	30 %	30 %	30 %

*For these calculations more sophisticated "costing methods" like "present discounted value" should be taken into consideration, e.g. Wagner, 1972.

These, admittedly fictional data show that a totally automatic measuring system only makes sense if large numbers of determinations have to be carried out in one place and results have to be known as quickly as possible after sampling.

Vinyl chloride sampling and analysis is such an example. In the day-to-day practice of the industrial hygienist, however, this is often not strictly necessary. At the state of the art the most logical course to be taken would be to separate the sampling operation from analysing the sample, which would mean that samples are collected and sent to central analysing facilities. Calculations along the lines pointed out here show that this approach should have an important bearing on measuring strategy and could give impulses to the development of new automated instruments.

APPENDIX 1

CONCEPTS DESCRIBING THE QUALITY OF MEASUREMENTS

To describe the quality of measuring methods a number of concepts is used.
Important ones are given below:

Repeatability   - is the difference between measurements carried out
approximately at the same time with the same instruments
by the same person determining the same property of the
same object (ISO Standard).

Reproducibility - is the difference between measurements, carried out at
different times, with different instruments, usually of
the same type, by different persons determining the same
property of the same project (ISO Standard).

Precision   - is the magnitude of the deviation of a series of
measurements. To have practical significance, the value
of the deviation is expressed as a relative figure of the
arithmetical mean of the measurements. It defines the
interval I in which the result of an independent
measurement with a certain probability P falls. The
concept is applicable to both repeatability and reproduc-
tibility. Quantatively it is expressed in the following
way:

$$\frac{100 \sqrt{2}}{\bar{M}_A} \frac{t_p}{\sqrt{n}} \sqrt{\frac{\Sigma_{i=1}^{n} (M_{iA} - \bar{M}_A)^2}{n - 1}} \qquad \text{see figure 5}$$

n = number of independent measurements;

t_p = the student factor for the required probability and
for instance for P 95 % has the following
magnitudes as a function of n - 1.

n - 1	5	10	15	20	25	50
t_p	2,57	2,23	2,13	2,09	2,06	2,01

Accuracy   - is the difference between measured value and true value
(IES, 1980).

Resolution   - is the smallest difference of the measured property which
can still be quantitatively distinguished.

Time constant and bandwidth

  - The way an instrument follows sudden changes in magnitude
of the property to be measured can be derived from its
response to a step function (Figure 4), FRETTER, 1968;
CANNON, 1967.

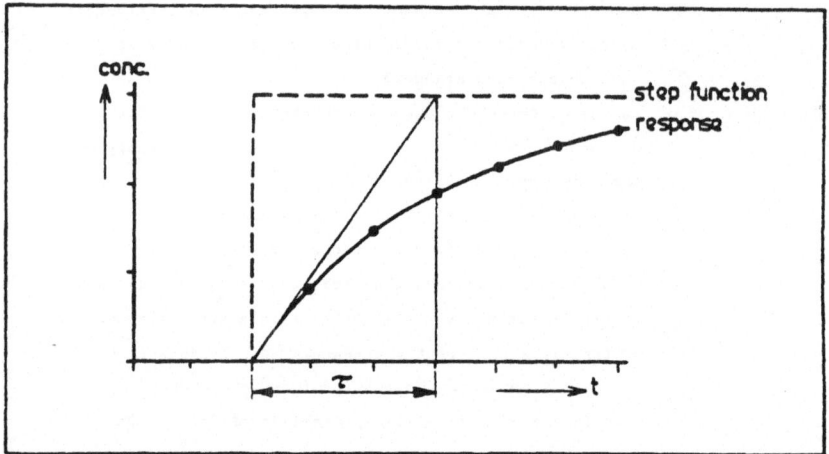

Figure 4. Response of an instrument to a step function.

Assuming that the instrument behaves at first approximation as a first order system, the ability to follow changes is then described by τ, the time constant, or translated into a sinusoidal change by

$$H = \frac{1}{2\pi\tau} \qquad\qquad H = \frac{1}{2\pi\tau}$$

H is the band width of frequencies in Herz, at the same time it is maximum frequency of concentration fluctuations to which the instrument can respond if τ is the same time constant in seconds.

<u>Lower detection limit</u> is the smallest measured quantity which can be distinguished from zero.

Summary of some of the concepts described so far

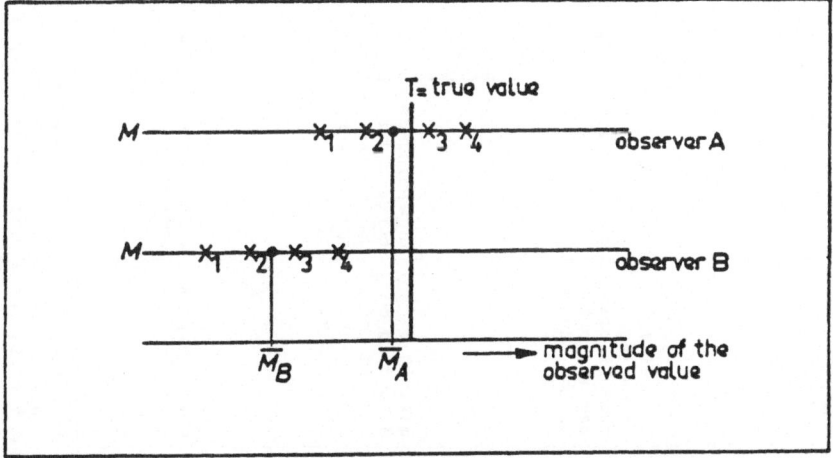

Figure 5.   Illustration of repeatability, reproducibility and
            accuracy.
            (M_A and M_B are the mean values of observations
            M_{iA} and M_{iB} respectively . i = 1,2,3,4, etc.)

The repeatability of the method is calculated from the
results M_{1A}, M_{2A}, M_{3A}, M_{4A}, M_{1B}, B_{2B}, M_{3B}, M_{4B}.
The reproducibility is determined from the results of both
M_{iA} and M_{iB} series of results.
M_A - T and M_B - T finally is an indication of the
accuracy of the method used, see Figure 5.

APPENDIX 2

Type of instrument	Instrument determines particles with aerodynamic/optical equivalent diameter	Reproducibility	Accuracy	Sampling time	Price	Remarks
1. Particle concentration is determined by the single particle optical counter by measuring frequency and intensity of light scattered by the particles which pass the instrument	0.3-8 μ	40 %	40 % depending on cut-off point and lay-out of the device	continuously	ECU 8 000 - 12 000	In the range 0.3-8μ a size distribution can be obtained relatively easily and continuously. The instrument is often used in the 1 measurement/minute mode $\sim 10^{-2}$ Hz frequency band; but this is no technological limitation. Frequencies of 10 Hz and higher are attainable (Brillouin, 1956)
2. Mass of particles precipitated from a known volume of air in filter tape are measured in situ by β-ray attenuation	<15 μ	30 % depending on conc. and sampling time	max. 30 % depending on cut-off point and lay-out of the device	depending on conc. of dust in ambient air between 30 and 40 min	ECU 10 000 - 12 000	The cut-off point can be chosen and time resolution can be modified by technological modification; e.g. size selecting equipment, suction speed and volume, etc.
3. Mass of particles precipitated by a high volume sampler from a known volume of air on a filter are determined by a separate weighing operation, carried out e.g. in a laboratory	<60 μ	15 %	can be approx. 15 %	time average over many hrs	ECU 4 000 - 10 000	Highest frequencies are lower than 10^{-3} Hz (sampling time half an hour). Highest frequencies are in practice generally 10^{-5} Hz (sampling time 24 hrs)

Nos. 1 and 2 are in principle fully automatic instruments. The quoted prices give orders of magnitude valid for the Netherlands in 1980. They give orders of magnitude only and no doubt considerable rebates would be obtained if large numbers of these instruments would be ordered. To 1 and 2 costs for electronic equipment should be added when it is assumed that data are stored on magnetic tape. These costs are estimated to be ECU 3 000.

References

BRILLOUIN, L. (1956)   Science and information theory, p. 97, New York, Academic Press.

CANNON, R.H. (1967)   Dynamics of physical systems, Chapter VI, New York, McGraw Hill Book Company.

FRETTER, W.B. (1968)   Introduction to experimental physics, Chapter I, New York, Dover Publication Inc.

IES Testing Procedures Committee, Journal of IES January 1980, p.78.

ISO Standard ISO/Dis 5725. This is still a draft and treats precision of test methods - Determination of repeatability and reproducibility.

WAGNER, H.M. (1972)   Principles of operations research, Chapter XI, London, Prentice/Hall International Inc.

MULTIDISCIPLINARY APPROACH TO PREVENTION AND HEALTH PROTECTION
BY MONITORING: ROLE OF INDIVIDUAL DISCIPLINES. THE COMPUTER
SCIENTIST: RECORD KEEPING BY COMPUTER I.

H. MALKER (SWEDEN)

Summary

*The purpose of this paper is to present a theoretical survey
of the construction of an information system that includes
data on occupational exposure to hazardous agents. To illustrate the theory, practical experience from the construction
of an exposure register of lead workers is described. Finally,
some of the results obtained with the "lead register" and some
of the problems that remain to be solved, for example coupling
of measurements from ambient monitoring and from biological
tests are discussed. What is not discussed in this connection, are the highly sensitive questions relating to
confidentiality.*

Introduction

Data may be collected for many reasons, from haphazard accumulation of documents in the belief that "they may come in
useful" to strictly structured registers with clearly defined
aims. The availability of individual data and of aggregated
data in the form of tables, diagrams, etc. has been simplified, and in some cases become at all possible, by modern
computer processing. One of the fields in which a multitude
of "hard data" traditionally are produced, but in which the
structuring, storage and processing of such data are still
relatively undeveloped, is work environment.

Measurements of exposure to injurious agents have hitherto
been directed towards preventive measures. In order to use
the data for other purposes, they must be structured, verifiable and comparable in place and time. One consequence is
that the methods of measuring and the general approach must
be reproducible and that classification and coding must be
according to uniform norms.

Those responsible for questions of work environment must
ensure that there are channels of information which permit
checks on this environment, and that these channels can be
utilised in decisions of priority for counter-measures. It
must also be possible to record effects of counter-measures
and to confirm observations by various use of hard data. One
instrument for achieving these aims is an individualised risk
register, which can be linked to correspondingly individualised disease registers, so as to create what can be called
an aetiological information system. By this is meant a systematic specification of individualised information concerning the effects as well as the possible causes of occupational diseases.

If such information on occupational risks is to be effectively utilised, for instance in epidemiological studies, it
must be on an individual basis. To permit linkage of information between different systems, identification must be
possible. This can relate to persons, firms, places of work,
branches of industry -economic activities - and types of
occupation.

As an aid in disease prevention, an exposure register can
give:
- early alarm signals concerning potential
  hazards
- improvement of facilities for follow-up and
  for comparisons between different industries,
  etc.
- data to be used in assessing, for instance,
  threshold limit norms.
In addition, such planned record-keeping can
- be integrated in local measures against
  occupational disease through the investigations connected with data collection, and
  through clear surveys of stored information
- form part of a system of screening and/or
  periodic checks in compulsory health surveillance

- be included in a system of aetiological information
- constitute a background register for theoretical and practical research.

The exposure register must contain data from individuals and
from workplaces expressed as "times and quantities". These
data derive mainly from biological tests, medical examinations and ambient monitoring.

To meet the requirements of register users, it must be possible to aggregate and present the stored data at different
levels. Data can then be processed in linkage with, for instance, general disease registers - cancer, causes of death,
congenital malformations and other clinical registers. These
linkages are to be regarded as part of general medical surveillance and as a means of utilising the other registers,
for example in evaluating warning reports.

An exposure register is feasible only in circumstances where
it is known or strongly suspected that there is a cause-and-
effect relationship between hazard and health (1,2,3).

Individualised, nation-wide and computerised registers of
exposure to occupational hazards have long been in demand but
do not as yet exist in any country. For maximum effectiveness of such registers, unique civic registration numbers are
almost a prerequisite.

Planning and constructing an information system - a model

In the construction of an information system there are certain basic aims:

- that the data be readily available for specified purposes
- that the various users of the system be provided with relevant information
- that the quality of the information be appropriate for the purpose of its use.

These aims presuppose careful and specific planning. But the system must also be adaptable, so as to permit modifications for future fields of use which were not envisagable in the initial planning.

Planning and construction of an information system can be divided into four phases.

In the first phase a number of theoretical aims are established. The following factors must be taken into account:
- the prospective users of the system and the purposes for which it will be used
- the target population
- the required data
- the form, detail, aggregation, etc. appropriate for presenting the information from the system.

Phase 2 involves investigations of:
- which data are easily accessible
- which additional data may be desirable for various purposes
- what must be the limitations for the target population
- whether certain data must be excluded, e.g. because their quality cannot be established, or because they are incomplete or involve too much expense.
- whether data shall be obtained by compulsory or voluntary collection, or possibly from linked runs with other information systems
- possibilities of data-checking from one or more sources
- the suitability of existing classifications and the need for supplements
- the identification forms already used in other information systems and how far these are acceptable for present purposes.

Phases 1 and 2 involve charting of possible areas of use.
This is necessary so that the system can gradually be extended from a basic framework to the level that remains economically defensible.

In phase 3 the alternatives remaining after completion of
phase 2 are ranked, taking into account both degree of
desirability and cost.

In ranking the information to be computer-processed (phase 3)
one must also decide how much of the residual data shall be
stored and what form this storage shall take. The demands of
rapidity of access must be considered, for instance if an on-
line system is required for some or all of the data, or if
periodic input and/or output will be adequate. The technical
programme proceeds from the decisions made on these points.

A pilot study of the system constitutes phase 4. It is most
important that all the potential users shall have received
adequate training and instruction. Many runs are made in
this pilot study.

The lead register - an example

In 1976 a Swedish project was launched to develop a system
for elucidating associations between occupational environment
and health. One step in this project is the construction of
registers to record data on exposure to various hazardous
agents. In a trial stage, four such registers are being
evolved at the National Board of Occupational Safety and
Health, with records of persons exposed to lead, styrene,
quartz or asbestos.

At the start of the project it was agreed to construct a
separate register for each of the hazardous agents. This
implied a significant limitation, in that a single register
could not in every case cover the total occupational exposure
of individual workers.

The immediate aims are to investigate how the presentation of register information at different levels can assist in prevention of occupational disease and to gain practical experience of computerised collection, storage and presentation of data on occupational exposure. The needs of the register users in both short and long term will also be analysed. Proceeding from these needs, from the nature of the process which carries the occupational hazard and currently available experience of computerised information systems in this field, it is hoped to evolve a model for computer-aided handling of data on exposure to occupational hazards.

This model will form a basis for suggestions as to principles for recording, storing, processing and feedback of such data on local, regional and national level, with constant regard to flexibility necessitated by differences in users and circumstances and by prospects of enlarging the basic system or systems.

At the National Board of Occupational Safety and Health, work on the project was initially concentrated on evaluating various types of output data. As regards workers exposed to lead, the Board decided to conduct a trial in concerns with compulsory checks of lead levels in workers. Routines for collecting these measurements were already in operation. The main reason for the choice of lead to pilot the project, apart from the legislation on medical surveillance, was the relative simplicity of coupling between input data and practical environmental measures.

Experience from the trial with lead exposure is being utilised also in constructing the other registers included in the project, i.e. of exposure to styrene, quartz and asbestos. One objective of studying multiple agents is clearer evaluation of how to register measurements from ambient monitoring and how to relate the measurements to groups of individuals. Particular attention has hitherto been paid to the efficacy of feedback.

The objective in this type of data collection is that it should lead to, or maintain preventive measures of individual, local, regional and national levels. The model further satisfies aims in the existing statistical production, for instance in long-term planning and various investigations and research. The time-table for the project involves analysis and formulation of suggestions for fixed routines no later than the beginning of 1982.

Figure 1 outlines the information flow in the "lead register".

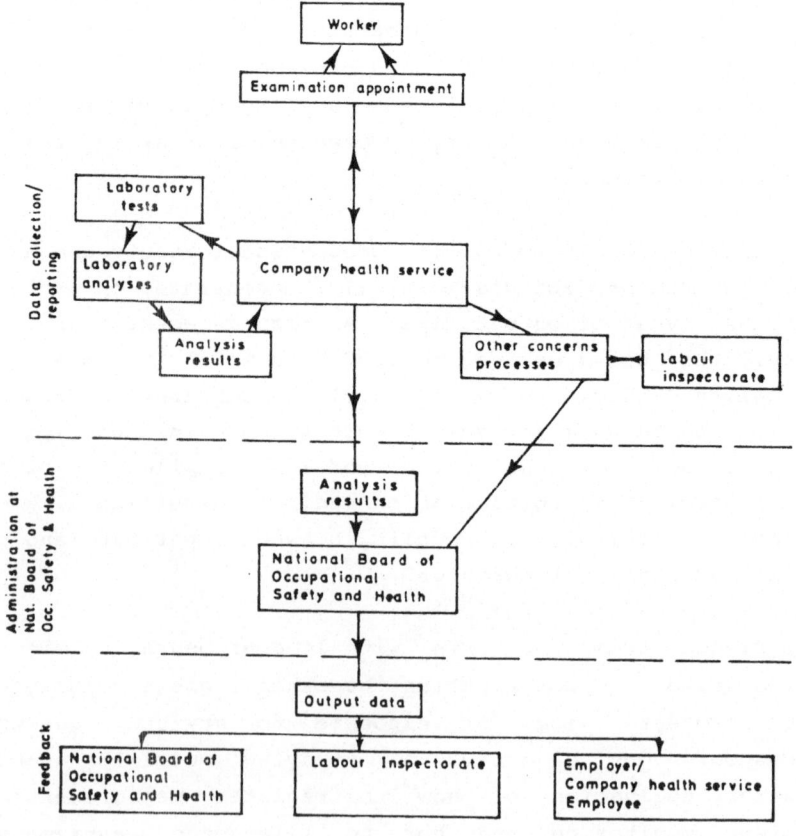

Figure 1. Information flow in the "lead system"

The projected system differs from many others previously employed in that the receiver of data - the register - functions as a service unit for the deliverers of data, to be used in their field work, so that use of these data is not confined to presentations of statistics, research, etc, at annual or other regular intervals.

Table 1 presents the prospective users of the information system and the functions the system is intended to assist.

Table 1. Users and use of the register

Register users	Functions to be assisted
Lead-exposed workers	Information, instruction, own measures to reduce exposure.
Managements, safety delegates safety committees	Planning of safety measures, short-term and long-term, and follow-up of safety measures.
Company health services	Duties of doctors and safety engineers in general, and reporting routines to National Board of Occupational Safety and Health.
Labour inspectorate	Planning and ranking of inspections and follow-up of safety measures.
National Board of Occupational Safety and Health	Check system for compulsory medical surveillance, used in formulating threshold limit values. Formulation of safety rules Follow-up of safety observance. Contributory analyses of register data.
Labour-management representatives	Comprehensive discussions of occupational environment.
Researchers, investigators	Background register.

In the continuation of the trial in lead workers, the routine for data supply were analysed and improved. The basic concept then was that the computerised system should as far as possible facilitate the reporting.

The "lead register" is designed to contain both biological
and technical data, if such data are available. In
order to satisfy the users' requirements, the information
within each concern must be registered both for
individuals and at some group level for workers with
approximately equal exposure to lead. In addition, it must
be possible to aggregate data over concerns and occupations.

Definition of target population

The ideal target population for a register of exposure to
some injurious agent consists of all persons who have been in
contact with the agent. That such an ideal population is
inaccessible with regard to lead exposure is due to the
following factors.

i) It is not even theoretically possible to reach
all persons who have had contact with lead at
some time and in some form. The target population must be restricted to those with occupational lead exposure.

ii) There are practical limitations also in coverage of this restricted target population. One
limiting factor is non-totality of compulsory
medical surveillance.

Financial considerations may impose further limits on follow-
up of some lead-exposed persons. The target must therefore
be constituted from and confined to a practically available
population, though this may not even include all persons with
heavy exposure to lead. In accordance with Swedish
legislation, only firms with more than five employees and
with access to an inspecting medical officer can be covered
by the lead register. Corresponding caution must therefore be
observed in use of the register for assessments on nationwide level.

Collection of data - "dropout"

Data collection for the lead register has hitherto been based on compulsory delivery. Some enquiries have been received from firms which are not covered by the existing legislation but wish to deliver data to the lead register. Since voluntary participation may be selective, however, and thus distort composite information, such data must be separately handled. This is of course regrettable when the purpose of a register is to be as all-embracing as possible. "Dropout" is in practice a major problem.

Current regulations stipulate that data concerning lead content in blood and ALA in the urine of lead-exposed workers shall be submitted to the National Board of Occupational Safety and Health. The lead register project is at present largely limited to these biological tests. Data from ambient monitoring of lead levels are voluntarily submitted by managements and are manually processed as complementary information.

Factors influencing the quality of the register

In formulating the requirements for quality of the important variables in a register, several factors must be taken into account. These are:
- the register's objectives
- requests to the register
- quality of all variables ("total quality").

Two extremes of objectives for a register are conceivable.
    i) "Crude" studies, i.e. in which the purpose only is to detect any major differences between, for instance, observed and expected rates or to detect approximate trends. These data can function as warning signals. The demands on quality of data can then be relatively low. It is only necessary to know how

the error in the most important variables is
distributed among the various background
variables and how such errors may influence
different results. This can be evaluated by
random sampling. For blanket analyses from
the lead register, this level of ambition
should suffice.

ii) At the other extreme is register searching at
individual level. Many studies of this type
require groupings of relatively few workers,
for example according to level of lead dose.
Accuracy in identification and other data must
then be high, particularly as the register
users, and thus recipients of feedback, include individual employees, safety department
staff, etc.

If a register is much in demand, particularly for practical
and theoretical investigations of varying types, it is advisable to concentrate on quality of the data. If this is not
done, users of the register will have to make their own
quality analyses, which may be of variable value. A formal
"description of contents" should therefore be obligatory for
all such registers. We do not yet know what the demands on
information from the lead register will be. Work is at
present in progress on a "description of contents" which,
inter alia, will present the various methods of analysis
underlying the data and their comparability. It is hoped that
in time this description will include also factors such as
work processes, use of protective equipment and changes in
working conditions over the years in specified occupations.

The quality of data is influenced by methods of measurement
and analysis, by difficulties in classification and coding,
and by punching errors, etc. Instead of concentrating on
reliability and completeness of certain "hard" variables such
as identification, it is often a better use of resources to
seek out the defects in other variables such as diagnosis,

occupational classification and domicile and to elucidate
the distribution of these defects and their significance for
studies of various types. A register that is "complete" in
the sense that all relevant persons are included and certain
variables such as identity data are correctly entered can
sometimes give a deceptive impression of the quality of the
other variables. The continuous checks of quality and com-
prehensiveness that should be a part of the routine running
of registers should preferably help to reveal how defects in
quality can affect investigations of important background
variables that are not included in the register. The lead
analyses may only be performed by laboratories approved by
the National Board of Occupational Safety and Health, one
reason being to maintain the quality of the lead register.
As the examined workers are among the recipients of feedback
data, errors of coding, etc. are quickly detected.

Identification data

There are two types of identification:
- person identification
- risk identification

Individual identity numbers greatly facilitate individualised
follow-up. Since 1947 each resident in Sweden has a civic
registration number, which is used in all connections. These
numbers permit linkage between registers and thus also an
aetiological information system. The significance of an
aetiological information system is primarily that diseases
with long latency periods, such as cancer, can be traced in
relation to other factors. Such tracing can be prospective
or retrospective. By linkage between different exposure
registers, mixed exposure can be elucidated.

Exposure to injurious agents can be expressed with varying
precision, from a simple statement of occupation to
individualised data on factor(s); duration and intensity of
exposure. On a nationwide level the most common data

presently available are occupation, economic activity and
region. These data even in combination, give only a rough
impression of the occupational hazard. Uniform norms of
classification are required for general background information and for nationwide and international comparisons. As
occupational classification the lead register uses a Nordic
modification of the international system (ISCO). But as this
classification is not useful for planning safety measures at
local level, each worksite also uses a grouping according to
level of exposure. These are specifically internal codings,
stated in plain text and unsuitable for nationwide comparisons. In the register each concern is coded and also the
industry - economic activity - to which it belongs. Thorough
consideration of identification and classifying systems at an
early stage of register construction can save the heavy
expense involved by late-stage changes.

Presentation of output data

In presenting numerical data, diagrams are usually superior
to other methods. Information from the lead register is
issued whenever possible in diagrams, supplemented by tables
so as to give details such as the range of observed values.
Output from the lead register is exemplified in the
Appendix.

Input

An information system can function well only if the suppliers
of data feel that the system well repays the time and expense
involved in collecting these data. Input routines with periodic laboratory reports and ambient monioring are simplified
by computer processing. In earlier manual systems, up to
four forms were required to convey information from sampling
to laboratory, back to doctor and management and then to the
Board of Occupational Safety and Health. For the new system
a pre-printed form to be used throughout the data flow is
under test. All the relevant information, including results

of the latest tests, is thus accommodated in the same form.
Office work is further reduced by details such as pre-printed
labels for test tubes.

Feedback

Much of the recent criticism about data collection, in
Sweden at any rate, stems from the data suppliers'
feeling that such routines are not meaningful for them,
and this affects the quality of the information. Clear
presentation of objectives is therefore essential.

Figure 2 sets out the model used in the trials with occupational exposure registers.

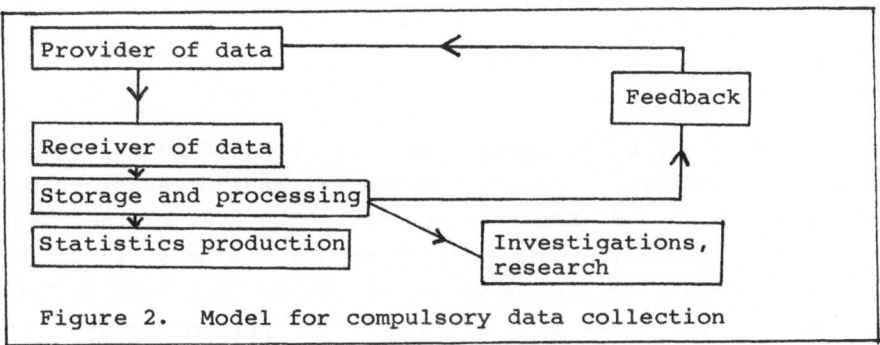

Figure 2. Model for compulsory data collection

Direct feedback to the providers of data is made partly as
acknowledgement of the received information. It is presented
as specifications of immediate interest to the respective
functions. This extends the access to output information and
should help to speed up measures resulting therefrom, such as
modifications of occupational environment. (Further details
are given in the Appendix).

It is important that the register users themselves decide the
frequency and form of feedback, though this makes heavy demands on the flexibility of the system.

Information and instruction

In evolving an information system, it is important to proceed by stages and to evaluate the system first on a partial population. Information and training of the persons who will participate in the trial are likewise important. As regards exposure registers, interest must then be focused on the specific hazard, its possible effects and the preventive measures that can be taken by employers and workers. The investigations necessarily involved in collection of data mean that the persons exposed to occupational hazards become more aware of their risks. When there is also data feedback and information around it, one may expect an increase of interest in all parties, including companies, and safety committees, that should result in environmental improvements, and sometimes even in individual habits.

Finance

The cost of one analysis for lead in blood is at present about 150 Swedish kronor. Technical environmental checks cost around 2,000 Swedish kronor. The cost of the "lead register", including data collection and feedback, is difficult to estimate in the construction stages, but will probably be in the order of 5 Swedish kronor per worker and test occasion. Computerised output of diagrams, tables, etc., which otherwise would be done by managements, company health centres, labour inspectors and the National Board of Occupational Safety and Health should, with the current extent of the lead register (c.2.000 workers with an average 3 medical examinations per year) result in a saving of two manpower years for each year of operation.

It is the build-up of an information system that is expensive, not its routine running or maintenance. If great care is not taken in construction phases 1 and 2, mistakes detected in the later phases will be very expensive to correct.

Results and continuation of the work

The model for an information system that is being developed for registration of occupational exposure to hazardous agents is relatively crude. In principle, therefore, it should be applicable to most of such agents as regards both data processing and information requirements of interested parties.

It is hoped that from this model will be evolved information systems with peripheral routines for rational handling of data on occupational exposure, possibly with the aid of electronic processing. Though it is not yet possible to predict the technicalities of computerisation in this connection, it would seem appropriate to aim for a general base upon which various exposure registers can be built up in separate systems. The common base must include data such as identity numbers that will permit exchange of information on both exposure to and effects of the different agents.

Another important reason for a general base is that, in order to cover hazards with long, as well as those with short latency time, registers must remain useful for at least 10 to 20 years. And, as already pointed out, the base should serve also for new demands which can be expected to arise but are difficult or impossible to foresee when the system is established.

The model comprises parts of the following functions in the prevention of occupational ill-health.

Registration of data from:
- ambient monitoring
- biological tests
- medical examinations/inspections, relevant background information e.g. on various risk indicators.

Handling of data
- analyses of test results and calibration and checks of their reliability, checks of laboratories
- assessment of results from spot measurements and samplings
- registration and storage of analyses results and other information in a coordinated exposure register.

Data processing
- processing and presentation of information from data stored in the exposure register
- coordinated processing with data from disease registers, etc. and presentation of linked information.

The lead register has hitherto been very well received by those involved in the evaluation and by other contacts. Most of them report an increased interest in the occupational environment. This may be one of the reasons why levels of lead in the blood have fallen in some workers, or even groups of workers, even when counter-measures have not been intensified.

In the few instances in which data from both biological and ambient monitoring could be linked in groups of workers, the correlations hitherto have been poor. The two measurements presumably are mutually complementary. In order to elucidate how linkage between biological and ambient monitoring can be utilised, studies are also being made on workers exposed to styrene or other agents. The following are among the problems for this extended analysis.

- How should linkage be made between data from biological and ambient monitoring of occupational exposure to hazardous agents and effects of these agents? Should, for instance, the technical and biological data be presented in a single diagram, and in such case what should be the chronology of linkage?

- How should data from non-individualised monitorings be related to individual workers?
- What peripheral information is important? Exposure to more than one occupational hazard? How should such information be registered?
- Can access be obtained to disease registers other than those centrally compiled, such as regional patient registers? How in such cases, are problems arising from "dropout" due to population movements, etc. to be dealt with?
- How can a meaningful specification of input data quality be obtained, and how should it be presented to users of the register?
- What will be the short-term and long-term requirements of different register user categories in regard to output data, and how shall the data be presented? Users in this connection are individual workers, managements, company health services, Labour Inspectorate, Board of Occupational Safety and Health, occupational medicine clinics, trade unions, employer organisations, researches, etc.).
- How should a general, logical register structure be formulated?
- How should the techniques of laboratory analyses and the results of checks on laboratories be registered?
- How should changes in industrial production be registered?

Since agent-specific exposure registers will be limited to known or strongly suspected hazards, they must be supplemented by general observations in "aetiological information systems" recording data such as disease, occupations, industries, domicile, etc., so that indications of hitherto unknown occupational hazards can be recognised as early as possible. Further penetration will then be required to clarify possible "new" associations (4).

References

1. Report from the Working Group on Epidemiological Surveillance Systems 20 October 1978.

2. Epidemiological Surveillance of Long-Term Health Effects of Environmental Hazards, Report on a Working Group 24-26 September 1974.

3. Principles and Practice of Screening for Disease, J.M.G. Wilson and G. Jungner.

4. Etiologiska Informationssystem, B. Malker, H. Malker, Nordisk Foretagshalsavard 1979, 2, 123-134.

Appendix

The output data from the "lead register" are intended for:
    managements and lead-exposed workers
    the Labour Inspectorate
    the National Board of Occupational Safety and Health
    trade unions
    others, including researchers

Most output data are distributed once monthly during the trial period. The number of documents per month varies widely, depending mainly on the length of the interval between inspections and the intensity of sampling. Apart from the inspection documents, the volume of output data is determined by other suppliers of input-management, company health services, safety committees, etc.

Spot checks of completeness and accuracy are made at the National Board of Occupational Safety and Health before reports are issued. These checks cover all types of output. The frequency of output is determined by the register users.

The following are examples of output data that are available in the trial period.

- INSPECTION SHEET, which collectively presents the results from a biological sampling session. This is the doctor's receipt for delivered data.
- CASE SHEET, showing all the test results in an individual worker. The main use is to satisfy enquiries from the examined person.
- CASE DIAGRAM, illustrating these individual test results in relation to time. This diagram is delivered to the worker himself and to the doctor.
- COMPANY SHEET, which reports in internal code the results from a number of biological sam-

pling occasions. These are tabulated data
and show "group" developments chronologically.
The recipients are managements, company health
centres, safety representatives and Labour
Inspectorate.
- COMPANY DIAGRAM, illustrating the above data.
  The recipients are as above.
- MISSED TEST DATE, notification that tests have
  not been made within the appointed time.
  Intended primarily for Labour Inspectorate as
  an aid in surveillance.
- NOTIFICATION OF EXCEEDED THRESHOLDS, showing -
  when necessary - in how many persons the biological test readings exceeded norms specified
  by the National Board of Occupational Safety
  and Health or by managements. This is intended primarily for Labour Inspectorate, but
  many managements have shown interest in it and
  receive it on request. The figures show in
  which companies there is greatest lead risk.
- COMPANY LIST, showing which companies in a
  labour Inspectorate district are included in
  the trial.
- STATISTICAL REPORTS, with the results of
  biological tests distributed according to a
  number of variables. These reports are
  primarily intended for the National Board of
  Occupational Safety and Health and the Labour
  Inspectorate, but they are also available for
  others. Some of the involved companies have
  received them on request.

In addition there are appointments lists and
records sheets.

The National Board of Occupational Safety and
Health receives interim data when necessary.

MULTIDISCIPLINARY APPROACH TO PREVENTION AND HEALTH PROTECTION
BY MONITORING: ROLE OF INDIVIDUAL DISCIPLINES. THE COMPUTER
SCIENTIST: RECORD KEEPING BY COMPUTER II.

P. WOLKONSKY (USA)

Summary

*Standard Oil Company (Indiana) has developed a comprehensive
computerised occupational health recordkeeping system that
has been in use throughout the consolidated company for five
years. The system's primary focus is the handling of a large
data base that allows correlations to be drawn between
disease and medical findings, work history and environmental
exposure, accident information, and demographic factors such
as social and workplace history.*

*Because the data are drawn from a heterogeneous, normally
healthy population, epidemiological studies that evaluate
these data may be applied to the public as a whole, as well
as to the petrochemical industry. The four areas from which
data are drawn are medical examinations, visits and immunizations; safety reports of accidents; corporate personnel
files; and industrial hygiene and toxicology surveys and
studies.*

*This paper discusses the data and the method by which they
are collected, system security measures to prevent access by
unauthorised parties, and system reporting capabilities.*

Corporations have an obligation to each individual employee,
and a responsibility to the work force as a whole, to provide
a safe and healthy work environment. For decades, Standard
Oil of Indiana has met this responsibility by employing
medical, safety and industrial hygiene professionals to
provide the services necessary to assure the good health and
safety of its employees.

Interaction among the various groups of the responsible
departments is vital, and the amount of information generated
by each group is tremendous. Table 1 sets this out. In
order to assume successfully the responsibility for safety
and good health, all these pieces of information must be

readily available for retrieval and analysis; with a large
and widely-scattered employee population, such as that of
Standard Oil, computerization is the only feasible method to
assure that these data are indeed available.

Table 1. 'Health Data' Within the Company

Employee
Job history
Location codes
Sickness and disability

Claims
Workmen's Compensation payments
Death certificates
Internal cost reports

Medical
Personal and family history
Physical examination
Laboratories
Immunizations

Industrial Hygiene
Personal samples
Area samples
Potential exposures by location
Exposure levels

Toxicology
Animal research
Materials safety data sheets

Safety
Accident data: personal actions
Physical conditions
Supervisor data
(D.O.T. data)

Accordingly, almost nine years ago, the decision was made
that Standard Oil would establish its own computerized
occupational health system, since there were no acceptable
systems available at that time. The primary focus was to be
a system that would handle a large data base and would allow
correlations to be drawn between disease and medical findings, work history and environmental exposure, and demographic factors such as age, sex, social history and race.

During development, a number of objectives was set forth.
The system would have to provide a good data base that could
be used for participation in epidemiological studies that

could be applied to the public as a whole, as well as to a particular industry. Other objectives included management of medical claims and long-term disability programmes, identification and evaluation of high-risk employees, production of union-required occupational illness and injury reports, response to governmental inquiries and aid in litigation cases, as well as preparation of special internal reports.

The system is designed to collect data from four sources: medical department examinations and visits, safety information in the form of accident reports, employee information supplied through the corporate personal system, and various forms of industrial hygience and toxicology data.

The medical module, in operation since December of 1975, allows storage and retrieval of data from preplacement examinations, required and voluntary periodic examinations, visits to the medical department and immunisations; it includes personal/family history, physical examinations, visits, (illness/injury data, immunisation, physical capacity, death certificates, prior diagnosis. The examination types are periodic voluntary, periodic required, preplacement, expatriate, expatriate tropics) repatriate retirement, disability, limited and surveillance. The medical history is recorded on special mark-sense forms by the patient and reviewed with him by the physician; other data are recorded on appropriate mark-sense forms by the physician or nurse administering that portion of the examination or visit. These forms become the source document for the medical record. By having the medical professional record the information directly on the computer input sheets, the possibility of error in transcription, for example by keypunching, is eliminated.

When the exam or visit is complete, the forms are forwarded to a designated medical department terminal for processing. There are eight such locations spread over our operating territory in the United States. Each of these location terminals has an OpScan optical reader and Anderson-Jacobson printer, acoustically coupled to a telephone linkage to the main computer in Chicago. In all cases, the terminals are housed within medical departments and are operated by nurses or medical secretaries. When the forms have been processed, they are returned to the originating location for filing in the medical chart.

As the data are entered, a complex series of "edit checks" for syntax, logic, completeness and range is performed by the computer. The first level makes certain the data are complete - if the required field is four digits long, there must be four digits entered. The second level checks to assure that all tests designated as required have been done. These may be tests required with every examination or required at specific intervals. For example, if a certain individual has not had an upper GI series after an interval specified, the terminal operator is notified immediately, and the medical department can schedule accordingly.

The third type of edit check tests the value of a numeric test result against two types of ranges. First, the value is tested to see if it falls within a clinically normal range. If it does not, it will be flagged on the computerized examination summary as "abnormal". Second, if the value recorded is clinically impossible, the information is rejected and the terminal operator notified. Unlikely as it might be, the operator may find, upon investigation, that the recorded value is indeed correct; in this case, the range controls may be overridden.

Safety engineers provide the data for the second module of our occupational health system. At Standard Oil, the Safety Department is responsible for fire protection and mechanical safety, and so our input takes the form of Accident Reports. The data can then be extracted to provide specific safety information, such as which units at a certain location have the highest accident rate or what is the most frequent type

of accident; or the data may be correlated with medical
information in order to answer questions such as what types
of injuries are involved.

Table 2. Accident/safety module

Records Data on Line Into System

Two Part Mark Sense Form

Location Override	CAS Registration Number
Time and Date of Accident	Other Hazard
SS No. of Injured Employee	Equipment Involved
SS No. of Supervisor	Payment Amount
Accident Type	Traffic Accident Type
Accident Cause - Non Traffic	Traffic Accident Cause
Activity	Contents of Vehicle
Weather	
Claim No.	

No matter how good an occupational health system is in and of
itself, it is still highly dependent upon a strong employee
information system. Standard Oil has such a system, and we
do not duplicate effort by maintaining full employee information records within the medical system. Personnel data, such
as age, sex, race, social and work history, are maintained
and updated by the corporate personnel system; and only those
pieces of information we need for identification and demographic study are passed to the medical system's employee
file.

The medical information that we have been discussing is
intensely personal, and the employee has a definite right to
be assured that that information will be kept private.

The physician-patient relationship is one that is necessarily
based on trust. The physician must trust that the patient
has the confidence to provide full history, including social
and family history as well as personal medical history.
Determining the cause and course of disease and obtaining

good treatment results depend upon this two-way trust. In
order for the employee to derive maximum benefit from a corporate medical programme indeed, for the employee to remain
in the voluntary corporate medical programme he or she must
be assured that the physician-patient relationship will be
upheld, and that the data that are provided in confidence
will not fall into inappropriate hands.

More than fifteen years ago, as a positive statement supporting the medical department's role in providing preventive and
emergent health care to its employees, Standard Oil adopted a
written policy on confidentiality of medical information. It
is strict, considering all medical information (with the
exception of that exempted by statute) to be privileged and
requiring that that information be maintained in confidence
among company medical personnel. Functional information,
such as the ability to return to work, is the only information that may be made available to management.

Recently, a rule promulgated by one of our government
agencies, the Occupational Safety and Health Administration
(OSHA), has forced us to alter that policy. If the employee
has so authorised in writing, we must now make available that
employee's medical record to any designee specified. In
addition, OSHA now has access to all information requested
through proper protocol, with or without the employee's
consent.

Aside from this very important issue, extensive safeguards
have been built into Standard Oil's computerised occupational health system to prevent access by unauthorised
individuals. These safeguards pertain to all information
stored within the medical department computer system and
include secure terminals, an answer back system, a sign-on
procedure, multiple files and coded responses.

As has been stated, every terminal is operated by an employee
of the medical department who has been given a sign-on code

and a password that is to be kept secret; either or both of these codes may be changed at any time. In addition, each terminal is "hard-wired" - that is, the main system will accept data or return information only if the requesting terminal is one authorised to process the data requested. Only the central terminal in the General Office in Chicago has access to all information in the data base.

Further, the method by which data are stored includes a series of built-in deterrents to violations of security. First of all, employee or personnel information is not stored with the medical data, but is maintained in a separate file, and no identifiers such as employee name are connected directly to the medical files. A third file supplies the bridge between the employee and medical files. It is comprised of name, address, and social security number only. As with all our files, the social security number is the only common data element, and as another security measure, it is scrambled in all cases. Therefore, if someone were able to penetrate the medical files, that person would be unable to identify any of the records without the key to the bridge file.

However, precautionary measures do not stop here. Even if one could identify a record as being that of a certain individual, the data contained in that record are not easily read and interpreted. In many cases, the data elements are stored in a six-digit grid format. For example, one of our history forms asks the patient, "Have you ever had measles?" The patient may answer in the affirmative by marking the appropriate indicator on the form, and the response will be stored as "133126".This means that a positive answer was given to the question located on form 13, column 31, line 26. Without access to a Translation and Code Table, or TACT file, not only the answer, but the question itself, could not be determined by the entry in the data file.

In addition, since the medical files contain numeric as well as positional data, all numeric data, such as laboratory test results, are stored in a specific order in the internal records. This means that an unauthorised interrogator would have to be familiar not only with the programming itself but also with the layouts of those internal records in order to be able to identify individual results.

In addition to the specific programme controls, there are the usual administrative procedures designed to preserve confidentiality of computerised data. As with all other medical records, all input forms and subsequent sensitive reports are kept under lock and key in secure medical departments - nowhere else.

The reporting capabilities of the system are extensive and provide off-line reports on exmination schedules, examination notices, activity and a TACT file print. Currently, periodic reports generated include activity evaluation and quality control. Requiring standardised data helps to ensure that, as an example, uniform examinations are being performed. Periodic testing of the quality and quantity of the data points out those locations that may not be adhering to departmental guidelines or procedures.

The first two areas discussed, medical and safety, fall under the direction of the Medical Director, and information is supplied directly to the system by the medical and safety professionals; the third, employee information, is updated to the occupational health system on a monthly basis from the corporate personnel files; the fourth regarding environmental factors is not, at this time, directly available due to organisational separation of departments.

At Standard Oil, industrial hygiene and toxicology are functions of another department, Environmental Conservation and Toxicology, or EC&T. Relevant data are computerised within the Environmental Conservation and Toxicology group, and we in the Medical Department rely upon them to ensure the integrity of those data.

Development of the EC&T Information System is in the infant stage, and attention is now being directed toward identifying future needs. Among these are the capability to update information, such as that gained from industrial hygiene surveys, and already stored in the system. Provision must be made for ad hoc reporting in addition to fixed-format reporting, and a critical area is ensuring the availability of data in such a manner that it may be readily correlated with data in the Medical History System.

The latter correlation requires also sound data in one more area, namely, workplace history. Ability to identify a single workplace with a potential hazard means little if the employees associated with that workplace cannot also be identified.

When fully developed, each employee will be assigned a detailed location code. If those location codes are sufficiently well-defined, we can simply ask the computer to list all employees who have at any time, past or present, worked in that particular location.

Standard Oil of Indiana has an occupational health programme that is continually changing and growing to address the issues of preventive and emergent health care (FIGURE K.); and coordination is the key. Strictly administered policies, carefully tested procedures, and good communication channels among the various departments will assure that our success will continue.

MULTIDISCIPLINARY APPROACH TO PREVENTION AND HEALTH PROTECTION
BY MONITORING: ROLE OF INDIVIDUAL DISCIPLINES, LABOUR
INSPECTORS/COMPLIANCE OFFICERS I.

J. D. G. HAMMER (U.K.)

Summary

*This paper briefly outlines the role of the Labour Inspector/
Compliance Officer and his relationship with employers, trade
unions, the general public, the legislature and other specialists, describing the ways in which he makes use of ambient
and biological monitoring in his work. Some observations are
made about the nature of this work and examples are given of
the way in which he handles ambient and biological data in
practice. The paper concludes by setting out what the Labour
Inspector/Compliance Officer (LI/CO) expects from the legislature, scientists, hygienists, doctors, industry, commerce,
the trade unions and public authorities in their consideration and use of ambient and biological monitoring if his work
as an inspector is to be effective.*

Scope

Unless the sense otherwise requires "ambient monitoring" is
taken as including:

i) measurement of exposure of individuals by personal
   monitoring;

ii) measurement of process control by strategically
   placed background monitors;

iii) use of automatic continuous monitoring with recorders for both personal and background monitoring.

In general the Labour/Compliance Officer will make use of the
first two methods although employers will have to use the
third method for particular substances. Whilst this paper is
concerned solely with monitoring within the workplace, it is
throughout assumed that adequate consideration will be given
by the LI/CO to the emission of toxic substances to the
outside environment and that he will liaise with authorities
responsible for the control of such emissions.

General considerations

The Labour Inspector/Compliance Officer operates at the point
at which law, science and practicalities of production meet.
Although an enforcer of the law his concern is to translate
and interpret that law in the light of current knowledge and
with an eye to the practicalities of industry and commerce.
Although aware of the state and the development of scientific
and medical knowledge, he cannot wait for greater certain-
ties, for theories to be tested, for techniques to be developed. He has to make prompt decisions to take action or not
to take action, to give advice or not. The LI/CO stands
independent of industry, of employers and of employees each
with their own particular interests and priorities. Although
it is the employer who is primarily responsible for solving
any problems created by the processes and chemicals used in
the undertaking, the role of the inspector is not that of a
mechanistic enforcer such as the traffic warden responsible
for preventing parking offences. Rather, the LI/CO is one
who understands the genuine concerns of employers and
employees, maintaining his distance only in his independence
of judgement.

The role of the labour inspector/compliance officer

The role of the LI/CO is to make judgements:
- not judgements in a legalistic sense, for that
  is the role of the judge but, in relation to
  the law, the judgement as to whether to invoke
  formal enforcement procedures at that stage;
- not judgements in a medical or scientific sense
  on the primary scientific or medical evidence,
  but judgements about whether ambient or biological monitoring is appropriate and practicable
  in the situation and what weight and interpretation to attach to the results;
- not judgements on the philosophy of the employer or the social utility or economics of the

product or service, not judgements on the fears
of employees whether for their health or for
their jobs, not judgements on the fears or
aspirations of society;

- but judgements, made in the light of all these
factors aimed at the improvement of working
conditions both in the short and long term.

It is not always appreciated that for the LI/CO the decision
not to act, to allow things to run for a bit, to await
developments or further experience is just as difficult as
the decision to take action on the basis of monitoring
results. It can of course be argued that the legislature
passed the law and if the LI/CO has assessed some risk
(perhaps unquantified and unquantifiable at that stage) then
he has no option but to take a clear lead and make decisions
no matter how hard they may be; it is for society, the
company and their employees to take the consequences. There
will of course be circumstances where such clear and unequi-
vocal action is called for and is entirely right. But in
more cases the exercise of the inspector's balancing judgement in reviewing the result of ambient and biological
monitoring is unavoidable:

- the law is much more likely to be cast in
general than in specific terms;
- the scientific and medical evidence is unlikely
in most cases (and certainly not in the case of
most potential carcinogens or of new formula-
tions) to be incontestable;
- the economic and social pressures whether from
employers or trade unions or the general public
may well be more powerful than, and certanly
different from, those envisaged by the legislature concerned with principles rather than with
particular circumstances.

In the light of these issues the responsible inspector has to decide what his immediate and long term objectives are for the improvement of any particular workplace. Having decided on his objectives there are several courses of action open to him.

First if the firm is cooperative and shares the inspector's concern then it may be sufficient that the monitoring results are explained and that firm advice is given as to the improvements which are to be implemented.

Second, if there is any doubt as to the willingness of the management or of the workers to cooperate in securing the necessary improvements then the inspector will wish to negotiate a formal agreement with defined time limits and with specifically stated objectives. In Great Britain such an agreement often takes the form of an Improvement Notice or Prohibition Notice, the advantage of this course being that there is less room for misunderstanding and less room for subsequent excuses as to why changes or improvements have not been made.

A further reason for their success is that the recipients of the Notice are liable to be prosecuted in a court of law if the terms of the Notice are not complied with.

Third, the inspector may have recourse to a court of law without recourse to Notice procedures. More often than not going to a court of law is not the most efficient way of securing improvements either in individual premises or in a wider context in industry at large. For one thing court proceedings are seen to be punitive and therefore somewhat negative. Again, the outcome of a legal battle is not predictable and if the inspector should lose in court he may finish up in a weaker position in the short term with no remaining resources for securing improved conditions. Alternatively, he may win his case perhaps securing a harsh penalty or even the closure of the plant and the effect of

such a judgement may be seen by others as economically or
socially more damaging than the health hazard which gave rise
to the judgement. This can lead to pressure to revise the
law, reducing the level of protection.

The labour inspector's/compliance officer's contribution from practical experience

The practical experience of the inspector is an essential
ingredient in the recipe of control of exposure through
monitoring systems. His knowledge of industrial processes
will enable him to make comparisons, to understand production
pressures, and to reconcile situations where the results of
ambient and biological monitoring seem to indicate that the
workers are healthy in spite of atmospheric conditions, or
the converse.

His experience will allow him in some processes to use
monitoring as confirming evidence that the system of work he
has observed is unsatisfactory; for others the results will
demonstrate the existence of risk suspected but not apparent
to the eye or nose only.

Only his knowledge of the process will alert him to the fact
that because it is cyclical, emissions may be higher at
certain times in the cycle. Again, the process may give rise
to much greater levels of air pollution and much greater risk
of inhalation or ingestion during intermittent and allegedly
unforseeable processes such as cleaning, maintenance or
breakdown. The inspector therefore has to satisfy himself
that not only he, but also the employer, has taken account of
all phases of the process and all circumstances. In the case
of biological monitoring this means ensuring that account is
taken not only of process workers, but maintenance workers
who may be at risk or labourers who dispose of waste
material.

His experience will tell him when the levels detected by monitoring are likely to be improved by tinkering with ventilation systems or procedures, or whether some radical change to the process needs to be encouraged.

Such changes may range from the relatively obvious such as enclosure or wetting, to alternative means of batching and charging additives, to alternative mechanical techniques for operating a plant or rearranging the flow of work. For instance, the provision of conveyors in foundries, in addition to any production benefits, greatly facilitates the control of dust during knockout and fettling. Other changes may be more fundamental, extremely costly and perhaps only realistically implemented in the course of decades. Examples are the replacement of the Soderberg cell process in aluminium smelting by the pre-baked anode process which gives rise to less fume in addition to providing a higher standard of control, or again the rebuilding of coke oven batteries to incorporate sequential charging, also giving better fume control. On the other hand some of the practical problems are extremely mundane though the solutions are also sometimes relatively expensive and no less difficult to achieve. For example, in the cotton textile industry traditional methods of removing dust and "fly" from machines by brushing or "flapping down" using pieces of cardboard can only be discouraged if vacuum cleaning plant is installed and used in their place. In the ceramics industry once one has solved the problem of controlling dust during raw material preparation and fettling, the main source of atmospheric pollution and inhalation of silicious material is found to be the evolution of dust from the operative's clothing and from the floors where spilt clay and slip is dried and finely ground by the passage of wheels and feet. Thus the analysis of ambient air samples can lead the inspector to become involved in questions of clothing design and floor cleaning methods.

His experience of past problems leads him to the consideration of building design, for instance how to facilitate the dispersal of carbon monoxide from multi-storey car parks or public transport depots, matters sometimes inadequately considered by architects.

Sampling may also be used by an inspector to demonstrate the need for improvement in the maintenance of plant. Ventilating equipment originally of adequate capacity may deteriorate rapidly in the presence of heavy fume and dust concentration, and this will be revealed by monitoring and the use of other detection techniques such as the "dust lamp". This has for instance been demonstrated in the rubber industry where rapid deterioration of exhaust ventilation at the mixing plants has been shown to be the cause of major contamination of the workroom atmospheres.

From his practical experience the inspector also has to be aware of the possibility of samples being affected or being atypical, whether because of different working methods adopted by different workers or by deliberate falsification, though this latter process has to be done discreetly if the inspector is not to reject the results as wholly aberrant or due to equipment failure.

The LI/CO's experience will enable him too, to judge broadly the quality of efforts made by the employer to monitor conditions in his premises - a judgement which is important not only in interpreting the results, but for insight into general attitudes to worker protection. He will be helped by his experience to decide how far he can rely on the employer's data, and when to call upon his own resources for monitoring.

In reviewing the effect of results from ambient and biological monitoring the LI/CO has to have his eye on further technical developments, for instance the assessment of results obtained at different designs of foundry fettling branches devised to meet particular needs, should enable him to draw together for the guidance of the whole foundry

industry guidelines on which designs are in practice the most
effective for particular sizes and shapes of casting. He has
to accept that sometimes a technique which appears theoretically and in controlled experiments to promise immense
benefits, turns out to be disappointing in practice.

The labour inspector's/compliance officer's practical needs

First of all, if he is to fulfil his role effectively, the
LI/CO needs law which is progressive - that is law which is
on the one hand flexible and adaptable to changing circumstances, yet on the other hand gives him a fair certainty of
success when he invokes it to require improvements. The law
should provide a framework of intent within which the LI/CO
can make his own judgements in the light of current knowledge. What the LI/CO does not want is law which is too
detailed and too simplistically absolute and which is
therefore unenforceable because its requirements are not
practicable.

Second, he needs not only to be aware of the current state of
scientific research and medical knowledge, but also if
possible to have available to himself, industry and the
courts agreed and published control limits, together with
guidance on the taking and interpretation of ambient and
biological samples so that he does not have on each occasion
to argue his case ab initio. It is particularly helpful if
there exists some sublegislative body, or bodies, representing scientific, industrial and inspectorate interests which
can weigh the changing evidence and produce such practical
interpretation and guidance, which, even if it does not stand
the test of time, will at least be regarded as helpful and
relevant in that decade.

Third, he must have available to him the services of hygienists for ambient monitoring and of medical personnel for
biological monitoring. He needs also be be assured that
techniques for making ambient and biochemical estimations are

broadly agreed and accepted within the scientific and industrial community.

Fourth, he needs to be au fait with current industrial practice. He must understand current hygiene problems in industry and also the latest technological developments.

Fifth, he needs to be functioning within an organisational structure which has a coherent policy toward the use and control of toxic substances, without which the exercise of individual judgements would lead to unacceptable variations in enforcement practice.

Finally, he needs tough powers of enforcement with which he can make his considered judgement effective.

The involvement of the hygienist and laboratory support

If the ambient air measurements are to be credible, then the Labour Inspector/Compliance Officer, who may well be a hygienist, must be personally involved in setting up the survey in the premises. He must use his knowledge of the practical problems and vagaries of the process and of people in deciding where and when and how the sampling should be undertaken and recorded. It is emphatically not simply a job for the technician, important as his role is in support.

The inspector also needs good facilities for the processing of monitoring samples which enable him to take rapid action where this is called for and to use the results in a dialogue with the employer and the employees. The exclusive use of a remote central laboratory can make this a very long-winded process. A possible solution is that adopted in Great Britain where in addition to providing general inspectors with initial diagnostic instruments we have seven multi-disciplinary specialists consultant groups spread across the country each with its own laboratory and scientific staff. The laboratories are equipped for analysis of inspectors' air samples by modern instrument techniques (atomic absorption spectrophotometry, gas chromatography, infra-red spectroscopy) and by methods of analysis that use the more traditional laboratory glassware, microscopes, etc. They perform the analyses of all but the most complex samples or the uncommon ones that require a particular kind of apparatus that they do not have. In these circumstances they rely on the back-up of the Research and Laboratory Services Division central laboratory. Each group is also provided with a mobile laboratory which can be used to carry to the site air sampling and analytical apparatus appropriate to the occasion. Where the general public is at risk the visible presence of an independent authority can have a useful presentational effect.

The central laboratory not only processes all the biological samples but also the more complex or unusual air samples using X-ray diffraction, mass spectrographs and electron microscopes - equipment too expensive to be duplicated in the field.

In this way the LI/CO can have access both to the rapid analysis of urgent and common samples and also to a laboratory which can develop the methodology of analysis.

Disclosure of air sampling results

Whilst other speakers are to consider the confidentiality of biological monitoring results, it is appropriate to suggest here that inspectors should not generally keep the results of their own ambient monitoring to themselves but should disclose them as soon as possible both to the employers and to the trade unions, accepting also the need to comment on and interpret those results, whether or not there is justifiable cause for concern. It may be necessary to explain why certain levels are "acceptable". It is preferable to be open with the facts and face the consequences of disclosure than for the inspector to use this information secretively as his personal property which, in the long run creates suspicion among employers, trade unions and the general public.

Conclusions

From industrial management and trade unions the LI/CO expects an understanding not only of the immense value but also the limitations of ambient and biological monitoring. He wants to see these techniques used to investigate problems, to identify plant and processes which require modification and improvement and to monitor standards of control. The LI/CO expects industry to feed the results of such monitoring into the consideration of new plant and processes. He expects both sides of industry to abjure the use of monitoring results for politico/economic ends. Above all, he looks to both sides of industry to cooperate with the LI/CO, with scientists, hygienists and doctors in making available their experience and results, to build up a greater national and international bank of knowledge both about solutions to practical problems in particular processes and industries, so that control techniques can be improved, and also about dose/response relationships so that hygiene standards can be modified and refined.

But equally the LI/CO looks to his fellow specialists with certain expectations. He would like to see further development of the concept of environmental and biological control limits which give practical guidance to industry and enable him as an inspector to make informed judgements and to act decisively. He looks to specialists for support in court or tribunal. He would like to see the further development of analytical techniques and he would wish for ambient and biological monitoring results to be used more systematically in relation to one another, in order to build up better documented knowledge of dose/response relationships. He hopes to see more retrospective and prospective epidemiological studies not only on a national but on an international scale which, when they properly combine ambient and biological monitoring results are convincing to industry, the trade unions, the courts and the legislature.

And in his work in the field the LI/CO hopes for an understanding of the constraints on his work in that he both
advises on and enforces the law in a world where account has
to be taken of economic costs, of practical production
problems and of people with their idiosyncrasies.

MULTIDISCIPLINARY APPROACH TO PREVENTION AND HEALTH PROTECTION
BY MONITORING: ROLE OF INDIVIDUAL DISCIPLINES. LABOUR
INSPECTORS/COMPLIANCE OFFICERS II.

D. RHONE (USA-OSHA)

Summary

*This paper presents a description of the occupational
health programme administered by the Occupational Safety
and Health Administration (OSHA), of the U.S. Department
of Labor. The paper discusses the agency's major functions
and the duties and responsibilities that the compliance
safety and health officer (in this case an industrial hygienist) assumes in the execution of those functions. The
requirements mandated by the agency's new health standards
are examined, and particular attention is given to the
crucial role that both ambient and biological monitoring play
in assuring adequate worker protection from workplace health
hazards and the challenges inherent in an effective
occupational health programme outlined.*

OSHA's Occupational Health Programme

The Occupational Safety and Health Act was passed into law in
1970 with its major goal being to assume safe and healthy
workplaces for all Americans. OSHA is the agency established
to ensure enforcement of this law. In order to carry out its
mission effectively, OSHA has engaged a highly trained, professional staff of Compliance Safety and Health Officers
(CSHOs). Although a vigorous cross-training programme has
been initiated to assure that compliance officers are knowledgeable in both safety and health disciplines, safety
specialists continue to have primary responsibility for
investigating safety hazards and industrial hygienists are
charged with the conduct of health inspections and the
enforcement of health standards.

The role of the industrial hygienist

As a minimum requirement, industrial hygienists must have a
Bachelor's Degree in Industrial Hygiene or a related field,

or four years of progressive, technical industrial hygiene experience. In addition to these basic requirements, many of the agency's industrial hygienists have graduate degrees in industrial hygiene or environmental health.

Since the topic of this paper is the agency's occupational health programme, the following discussion will focus on the various duties of the industrial hygienist/compliance officer. It should be remembered that OSHA attempts to achieve the goal of safe and healthy workplaces not only through compliance inspection and standards enforcement, but also through such preventive measures as employer and worker education and by encouraging voluntary compliance. The industrial hygienist has responsibilities in all of these areas.

The principal responsibilities of the industrial hygienist/ compliance officer are to perform industrial hygiene surveys in the workplace and to enforce the health standards that have been promulgated under the Occupational Safety and Health Act.

In order to assist the industrial hygienist in the execution of these inspections and enforcement duties, and to assure uniformity, the industrial hygiene field operations manual was developed which sets forth OSHA's technical policy for the handling of health surveys and also lists the industrial hygiene practices and procedures to be observed in the conduct of these investigations.

Prior to opening an inspection, the hygienist reviews the traditional health hazards associated with the industry to be inspected. The sampling methods to be utilised and all standards that may be applicable are also studied.

The initial phase of an inspection is referred to as a "walk-around" and its primary purpose is to identify potential health hazards in the plant. This identification of

potential health hazards requires that the industrial hygienist collect all available information on the plant processes,
obtain a listing of all chemical substances used and all
physical hazards present, determine the duration and frequency of cyclic work processes, survey existing engineering
controls, review the employer's air and biological monitoring
results, and screen potential exposure areas by using a
variety of direct reading instrumentation. Upon completion
of the "walkaround" phase of the investigation, the hygienist
will evaluate the above data and make a determination as to
whether or not full shift sampling is warranted.

Because OSHA is a law enforcement agency, its policies on the
conduct of industrial hygiene inspections dictate that the
industrial hygienist must assure that all inspection activities are adequately documented and that all violations found
during the investigation can be supported in a court of law.
Consequently, in most cases the hygienist must perform full
shift air sampling in order to document an employee over-
exposure since most of OSHA's permissible exposure limits
are expressed as eight-hour time weighted averages. Additionally, most air samples must be taken in the personal
breathing zone, defined as a sphere, approximately two feet
in diameter, surrounding the head - since these samples would
most closely approximate actual employee exposure. Area
samples may be taken to identify exposure sources and to
assist in the determination of the effectiveness of, or the
need for, engineering controls.

When sampling results indicate that employee over-exposures
exist, the Occupational Safety and Health Act mandates that a
citation be issued to the employer. This citation lists the
alleged violations of the Act, may carry penalties depending
upon the seriousness of the hazards, and sets a time limit
for the abatement of the violation. In most cases, OSHA's
position is that personal protective equipment (respirators
or hearing protectors) is acceptable only as an interim
abatement measure and that final abatement of the hazard must

be accomplished through the institution of engineering or administrative controls. One of the most important reasons for
not accepting personal protective equipment as a final abatement measure is that it places an undue hardship on the
employee to control his exposure, rather than controlling it
at its source. In addition, respirators and hearing protectors require proper fitting to ensure effectiveness. It
is frequently difficult to enforce their use and the fact
remains that once the employee removes the protective equipment he will be exposed. However, personal protective equipment would be an acceptable abatement method if no other
feasible controls existed. However in most cases feasible
engineering controls are available such as the installation
of additional ventilation, the substitution of less toxic
materials or the isolation of the process that is causing the
exposure, installation of sound barriers, as well as
administrative and work practice controls.

Because OSHA insists upon the use of engineering controls as
a first line of defense to protect against health hazards, it
has been necessary for the agency to establish a competent,
diversified and informed technical support section. In addition to an an in-house staff of engineers, physicians and
industrial hygiene experts, outside experts are frequently
consulted in attempts to develop feasible solutions to
difficult technical problems. This is also the case during
the promulgation of new standards in that OSHA solicits
comments from medical and toxicological experts concerning
safe exposure levels, and information from engineering
experts, labour groups and industry groups as to the
feasibility of controls to achieve these exposure levels.

In some instances, OSHA has even been instrumental in the
development of new control technology. One of the best
examples of this is the results that were brought about by
the Vinyl Chloride Standard. When the Vinyl Chloride
Standard was promulgated setting a permissible exposure limit
of one ppm, the entire plastics industry complained that it

was impossible to control exposures to this low level.
However, necessity again became the mother of invention and
within a few years, the technology was developed that would
keep employee exposures below the permissible limit and
result in more efficient production.

While the agency does encourage the use and development of
new technology to eliminate health hazards, it is also flexible, and is aware that in some instances feasible controls
are not available. In such cases, a very stringent personal
protective equipment programme is required in order to provide maximum employee protection. There are also instances
where due to other limiting factors, an employer cannot comply with an OSHA regulation. In that situation, an employer
may be granted a variance, provided that the employees are
provided protection equal to compliance with the standard in
question.

Finally, the industrial hygienist also plays an essential
role in the processes that follow the issuance of a citation.
Perhaps the hygienist's most important function at this time
is the evaluation of the employer's proposed abatement plan
and its effectiveness in controlling exposures and protecting
employees. However, should a citation be contested by an
employer and the case proceed to a hearing, the industrial
hygienist assumes an equally important part as a chief wit-
ness and must be able to present legally sufficient testimony
as to the findings of an inspection.

Although the compliance activities described above are the
hygienist's primary occupation, education of workers, employers, and the general public are also part of his duties. In
addition, should a violation of another regulatory agency's
standards (such as the Environmental Protection Agency) be
observed during an OSHA inspection, the condition is referred
to that agency for corrective action. Therefore, the industrial hygienist helps to assure a healthful environment for
all through his compliance activities in the workplace,

programme support efforts, and awareness of hazards outside the workplace.

The new health standards

Currently, OSHA has adopted permissible exposure limits for approximately 400 substances. For the majority of these sub-stances the permissible exposure is all that is regulated, although possible ingestion hazards or skin absorption problems would be addressed. For the most part, the other aspects of a good industrial hygiene programme were not addressed.

However, in the past few years, OSHA had issued several major expanded health standards, such as coke ovens, acrylonitrile, inorganic arsenic, cotton dust, and lead. The issuance of these standards has brought about a significant change in the realm of OSHA's enforcement capabilities. These new stan-dards all have similar requirements. In addition to estab-lishing a permissible exposure limit and requiring respective engineering controls, these standards require that the employer perform routine environmental monitoring. Also, overexposed employees must be provided with adequate hygiene facilities, protective work clothing, and proper medical surveillance. The employer must maintain an effective medical surveillance programme to monitor the workers' health. Thus, the existence of serious health problems due to workplace exposures can be determined, and appropriate preventive measures can be taken to assure that these health problems are not aggravated by continuing exposure.

By far the most important aspect of these standards is the agency's philosophy that by educating the workers and making them aware of the facts, they will be better able to assist in controlling their workplace environment. Consequently, these new standards require that the employer notify the workers of their exposure levels and of the results of their medical exams and biological monitoring. These standards

also require the employer to develop training programmes
for all exposed employees, to inform them of the health
hazards associated with the substance, the proper work practices to be used to minimise exposure, and other requirements
of the standard. Thus, for these new standards, worker
education plays a crucial role in implementing a complete
industrial hygiene programme.

Biological monitoring vs. environmental monitoring

It seems appropriate at this time to discuss some of the
controversy that arose during the promulgation of the lead
standard in regard to whether or not biological monitoring
alone could adequately protect workers exposed to lead.
Several different opinions were presented and evaluated by
those responsible for developing the standard. When the
final standard was finished, the decision made was that evaluation of the plant environment is best and most directly
accomplished through a comprehensive industrial hygiene
survey. This includes the use of traditional industrial
hygiene methods: air monitoring to determine the sources of
exposure; biological monitoring; reviewing the adequacy of
the engineering controls already in place; and evaluating the
progress made toward implementation of new controls.

Since OSHA believes that control of an air contaminant is
best accomplished at the source, background environmental
monitoring provides a direct measure of the effectiveness of
the controls. The end result of engineering control technology - the workers' actual exposure - is thus determined
through methods designed to prevent chronic lead related
disease: airborne monitoring first, and biological monitoring
second.

Biological monitoring (blood leads) is helpful in determining
problems in individual workers, and may demonstrate that the
employee is exposed to an ingestion hazard, in the circumstances when his air monitoring results indicate that he is

not exposed to excessive lead-in-air levels. However, there are several drawbacks to relying totally on biological monitoring results for enforcement purposes. One problem is that excessive lead exposures do not necessarily result in immediately significant blood lead levels. Therefore, workers may be exposed for a considerable length of time before the biological monitoring results revealed these exposures. Another consideration is that low blood levels could be achieved solely by the use of respirators and the employer could thus circumvent the problem and not institute engineering controls. All of this discussion leads to the conclusion that for OSHA standards, air monitoring has been determined to be the primary method of evaluating worker exposure, and biological monitoring is an integral supplement in assuring the continued health of the worker while a potential for adverse exposure exists in the workplace.

Conclusions

OSHA's emphasis on occupational health hazards during the past five years has resulted in many insights into the problems facing any agency charged with the reduction of occupational disease.

First and foremost, education of the employer and employee is the greatest challenge facing the health professional. OSHA is now evaluating the results of our funding of non-profit organisations (employer-employee groups, and universities) to determine if these educational efforts are effective. We believe the worker must have the right to review those medical records and environmental monitoring results which the employer possesses, and we require this through federal regulation for all hazardous substances. We further believe that a worker should be informed of the hazards and related chemicals to which he is exposed - a practice not common in the United States - and we are developing regulations to address this issue.

Second an effective method must be developed to deal with
broad classes of hazards, rather than with each one individually. The health community has recognised thousands of
hazardous exposures in the workplace which should be
addressed by an agency charged with worker protection. OSHA
has initiated this effort with a broad method of identifying
and classifying occupational carcinogens for future
regulation.

Third we must review the toxicity of new chemicals before
they are introduced into the workplace. Our sister agency,
the Environmental Protection Agency (EPA) has begun this
effort with the pretesting requirements of the Toxic Substances Control Act. A plan to test the thousands of industrial chemicals now in existence is also critical. We need
no further tragedies as those associated with vinyl chloride,
asbestos, organic pesticides, and coke oven emissions.

Fourth the government must develop better incentives for the
prevention of occupational disease. The delayed impact of
latent disease belies the importance of preventive actions.
Incentives, other than enforcement of standards, workmen's
compensation, and disability insurance, are necessary. As
safety and health professionals, we must improve our ability
to demonstrate that safety and health are cost effective.

Finally, we must continually feel the pulse of society's
perception of workplace risk and benefit. In OSHA, we have
"opened up" the regulatory process to encourage public participation in decision making. We have recognised that regulation of workplace conditions is a function of the pressures
which our society creates. Our role in government includes
the responsibility to present our society with all of the
data and uncertainties necessary for public decision making.
This must be done as part of the process of educating the
public, which is critical to our success.

Thus, the rule of our OSHA staff, safety and health professionals, is to continually strive to promote hazard prevention through the unbiased application of their training,
through the enforcement of standards, education of the workforce, and constant awareness of the public's need to know
the basis for determining acceptable levels of risk in the
workplace.

MULTIDISCIPLINARY APPROACH TO PREVENTION AND HEALTH PROTECTION
BY MONITORING: ROLE OF INDIVIDUAL DISCIPLINES. MEDICAL
INSPECTORS/MEDICAL OFFICERS I.

P. LANDRIGAN, J.K. BAINBRIDGE AND J.M. MELINS (USA-NIOSH)

Summary

The practice of occupational medicine in the United States
relies increasingly upon epidemiology. Sixty-four percent of
physicians in the National Institute for Occupational Safety
and Health (NIOSH) are trained in epidemiology, and the
number of physician-epidemiologists in NIOSH has increased
since 1976 from 11 to 29.

In this presentation, we describe the expanding role of
physician-epidemiologists in occupational medicine in the
United States. In NIOSH, physician-epidemiologists now play
a central role in the conduct of epidemiological studies
covering entire industries, and in retrospective cohort
mortality studies, in case-control studies, and in cross-
sectional medical studies as well as in Health Hazard Evaluations. The field of occupational epidemiology is only in its
infancy.   It will expand considerably during the next decade
as countries shift resources from such traditional public
health activities as the control of infectious diseases and
the protection of maternal and child health to major efforts
to identify and prevent mortality and disability among the
most productive part of their nation's workforces.

Introduction

Epidemiological techniques which were developed to define,
analyse, and prevent such infectious diseases as cholera, (1)
measles, (2) smallpox, (3) and tuberculosis (4) have proven
to be extremely useful in the understanding and control of
occupational disease. (5-9) Epidemiology has been used to
establish the aetiology of acute workplace illness, such as
kepone poisoning, (10) to follow the course and define the
risk factors of major, continuing epidemics, such as asbes-
tosis (11) and byssinosis, (12) and to assess the significance of rare disease events, such as angiosarcoma of the
liver. (13) Epidemiology has come to be a discipline of
major importance in the practice of occupational medicine.

Physicians with skills in occupational epidemiology are
increasingly being employed in the United States by major
manufacturing firms, international labour organisations,
universities developing occupational medicine programmes,
State health departments and the Federal Government. Today
in the United States, the organisation with the largest
number of physician-epidemiologists involved in the study of
occupational disease is the National Institute for Occupational Safety and Health (NIOSH), a Federal research agency
established under the Occupational Safety and Health Act of
1970 to make recommendations to the Department of Labor
regarding workplace health and safety standards.

In the past four years the number of physicians in NIOSH with
formal training in epidemiology has increased from 11 to 29,
and the proportion of all NIOSH physicians with epidemiological expertise is now 64.4 per cent (Figure 1). In large
measure this increase was stimulated by the interest in disease prevention which followed passage of the Occupational
Safety and Health Act. Also, it has coincided with the
administrative joining of NIOSH with the Centre for Disease
Control (Atlanta, Georgia).

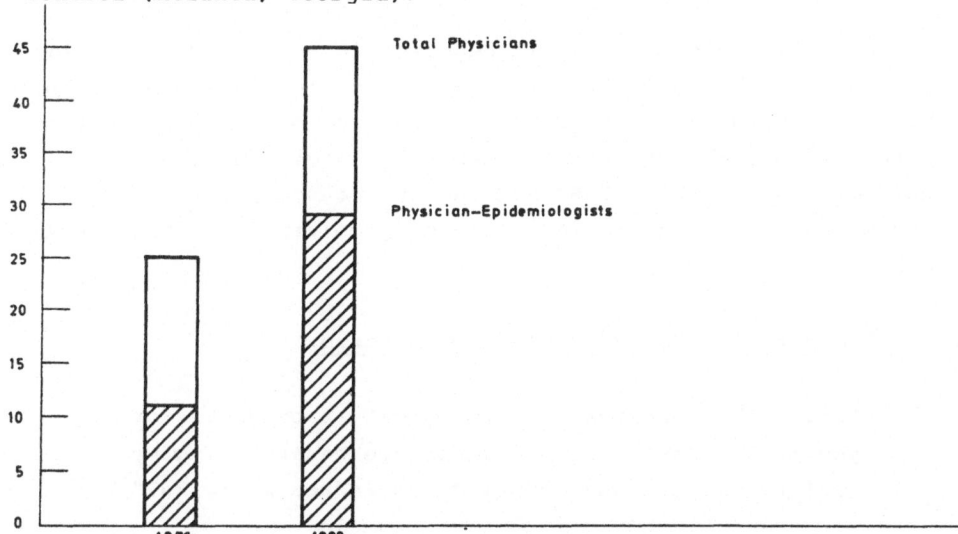

Figure 1.   Total Number of Physicians and of Physician-
            Epidemiologists. National Institute for
            Occupational Safety and Health   1976-1980

Field medical officers in NIOSH are now expected to exercise their clinical skills in a broad, epidemiologically defined context. They are expected to integrate their clinical abilities with their training in epidemiology. Thus, the focus of NIOSH investigations is no longer restricted to consideration of ill workers or of workers with known expo- sure to toxic chemicals or hazardous processes. Instead our physicians have become accustomed to evaluating the entire workforce of a plant or an industry - exposed and unexposed alike. Further, they have become accustomed to conducting their medical evaluations in close concert with our indus- trial hygienists so that their medical data might be corre- lated with environmental findings. This approach has enabled NIOSH medical officers to accurately define the prevalence and risk factors in various occupational diseases and to undertake relatively sophisticated dose-response analyses on even small groups of exposed workers. Such studies are essential in imputation of the aetiology of occupational disease, in recognising the spectrum of syndromes produced by occupational exposures, and in making recommendations or setting standards for limiting the exposure of workers to harmful substances.

In this presentation we shall describe in some further detail the role of physician-epidemiologists in the NIOSH Health Hazard Evaluation Program. Also, we shall present two examples of recent studies which illustrate the role of epidemiology within NIOSH and underscore the power of epide- miological techniques for solving problems in occupational disease.

The NIOSH Health Hazard Evaluation Program

"Are the chemicals, biological substances, or physical agents in my workplace hazardous to my health? If so, what can I do to reduce my risks?"

Under the provisions of the Occupational Safety and Health Act of 1970, NIOSH is required to help workers and employers to answer these questions. Thus when our assistance is requested by an employee representative, a union, an employer, or another Federal or State Agency, NIOSH is required to conduct an on-site investigation to try to determine whether the specific hazards in a particular workplace are potentially toxic in the concentrations used or found. The Congress of the United States had two intentions when it required NIOSH to perform this activity - which NIOSH calls its Health Hazard Evaluation Program. The first was to provide a service at no cost to employers and employees - particlarly to those in small businesses which comprise over 90% of workplaces in the USA - in identifying and reducing potentially hazardous working situations. The second intent was to provide a practical means for determining whether or not existing workplace standards were, in fact, protecting worker health. In order to understand the role of physician-epidemiologists in achieving these two purposes - which, by the way, may often be in conflict - we describe how NIOSH conducts health hazard evaluations, and discuss two of the more than two hundred investigations completed during the past year.

Typically, a Health Hazard Evaluation begins with a telephone call or a letter to NIOSH. In this initial contact, we attempt to determine whether NIOSH is the most appropriate agency to respond to the request, how soon we need to respond, and the types of staff which we will need to send to the workplace to conduct the investigation. Generally, a request will fall into one of two categories:
- either an unusual proportion of workers at a work site appear to be experiencing excess morbidity, disability, or mortality, the cause of which is unknown; or
- workers suspect that a particular chemical, biological substance, or physical agent in their workplace may be hazardous, but they do not know

whether or not there are potentially adverse
health effects resulting from their exposures.

NIOSH responds to most Health Hazard Evaluation requests by
sending to the workplace an initial survey team composed of a
physician-epidemiologist and an industrial hygienist. During
this initial visit, NIOSH staff discuss the request with the
employer and employees, observe relevant work processes, work
practices and work environment, take preliminary environmental samples, review work history and medical records and
privately interview workers who appear to be at risk of
exposure. At the end of this initial visit, NIOSH normally
makes verbal recommendations to the employees and employer as
to how to minimize potential exposure. Approximately 20% of
the investigations can be concluded at this point, with a
formal report being provided to the employer, employee
representative, and to the appropriate Federal Standards
enforcement organisation.

The types of investigations which can be concluded after a
single field visit are those in which workers are exposed to
only one or two hazards, where there are clear and time-
tested standards established for those hazards, and where any
illnesses in workers can be clearly related to the workplace
exposures. Unfortunately, most requests do not fall into
those relatively simple categories. Although in the early
years of the past decade, most requests were quite straightforward, employers and employee representatives are now
becoming more knowledgeable about workplace hazards and more
sophisticated in making requests. This change in the nature
of requests has been a major factor in the increased need for
physician-epidemiologists in the Health Hazard Evaluation
Program.

For those situations in which the NIOSH industrial hygienist
and physician-epidemiologist are unable to complete the
investigation during the initial field visit, the team
returns to NIOSH. Then following discussions with experts on

the alleged hazards or illnesses and a review of the scientific literature, the team prepares a protocol for a more
detailed epidemiological and environmental investigation.
These protocols would include such items as case definitions,
working hypotheses, definitions of control groups and
sampling plans. With the protocol developed, the team
returns to the workplace to conduct further environmental
sampling, to obtain medical histories and to conduct medical
examinations of exposed (and unexposed) employees, and to
review employee medical records. Following the analysis of
data from these additional investigations, NIOSH provides a
formal report to the employees, employer and appropriate
State and Federal Agencies. The physician-epidemiologist and
the industrial hygienists, as well as a wide variety of
support personnel must work together quite closely in developing such a report and in making a final determination as
to the hazard of the conditions and exposures in a particular
workplace.

The final report on a Health Hazard Evaluation, which
includes specific recommendations for action to protect the
exposed workers, must be posted in the workplace for a period
of 30 days. Although NIOSH does not have the authority to
force companies to improve working conditions, most NIOSH
recommendations are in fact implemented, particularly those
which are the least expensive. In most instances, this
implementation appears to be a consequence of collective
bargaining by employees and/or fear of subsequent legal
citation by employers. Also, all NIOSH evaluation reports
are transmitted to the appropriate enforcement agencies.
Approximately 65% of NIOSH requests come from employees (90%
of these from labour unions), and 35% from employers. Over
50% of NIOSH investigations conclude that a real or potential
health hazard exists.

Should the NIOSH team discover during a Health Hazard Evaluation that workers are experiencing illness or adverse health
effects for currently unregulated substances, or that adverse

effects are occurring at levels of exposure below existing
exposure standards, we would prepare recommendations for
revised exposure limits, for safer work practices, or for
increased environmental and medical monitoring, and would
provide this information to the appropriate Federal regulatory agency - Occupational Safety and Health Administration,
Mine Safety and Health Administration, or the Environmental
Protection Agency. In practice, however, such major
recommendations are made only infrequently, because (i) the
number of workers exposed to a hazard in a given workplace is
normally relatively small, (ii) workers are normally exposed
to several hazards simultaneously, and evaluation is
therefore difficult, and (iii) health hazard evaluations are
normally aimed at assessing the acute rather than the chronic
effects of workplace exposures.

Examples of health hazard evaluations

Two examples of recently completed Health Hazard Evaluations
should serve to illustrate the nature of NIOSH's health
hazard evaluation programme and the role of the physician-
epidemiologist in the programme. The first (12) involves an
assessment of lead poisoning in a lead-acid battery manufacturing plant in Bennington, Vermont. The second (13)
revolves around a request from teacher aides in the State of
Washington for NIOSH to determine if exposures from hand-
operated duplicating machines that use methyl alcohol could
cause adverse health effects.

In the first instance, the United Automotive, Aerospace, and
Agricultural Implement Workers Union (UAW) requested NIOSH,
in late May 1978, to evaluate worker exposure to lead and
other substances at a lead battery plant in Vermont. To
study symptoms and exposure, NIOSH conducted industrial
hygiene and medical evaluations and assessed the effectiveness of existing engineering controls for limiting worker
exposure. Over a period of three visits to the workplace,
personal and area air samples were obtained to measure lead,

arsenic, antimony, sulphuric acid, arsine, stibine, and
benzene-soluble polynuclear aromatic hydrocarbons. Blood
lead, erythrocyte protoporphyrin, urine arsenic, and blood
urea nitrogen concentrations were determined.

The industrial hygienist found that lead concentrations in
35 of 342 personal air samples equalled or exceeded the
previous OSHA standard of 200 μg/m^3; 93 equalled or
exceeded the NIOSH recommended standard of 100 μg/m^3; and
172 equalled or exceeded the new OSHA standard of 50 μg/m^3.
Arsenic concentrations were also found to exceed both OSHA
standards and NIOSH recommended exposure limits. On the basis
of those data, NIOSH concluded that a hazard of exposure to
lead and arsenic existed in the plant at the times of the
NIOSH visits and made recommendations to the company on
ventilation, work practices, and medical surveillance. This
example illustrates that it is possible in some situations to
utilise health hazard evaluations for establishing dose-
response relationships. The Occupational Safety and Health
Administration, when it revised the occupation lead standard
in 1978, relied quite heavily on numerous NIOSH health hazard
evaluations related to lead exposure in determining appropriate exposure limits.(15)

In April 1980, NIOSH received a request from the Public
School Employees Union of Washington State (16) to determine
whether exposures of employees to fumes from hand-operated
office duplicating machines (spirit duplicators) used by 84
teachers aides in 18 schools were hazardous. The union
wished in particular to know whether the methyl alcohol used
as a solvent in the duplicators was causing hazardous
exposures either by inhalation or skin absorption. Three
teachers' aides had died during the previous four years, and
the Union wished to know whether those deaths had been caused
by exposure to the duplicating machines.

To evaluate exposures, a NIOSH field team went to the schools
and measured methyl alcohol concentrations in the breathing

zones of a sample of the teacher aides. The team also evaluated existing control measures in 12 of the 18 schools, and administered a questionnaire to 66 teachers' aides and to an equal number of randomly chosen age- and sex-matched teachers. Also, death certificates and autopsy information were obained for the aides who had died between 1975 and 1979. Efforts were made to determine whether any other aides had died within the preceding 10 years.

The environmental sampling revealed that breathing-zone concentrations around 75% of the machines tested exceeded the NIOSH recommended 15-minute exposure limit for methyl alcohol. The physician-epidemiologist found that 45% of the teachers' aides had experienced adverse symptoms in the month before the study, compared to 23% of the teachers. Symptoms included blurred vision (23% aides v. 1.5% teachers), dizziness (30% v. 1.5%), headaches (34% v. 18%), nausea (18% v. 6%), and skin problems (11% v. 1%). Although the health data were the result of self-reporting and therefore subject to observer bias, the two groups showed comparable prevalence rates for symptoms unrelated to methyl alcohol exposure. There was no indication from review of the death certificates and autopsy reports that the aides' deaths had been caused by methyl alcohol exposure.

When NIOSH investigators constructed enclosures around six of the duplicators and used the existing exhaust systems, the breathing zone concentrations of methyl alcohol were reduced by 90-98% to levels well within NIOSH recommended exposure limits. Thus, NIOSH was able in three months to conclude that a health hazard did exist and was able to provide very practical recommendations for limiting exposure.

Because the possibility existed that similar duplicators were widely utilised in school systems throughout the United States, NIOSH went on to publish a summary article on the results of the investigation in the Centre for Disease Control's Morbidity and Mortality Weekly Report (circulation

90,000). (17) Further we are working with the National
Education Association to publicise the results in national
journals read by teachers and school administrators. This
example illustrated two points: first that epidemiological/
industrial hygiene techniques can often be used for rapid
identification and reduction of workplace hazards, and second
that a good programme for data dissemination can increase
greatly the utility and the impact of a Health Hazard
Evaluation.

References

1. Snow, J. On the Mode of Communication of Cholera (2nd
    ed.). London, Churchill 1855. Reproduced in Snow on
    Cholera. New York: Commonwealth Fund, 1936.
    Reprinted, New York: Hafner, 1965.

2. Panum, P.L. Observations made during the epidemic of
    measles on the Faroe Islands in the year 1846.
    Reproduced in Delta Omega Society, Panum on Measles.
    New York: American Public Health Association, 1940.

3. Foege, W.H., Millar, J.D., Lane, J.M. Selective
    epidemiologic control in smallpox eradication. Amer. J.
    Epidemiol. 94:311-315, 1971.

4. Rich, A. The Pathogenesis of Tuberculosis.
    Springfield, Illinois. Charles C. Thomas, 1944.

5. Hamilton, A. Exploring the Dangerous Trades. Boston:
    Little, Brown, 1943.

6. Legge, R.T. History of industrial medicine and occupa-
    tional diseases. Industr. Med. Surg. 5:30, 1936.

7. Figueroa, W.G., Raszkowski, R., Weiss, W. Lung Cancer
    in chloromethyl ether workers. New Engl. J. Med. 288:
    1096-1097, 1973.

8. Acheson, E.D., Cowdell, R.H., Hadfield, E., MacBeth,
    R.G. Nasal cancer in woodworkers in the furniture
    industry. Brit. Med. J. 2:587-596, 1968.

9.   Case, R.A.M., Hosker, M.E., McDonald, D.B., Pearson,
       J.T. Tumours of the urinary bladder in workmen engaged
       in the manufacture and use of certain dyestuff inter-
       mediates in the British chemical industry. Part I.
       The role of aniline, benzidine, alpha-naphthylamine,
       and beta-naphthylamine. Brit. J. Ind. Med. 2:75-104,
       1954.

10.   Cannon, S.B., Veazey, J.R.Jr., Jackson, R.S., Burse,
       V.W., Hayes, C., Straub, W.E., Landrigan, P.J., Liddle,
       J.A. Epidemic kepone poisoning in chemical workers.
       Amer. J. Epidemiol. 107:529-537, 1978.

11.   Selikoff, I.J., Churg, J., Hammon, E.C. The occurrence
       of asbestosis among insulation workers in the United
       States. Annals NY Acad. Sci. 132:139-155, 1965.

12.   Schilling, R.S.F. Byssinosis in cotton and other tex-
       tile workers. Lancet 2:261-265, 1956.

13.   Creech, J.L.Jr., Johnson, M.N. Angiosarcoma of the
       liver in the manufacture of polyvinyl chloride. J.
       Occup. Med. 16: 150-151, 1974.

14.   National Institute for Occupational Safety and Health.
       Health Hazard Evaluation 78-98-710, Globe Union Battery
       Plant, Bennington, Vermont. Cincinnati: NIOSH, July
       1980.

15.   Occupational Safety and Health Administration, U.S.
       Department of Labor: Occupational exposure to lead,
       final standard. Federal Register 43:52952-53014, 14
       November 1978.

16.   National Institute for Occupational Safety and Health.
       Technical Assistance Report 80-32, Everett School
       District, Everett, Washington. Cincinnati: NIOSH August,
       1980.

17.   Center for Disease Control. Methyl alcohol toxicity in
       teacher aides using spirit duplicators - Washington.
       Morbid Mortality Weekly Report 29:437-438, 12 September
       1980.

MULTIDISCIPLINARY APPROACH TO PREVENTION AND HEALTH PROTECTION
OF MONITORING: ROLE OF INDIVIDUAL DISCIPLINES. MEDICAL
INSPECTORS/MEDICAL OFFICERS II.

B. MORIN (FRANCE)

Summary

*Occupational health inspectorates, which were set up in
several countries in Europe during the first half of the 20th
century, have developed alongside occupational health services
and labour inspectorates and now constitute a well-defined
body whose role in protecting workers' health is rapidly
expanding.*

*In this the duties of occupational health inspectors and their
role in the various countries of the European Community are
outlined. Details are given of the part they play in assessing toxic agents through ambient monitoring at workplaces and
medical checks of workers exposed.*

Introduction

The tasks of occupational health inspectors at workplaces are
defined in terms of the overall aims of the labour inspectorate in preventing occupational hazards and improving working
conditions, and with reference to the aims of occupational
health services in their widest sense: i.e. fostering and
maintaining the physical, mental and social well-being of
workers to the greatest extent possible, preventing any
impairment of their health by working conditions, and adapting
work to the physiological and psychological capacities of the
individual worker. These goals imply very varied monitoring,
advisory and informational tasks, and lastly, study and
research activity which has been particularly well explained
in a 1968 International Labour Office publication on the role
of occupational health inspectorates.

Monitoring the application of laws and regulations

The basic task of occupational health inspectors is and has always been to monitor the proper application of legislative provisions and regulations concerning the protection of workers' health. More explicitly, checks are carried out to monitor the application of provisions relating to health at work, the organisation and functioning of occupational health services, protection against harmful substances, first aid, child labour, work involving handicapped persons and pregnant women, the prevention of occupational accidents and diseases. This task is carried out in conjunction with the labour inspectorates, which are advised by occupational health inspectors on all matters relating to occupational health.

Advice and information

This task of occupational health inspectors is particularly important, especially in small and medium-sized undertakings which make up the great mass of industry in western countries. This activity involves occupational physicians, employers and workers, and is aimed at publicising and explaining legal standards which are often very exhaustive and increasingly complex, in line with technical and medical progress. This role of occupational health inspectors is vital if agreement between labour and employers on measures for protecting health at workplaces is to be successfully achieved.

This activity is complemented by the preparation of special recommendations or rules in conjunction with labour inspectorates and safety and health departments.

Lastly, occupational health inspectors are very often involved in university education and in continuing health and safety training for occupational physicians, public health specialists, safety experts and paramedical staff.

Study and research

The simplest studies are surveys at workplaces which make up a large part of the work of occupational health inspectors, and are most often carried out in conjunction with labour inspectorates and the safety and health departments of sickness insurance offices. They are generally carried out within the individual company, industrial or commercial establishment, either during regular inspections or in the course of special inspections prompted by various circumstances such as:

- notifications of occupational accidents, occupational diseases or seemingly work-related diseases;
- complaints about working conditions;
- problems encountered in the running of an occupational health service;
- disagreements about a decision as to medical fitness, etc.

However, they may also have a wider field of reference, regional or even nationwide, when more general problems are concerned, like assessing the real extent of some particular hazard, the gravity of absenteeism due to sickness, or the consequences of new work methods, etc.

Two provisions are indispensable to such surveys: occupational health inspectors' right of access to undertakings, and the right to order or carry out additional workplace inspections in person.

These surveys are often the starting point for research carried out in conjunction with university institutes dealing with occupational health and with institutes specialising in health and safety, and are completed by increasingly numerous epidemiological studies. The latter require an information-gathering network which stretches from occupational

physicians to sickness insurance bodies; they deal with
notifications of occupational accidents, occupational and
work-related diseases, studies on the incidence of mortality
and morbidity by occupational branch or in relation to some
particular working condition.

Together these enquiries serve to provide information for
authorities and thus help towards bringing working conditions under public supervision by means of recommendations or
regulations.

Medical inspectors in EEC countries

The existence of the post of occupational health inspector
derives in practice from the fact that occupational health is
of public concern and therefore requires public supervision.
That goes a long way towards explaining the differences
noticeable in the various countries which make up the
Community.

In France for example, medical inspection of working conditions was given a progressively sounder footing following the
Law of 11 October 1946 relating to occupational health and
now includes a corps of forty regional occupational health
inspectors whose duties are precisely those described
previously. The medical inspectorate is a technical back-up
department within the Ministry of Labour and the Labour
inspectorates.

In the Federal Republic of Germany, supervision of occupational health received official recognition much later with
the Laws of 1973 and 1974. The duties of State occupational
health inspectors, which existed long before that, are of the
same type but imply more participation at occupational health
institute level in the Lander (education and medical examinations of workers at recruitment and check-ups thereafter).

In Belgium, medical inspection services have the same organisation and are part of the Ministry of Labour and Employment, although the 1965 legislation makes medical inspection at workplaces compulsory only for some categories of employers and workers.

In Ireland and in the United Kingdom, there are no statutory obligations concerning occupational health, but simply a collection of texts on health and safety at work. In practice occupational health services are only concerned with particular hazards. There are no medical inspectors; however some of the usual duties of the latter are fulfilled, for example in the United Kingdom, by the Employment Medical Advisory Service, which is part of the Health and Safety Executive.

In the Netherlands and in Denmark where the 1971 and 1975-1978 laws respectively provide for public supervision of occupational health, teams, which are not exclusively medical, attached to the supervisory authority are collectively responsible for the duties of occupational health inspectors. They are the College Voor Bijstand en Advies in the Netherlands and the Working Environment Council in Denmark.

In Italy and in Luxembourg, where the public supervision of occupational health is not legally compulsory, there are a number of doctors in labour inspectorates and in the Ministry of Labour.

Risk assessment : statement of the problem

Before considering the precise role of occupational health inspectors, we shall try to formulate the problem within our context by defining the term:

- "toxic agent" which will be understood in the usual sense in toxicology: i.e. the

combination of chemical factors, poisons or
substances which destroy or modify vital
bodily functions;

- "assessment" which will be understood as
  meaning "risk assessment", the fundamental aim
  of occupational health services, since these
  are responsible for protecting the health of
  the worker which may be adversely affected by
  working conditions;

- "workplace" which will be confined to the
  actual worker and his immediate surroundings.

This therefore excludes scientific assessment of the risk of
chemical substances, which is carried out prior to their
utilisation in industry, and the social assessment of risks
which depends on the attitude of society to these and for
which medical inspectors have no particular responsibility.
We will only consider the toxicological risk in connection
with its control at workplaces, where occupational health
inspectors can intervene directly within the framework of
their duties as a whole.

Monitoring the immediate surrounding of the workplace

The role of occupational health inspectors in this field is
only complementary to that of labour inspectors and safety
and health engineers from sickness insurance departments.

Occupational health inspectors must see that statutory or
regulation standards regarding chemical substances are
respected, must advise and inform both sides of industry and
occupational physicians on risks connected with exposure to
these factors, must participate in enquiries into exposure
levels following occupational diseases, must deal with complaints or those disagreements between occupational
physicians and heads of undertakings.

Biological monitoring of workers

The role of occupational health inspectors is much more
specific in this case. Naturally, they take part in conjunction with labour inspectorates in checks on the implementation of regulations and of national and even Community
recommendations (for example they recently began checks on
exposure to vinyl chloride), as well as investigations of
occupational accidents and diseases. In addition, along with
occupational physicians, occupational health inspectors work
to improve the biological monitoring of exposed workers and
apply epidemiological methods to the results. This
monitoring is carried out with two aims in mind.

i) Detection of adverse effects on workers by
- complete, systematic clinical examinations of
  all systems of the body;
- additional examinations of target cells and
  organs such as
  . blood count (e.g. for exposure to benzene
    solvents and radiation);
  . examinations of liver (e.g. for exposure to
    vinyl chloride);
  . X-ray bone scans (e.g. for exposure to
    fluorine);
  . multiple function tests, hypersensitivity
    tests, etc.
- study of the causes of mortality and morbidity
  amongst workers...

ii) Biological measurement of chemical substances
   and their metabolites, carried out on body
   fluids such as blood, urine and faeces, or on
   the whole body, e.g. for ionising radiation.

This biological monitoring is a purely medical task and
involves occupational physicians and health inspectors, who
are not bound to medical confidentiality in their dealings

with each other. Occupational health inspectors play an important part in carrying out epidemiological studies using all these data, especially as they act at regional level and belong to a nationwide corps.

These studies are the only ones enabling a cause-effect relationship to be surmised or demonstrated between exposure to chemical substances and the appearance of pathological or unusual phenomena. They ought to be undertaken especially for chemical agents newly introduced into industry, from the very start of production, by testing for acute and sub-acute toxicity as well as chronic toxicity and carcinogenesis.

If the toxicological studies which are carried out prior to the marketing of a chemical substance, and which are compulsory under the legislation of many countries, were to give rise to suspicions of a potential or possible toxic effect on man, registers could be drawn up, for these substances at least, of employees exposed, and data could be collected and collated on exposure levels, duration of exposure, symptoms and pathological phenomena observed and biological measurements taken. These medical registers would only be used by occupational physicians and health inspectors.

MULTIDISCIPLINARY APPROACH TO PREVENTION AND HEALTH PROTECTION
BY MONITORING: ROLE OF INDIVIDUAL DISCIPLINES. THE LAWYER:
LEGAL ASPECTS OF MONITORING, CONFIDENTIALITY AND THE WORKER'S
RIGHT TO KNOW I.

A. JEAMMAUD (FRANCE)

Summary

*The question of whether employees have any real right to be
kept informed of the results of ambient and biological monitoring may seem a surprising one to the person of 1980, and
even more so to those who attach any importance to improving
the protection of workers' health. Nevertheless, it is a
question worth asking, for, in countries which practise a free
economy, the point of departure is that no one - especially
not the employer - is legally obliged to give explanations to
those who are only in the firm to work because that is what
they are paid for. The countless legal standards, amassed
over more than a century, which aim to protect employees and
to guarantee them a certain amount of information, are merely
adjustments to the principles of a free economy, brought about
by the combined efforts of workers' demands, changes in prevailing attitudes and a better appreciation of the importance
of personnel management.*

*That is to say that if the authorities in our countries are
now, in their various ways, establishing what one might call a
'workers' right to information about their working environment; this prerogative will only be fully realised at some
time in the future because the principles of the economic
order are working against it. This basic tension underlines
the confrontation between conflicting legal attitudes. In
fact, certain principles accepted by contemporary social
legislations encourage a broad acceptance of the right to
information, while other legal standards impose a rule of
silence on those who carry out monitoring tests or are aware
of their results.*

*This paper therefore attempts to examine how, in the area we
are considering, the right of the workers to information is
established and strengthened and then to define the
restrictions imposed on those in possession of information by
the various obligations to secrecy.*

*In our arguments we shall take the example of French law,
while taking care to bring out the problems and difficulties
which no doubt arise in very similar terms in the other legal
systems of the EEC, given the common legal attitudes which
characterise the Community in one sphere - the social sphere -
which is so closely linked to the economic sphere, attitudes
based on principles which can only grow more similar as the
integration of Europe progresses.*

The existence of a worker's right to information

Even in the absence of legal texts which explicitly recognise a specific employees' right to information on the presence or the risks of the presence of toxic agents at their workplace, these employees can still have at their disposal either individually or collectively, legal channels for demanding and obtaining a certain amount of information in this field. We can therefore speak of their 'right to information' as a simple definition of this set of means - discussed below under the legal bases of the right to information: But, apart from these provisions which have been specially laid down by law, contemporary social law contains other elements which seem to encourage a broad acceptance of this right to information - discussed below under 'Encouraging acceptance of the right to information'.

The legal bases of the right to information

French law, for example, provides fairly precise legal frame-works for the ambient and biological monitoring of the working environment by determining the duties and powers of occupational physicians, factory inspectors or certain social security organisations. But it also gives the workers access to information on the results of this monitoring. The workers' right therefore results from a combination of powers and duties to inform conferred on (i) those who carry out or know the results of the monitoring and (ii) the function of workers' representative organisations within the undertaking. Similar combinations can probably be found in the other European legal systems (1).

Let us first consider the duties and powers to inform employees.

An obligation to inform lies firstly with the head of the undertaking. But it is rather implied in the rights and responsi-bilities of the workers' representative

organisations (see underline below) (2). The task of informing employees other than through formalised representative channels
rests with people who are more specialised in monitoring.
This duty lies essentially with the occupational physician.
For if the factory inspector is explicitly empowered to
impose certain checks (see below), he is not by law a source
of information for employees; this role is reserved for the
occupational physician who is informed, at the same time as
the inspector, of the results of the analyses ordered by the
inspector.

Similarly, if the social security regulations oblige regional
health insurance funds to communicate to the Labour Directorate the results of enquiries which they can decide to
initiate in certain firms or the information which they have
at their disposal on the dangers present in firms, they are
not required to inform directly either the employees, or even
the works medical officers.

According to the French Labour Code, the occupational physician is the 'counsellor' of the employees and the staff representatives, as well as of the head of the company, in matters afffecting the general hygiene of the establishment and
the 'protection of employees against all harmful effects', in
particular 'against the risks involved in using dangerous
products'. It is therefore his job to provide the workers who
are thus exposed with information on the toxic agents which
pervade the working environment, in order to carry out as
effectively as possible his duty as counsellor (3).

This information appears all the more legally binding as it
makes the occupational physician a vital cog in the monitoring of the presence of toxic agents and he is obliged to keep
records of the results: he must be aware of the nature and
the composition of the products used and the ways in which
they are used, as well as the results of all the tests and
analyses carried out at the workplace and on the products
handled or manufactured; he may himself request these tests

and analyses, against the wishes of the employer, if necessary, thanks to the support of the factory inspector or as a
result of the opinion he can give to the latter with a view
to compelling the employer to analyse the 'substances and
preparations which constitute a risk for the workers'.

While the legal texts do not state explicitly how this information should be conveyed, it is evident that the doctor,
during the 'personal consultation' which is part of every
statutory medical examination, can give each employee the
advice he thinks necessary in view of the toxic substances
present at his workplace and his state of health. Of course,
he can also provide such information when he is at the workplace. A legal doubt can arise only in connection with
information made available to the entire workforce of an
undertaking, a workshop or department and such information,
given the form of its presentation, may well need to be
explained in more detail. However, in practice, such group
information is presented in the form and by the institutions laid down in the legislation which also stipulates the
degree of detail to be provided concerning the various tests
of the working environment (cf. below).

It should be added that the law, by involving the occupational physician in the planning of safety training designed to
benefit certain workers, makes him more directly responsible
for providing information. Insofar as this training is based
on the risks to which the employee is exposed it would seem
that, in order to be effective, it should draw the attention
of each person concerned to the risks associated with the
possible presence of toxic agents and to the results of
recent measurements and analyses etc. In the course of such
safety training, the occupational physician, who is required
to have such information, would thus tend to become the chief
source of its disclosure to the workers.

Let us now consider the role of representative staff bodies.

There are many provisions of the Labour Code which make it a duty to provide, directly or indirectly, information on the toxicity of workplaces to a body generally representative of the workforce in the undertaking or to a more specialised institution.

The works committee plays a part in the search for solutions to problems concerning 'the working environment and physical work factors', which suggests that it is fully informed about measurements and analyses carried out by any agency whatsoever. However, it also has an advisory function in relation to the annual programme for the improvement of working conditions, the programme for the elimination of occupational risks and the draft plan for pay and conditions; these are documents which by their nature include information on the matters referred to or which cannot be discussed without such information being disclosed. All the more so, since the law requires the occupational physician to be present in an advisory capacity at meetings which have these subjects on their agenda.

However, the forum in which the employees' representatives are best placed to obtain information is the health and safety committee which is a feature of large-sized undertakings. In fact, the works manager, the occupational physician and the person, if any, responsible for the safety department are members of that body and its duties require its members, including those representing the employees, to be in possession of all the facts concerning toxic agents whose presence has been recorded at workplaces in the undertaking. It is this committee which assesses the occupational risks in the undertaking on the basis of information which the employer is required to supply and it also undertakes regular inspections of the undertaking and carries out enquiries into any accident or any occurence of an occupational disease.

Thus, under French law, it is mainly on the health and safety committee, with its wide-ranging terms of reference, that French employees can rely for information, although this is not formally recognised as a right in the field which interests us. The best way for the employees who are members of such committees to seek the application in their area of the statutory provisions which other aspects of the law seem to impose would be to seek a ruling to establish what information they are entitled to demand.

Encouraging acceptance of the right to information

The statutory provisions mentioned above are to be found in French law and are doubtless also a feature of the legislation of the other member countries of the European Community. However, quite apart from that consideration, Community law itself has to be taken into account.

If no mandatory act of Community social law - and this includes the 1962 Recommendation on occupational medicine - deals with the right of workers to know the results of measurements and analyses (4), there is, however, the Council resolution of 29 June 1978 on an action programme on safety and health at work (5). In fact, this document calls for the maximum amount of information to be made available to workers, since it considers one of the primary conditions for an increase in the level of protection against occupational risks to be 'the full participation of both sides of industry in preventive measures'. With regard to the more extensive monitoring of workers' safety and health, which it advocates, it states that 'efforts should be made to interest workers in monitoring within the undertaking, either by direct means or by means of existing bodies or institutions'.

While this document is at present no more than a guideline, it may be felt to have a certain 'doctrinal' influence (6) as regards the interpretation of positive standards. It is also worth noting that many European legal instruments, concerned

concerned to get away from the 'regulatory' (7) attitude
such as can be seen in ILO draft proposals (8), tend to
underline the part to be played by both sides of industry,
and consequently by employees, in protective measures against
occupational risks.

The Universal Declaration of the Rights of Man of 1948
proclaims the need to recognise each person's 'right to
health' (9). But it is not mandatory.

This is not the case in individual countries. In France, the
Constitutional Preamble in force since 1946 and which the
various jurisdictions regard as having the force of law
states that 'the Nation guarantees to protect the health of
all citizens'. Clearly it is inappropriate to talk of 'the
right to health' since each citizen does not have the legal
means to demand the provision of all things necessary to
safeguard his health. Nevertheless, the aim of substantive
law is to ensure that each citizen has the means to protect
his health. This is a material legal point (10) which can be
invoked in any discussions of the right of employees to be
informed of the results, measurements, analyses, or enquiries
relating to any health hazard to which they may be exposed at
work. Insofar as any improvement in health protection will
be in proportion to the information given to the interested
parties, it follows that the legal obligation to provide
information and the right to obtain it should be interpreted
quite widely. The problem is indeed not peculiar to French
law; recent studies of Belgian law indicate that it causes
even more concern in Belgium.

Thus, taken in conjunction with other features of the legal
system to which they belong, the fragmentary provisions which
serve as a basis for the employees' right to be informed
about the results of the tests we are concerned with should
require the information provided to be as comprehensive and
detailed as possible. While accepting this as the guiding
principle, it has to be admitted that other features of the

same legal system may have the effect of limiting the maximum dissemination of the fullest possible information. However, it is clear that these other provisions must be seen as merely setting limits or stating exceptions to the right to information, established in principle, and not as being of equal weight with this right.

Limits deriving from the obligation of confidentiality

Some provisions may entitle or require persons to withhold information in their possession.

Thus it seems that one obstacle to the employees' right to information is professional secrecy. However, medical confidentiality should really be the only limiting factor.

Professional secrecy and the workers' right to information

Professional secrecy is recognised to a greater or lesser extent in the legal systems of different free-economy countries, it being an important factor with reference to competition and new production. Manufacturing processes, even if they are considered of lesser importance, must also be included under the heading of professional secrecy (11), i.e. the right to withhold information which one does not wish to fall into the hands of a competitor, this right implying that employees at different levels of the undertaking have to observe certain obligations regarding secrecy. This right will therefore be at variance with certain rights to information. Thus the French Labour Code imposes an obligation of secrecy on persons who would, at the same time, be responsible for providing information on toxic substances at the workplace or be entitled to receive such information.

While the employer may be tempted to invoke the general principle of professional secrecy, in our view he would not be justified in withholding comprehensive information on health risks to which workers were exposed.

The confidentiality of information regarding manufacturing processes or the composition of products which the occupational physician or employee representatives may be required to respect (in French law this is stipulated explicitly) must not prevent the former from providing such information to the latter; since the employee representatives are obliged to respect the secrecy of such information they must by the same token be entitled to receive it.

But do these clearly stated obligations and, more generally, the rules regarding professional secrecy place an obstacle between the employees as a whole and the relevant information? We think not, for at least two reasons. Firstly, the interpretative principles referred to above mean that, in the final analysis, information on the presence of toxic substances may not be withheld from workers exposed to such substances. Furthermore, the fact that employees are under an obligation not to disclose the secrets of the undertaking (a stipulation of the French penal code which also provides for sanctions in the event of non-compliance) implies that they have privileged access to the information. It would therefore be wrong to refuse to provide them or to forbid others to provide them with such information on the grounds that it concerned manufacturing secrets.

Another point to be considered is whether persons external to the undertaking may obtain information from an 'insider' and if the latter can provide such information without being guilty of a civil or criminal offence. It is impossible to consider all such possible situations even if we were to restrict ourselves to French law alone. All one can say is that it seems likely that, given the general attitude to the question of professional secrecy, the disclosure of information by a person or organisation in a privileged position to persons or organisations external to the undertaking (e.g. a trade union organisation) would probably be considered a breach of civil law (at the very least an act of negligence). Thus an employer could presumably bring an action for damages suffered as a result of such irregular disclosures. On the other hand, in other cases and in view of the interpretative principles we have already mentioned, disclosure to someone outside the 'privileged' group ought not to be considered an offence.

For example, if there is in the undertaking no organisation representative of the employees or if the information required and authorised by law has not been disclosed within the undertaking, it seems quite legitimate for a trade union to ask for and to obtain, from the organisation which carried out any survey, the results of such a survey, even if the organisation concerned was merely authorised to make the disclosure and not ordered to do so. Moreover, it seems to us that, in order to protect the health of workers against occupational risks, trade unions representing the branch of industry to which the undertaking belongs should generally be recognised to have a right to such information, provided always that any misuse of privileged information thus obtained (wilful intent, negligence) would be open to the usual sanctions imposed by the civil law in such cases.

It ought in any case to be stressed that, in interpreting the right or obligation of non-disclosure, the emphasis should be on the limitations of such right or obligation wherever this would tend to restrict the disclosure of information concerning, inter alia, the presence of toxic substances at the workplace. Only medical confidentiality should be allowed to place any substantial limit on the right to information, since it protects the only interests which can be placed on the same level as the health of workers.

Medical confidentiality and the workers' right to information

By virtue of being a doctor, the occupational physician is obliged to respect medical confidentiality (13). The French Labour Code guarantees this confidentiality by means of regulations concerning the documents which the works medical

service has to keep and any breach of medical confidentiality
automatically leaves the occupational physician open to legal
proceedings under the civil or criminal code (14). Moreover,
the area within which the occupational physician is required
to respect medical confidentiality must be clearly defined in
order to strengthen his own position. Here again the principles of contemporary social legislation, whether national,
international or European, should have some influence.

According to the code of professional medical conduct operative in France, 'confidentiality covers everything which the
doctor has learnt in the exercise of his profession, that is,
not only what he has been told but also what he has seen,
heard or understood'. This is a wide-ranging definition
which seems to include under the heading of medical confidentiality all information on working conditions which he may
obtain in his capacity as occupational physician. Yet some
of this information would more appropriately be included in
the sphere of professional secrecy, such as information on
manufacturing processes or the composition of the product
handled. A clear distinction should therefore be observed
between these two spheres since professional secrecy should
in principle be subordinated to the workers' right to information while medical confidentiality should not be set aside
so lightly. Some would like to set the latter on a pedestal,
relying on its taboo effect to conceal certain matters, using
it as a screen in a way far removed from the real purpose of
medical confidentiality, but this tendency should be
resisted.

Since as few restrictions as possible should be placed on
the workers' right to information, medical confidentiality
should be held to apply only to cases where evidence of
the presence of toxic substances at work is obtained as a
result of a personal examination of a worker, i.e. the
requirement of confidentiality should limit basically the
propagation of information derived from biological monitoring of an individual. It should not, however, place an

absolute prohibition on such disclosure. The aim of confidentiality is to protect the private life of individuals but
this is no argument against disclosing information obtained
from the examination of employees if the disclosure respects
the anonymity of the persons concerned. For example, the
occupational physician will not be in breach of medical confidentiality if he informs the health and safety committee -
and the committee can in its turn so inform the workforce as
a whole - that a certain blood-lead level has been detected
in a certain proportion of the employees in an undertaking or
workshop, provided the number of employees referred to is
large enough to prevent individuals being identified (15).

Finally, it is recognised nowadays that medical confidentiality exists to protect the interests of the patient (16).
This explains why it is relatively and not absolutely
binding, in the sense that the patient, if he thinks it in
his interests to do so, may release the physician from his
duty of confidentiality (17). It is therefore conceivable
that, if an employee's medical examination revealed evidence
of the presence of toxic substances at his workplace, he
might explicitly release the occupational physician from his
duty not to disclose this information. However, while such a
measure would seem to ensure that the physician could not be
accused of any breach of either the civil or the criminal
code if he did disclose the information concerned, this is
not to say that he could be compelled to disclose it since it
is doubtless in the best interests of the employee to let the
physician decide whether the disclosure is advisable or not,
provided always that the latter is not required by law to
provide the information to others (e.g. as part of a statement of occupational diseases).

Conclusions

We think that the workers' right, as individuals or a group,
to information on the assessment of toxic substances at their
workplace is already well established in substantive law, as

can be seen from an examination of the provisions governing
the release of such information as interpreted in the light
of the principles underlying the legal systems in this part
of the world. The only limitations which should be imposed
on this right are those which derive from the need for
medical confidentiality, and any loose definition of the
latter should be resisted.

Notes

1.   For information on Belgian law, see: M. Sojcher-
        Rousselle, Droit de la sécurité et de la santé de
        l'homme au travail, Bruylant 1979, No. 186 (et
        seq.).

2.   In Belgium a personal report has to be drawn up on
        each employee exposed to dangerous products. This
        report is the responsibility of the employer and is
        prescribed by the terms of the Règlement général pour
        la protection du travail (General regulation for
        labour protection) which also requires general infor-
        mation on the risks to which employees are exposed at
        work (M. Sojcher-Rousselle, op. cit., Nos. 189, 223).

3.   It is worth observing that the Medical Council, which
        places great emphasis on medical confidentiality,
        sees this obligation to provide information in con-
        nection with counselling as a major duty of the occu-
        pational physician (Dr. J. Closier, 'Médecine du tra-
        vail et déontologie', Droit social, April 1980 p.17).

4.   The proposal for a Council Directive on the protec-
        tion of workers from harmful exposure to chemical,
        physical and biological agents at work (OJ No. C 89,
        5.4.1979), approved by the Council of Ministers in
        June 1980 (Bulletin of the European Communities,
        6/1980, 2.1.41 and 2.1.61), provides that workers
        shall be informed of the hazards arising from certain
        substances and products and of the results of expo-
        sure measurements and analyses carried out at the
        workplace.

5.   OJ No. C 165, 11.7.1978. The action referred to here
        was included in the Social Action Programme adopted
        by Resolution of the Council on 21 January 1974.

6.   Similar to the influence of the decisions of the
        Court of Justice of the European Communities (P.
        Bonassies, 'Une nouvelle source doctrinale du droit
        français: la jurisprudence de la CJCE, in Etudes
        offertes à P. Kayser, University of Aix-Marseille
        1979, Vol. I, p. 43).

7. For the British Health and Safety at Work Act of 1974
    and the Dutch draft legislation on safety, health and
    comfort at work, see M. Sojcher-Rousselle, op. cit.,
    No. 244.

8. M. Sojcher-Rousselle, op. cit., No. 245.

9. J.J. Ribas, M-J. Jonczy, J-C. Séché, Traité de
    droit

10. Already invoked in France in some controversial
    labour law cases. Cf: J-C Javillier, 'Une illu-
    stration du conflit des logiques (droit à la santé et
    droit des obligations): le contrôle médical patronal
    des absences en cas de maladie du salarie' Droit
    social 1976, p. 245.

11. S. Chamas, 'Le secret des affaires et le droit.
    Rapport général' in Le secret et le droit. Travaux
    de l'Association Capitant, Vol. XXV, Dalloz 1974, p.
    180. Luxembourg law treats manufacturing secrets in
    the same way as professional secrets in the strict
    sense of the term (P. Welter, Le secret des affaires
    en droit luxembourgeois'. op. cit., p. 319.

12. Liability either for damages or breach of contract.
    Breach of contract for example, in the case of the
    organisation to which an employer entrusted the test
    decided by him or required by the industrial medical
    officer.

13. In France this point has been made even clearer since
    the new Code of Professional Conduct of 1979 does not
    allow any special position to occupational medicine,
    which therefore has no exceptional status. See: J.
    Savatier, 'La médecine du travail dans le système de
    protection de la sante', Droit social, April 1980,
    p.6; J. Closier, 'Médecine du travail et déonto-
    logie', mentioned in (3) above, p. 16/17.

14. A. Jeammaud, 'Médecine du travail et responsabilité
    civile', Droit social, April 1980, p. 77 (specially
    pp 80-81).

15. This is to some extent the distinction which French
    law observes between individual medical records kept
    by the occupational physician, which must be kept
    secret (Art. R. 241-56 of the Labour Code) and the
    records of the undertaking, also kept by the
    occupational physician, but not considered
    confidential (Art. R. 241-58).

16. Art. 11 of the Decree of 28 June 1979 concerning the
    Code of Professional Conduct.

17. M.J. Mazen, 'Le secret des praticiens de la santé.
    Mythe ou réalite?' Gaz. Pal. 1975. 2 Doctrine p.
    468; D. Thouvenin, Le secret médical en droit
    français. Thesis University of Lyons III, 1977.

MULTIDISCIPLINARY APPROACH TO PREVENTION AND HEALTH PROTECTION
BY MONITORING: ROLE OF INDIVIDUAL DISCIPLINES. THE LAWYER:
LEGAL ASPECTS OF MONITORING, CONFIDENTIALITY AND THE WORKER'S
RIGHT TO KNOW II.

P.H. WEINER (USA)

Summary

*Workplace monitoring is an important tool for both regulatory
and investigatory purposes, assisting enforcement of existing
exposure limits and the accumulation of information necessary
for epidemiological studies. In a world of uncertainty,
where exposure limits are based on firm data for only a small
minority of substances, monitoring results can also be of
utmost importance to workers. Both environmental and biological data can help workers enforce existing laws, provide a
rationale for following stringent work practices, and assist
efforts to bargain collectively for a healthier workplace.*

*Workers in the United States are now achieving these rights
through regulation, but the right to know is more deeply
rooted in fundamental American values, as expressed in
American constitutional and common law, including the concepts of a right of privacy and a manufacturer's or
physician's duty to warn. This paper explores these rights,
and the countervailing interest in protecting trade secrets,
with regard to results of workplace monitoring.*

Introduction

The worker's fight for his or her right to know the results
of workplace monitoring is based, ironically, on our scientific ignorance and governmental uncertainty.

Millions of workers are exposed each year to doses of substances which may cause cancer, mutations in future generations, and birth defects. They work with no assurance that
government or industry will or can protect them from occupational disease. Most of the 70,000 or more chemicals in
commercial use were marketed without adequate pretesting for
their effects on human health. Today we have adequate data
for no more than 1% of them. Nor are risks readily apparent,
given disease latency periods of up to thirty years and the

extreme difficulty of either knowing the interactive effects
of several chemicals on a person or of tracing a disease to
specific exposures in the past.

Were we totally ignorant, the "right to know" would be empty
of meaning. To the contrary, however, we often have enough
knowledge to suspect a chemical's dangers. With that knowledge we could defer introduction of a new chemical but could
not, in an American legal system which protects owners of
chemical products until those products are proven hazardous,
sufficiently regulate an existing chemical product. It
should be embarrassing to acknowledge, in such stages of
regulatory uncertainty, that workers - or their bodies - have
often provided the key facts necessary to take decisive
action.

Thus it was only 13 worker deaths that finally spurred the
responsible regulation of vinyl chloride, despite mounting
toxicological evidence over a 30 year period. And it was
workers discussing their problems informally among themselves
that resulted in the realisation of dangers associated with
BCME and DBCP, despite antecedent toxicological clues that
simply had not been acted upon.

Worker knowledge of workplace exposures can thus be a vital
tool for collective self-protection during periods of regulatory inaction. Conversely, worker discoveries of patterns of
occupational disease have been a perhaps inelegant but certainly vital tool for arriving at scientific and regulatory
conclusions affecting the permitted use of various
compounds.

In addition, worker knowledge of exposures has been advantageous to workers, industry, and government alike in encouraging the use of and adherence to proper handling precautions
that might otherwise seem annoying or burdensome. And where
sufficient data exists on a given substance or product,
knowledge of exposures has sometimes resulted in collective
bargaining for a healthier workplace.

The reaction of industry and traditional health care professionals to the worker's demand to know the identity of
chemicals used in the workplace and the results of workplace
monitoring has often erred in two diametrically opposite
ways.

On the one hand, professionals have often denigrated the
worker's need to know, on the grounds that workers do not
have any expertise and could not improve upon the knowledge
and standards developed by the scientists and engineers.
Management occasionally expresses the fear that this information will "alarm" the worker unnecessarily, when we are
really uncertain scientifically regarding risk and effects.
The short answer to this argument is that history proves it
to be wrong, and that it is the ignorant rather than the
informed who are most subject to anxiety and malaise in the
workplace.

On the other hand, there are some who would transmute the
worker's "right" to know into a "responsibility" to know and
assume any risks that are known. The model is that of a
fully informed individual, choosing freely and effectively,
who would judge exposure hazards along with wages and hours
in deciding whether to take or keep a job. The worker would
thus make a personal risk/benefit decision about his or her
job, absolving the employer or manufacturer from some or all
responsibility for reducing exposures to a healthful level.
The problems with this model are manifest, including an inability to understand technical risk models (when they exist
at all), the psychological tendency to discount personal
risks derived from statistical probabilities alone, (1) and
the difficulty of assigning a present value to such risks as
birth defects in progeny. The same problems that cast grave
doubt on the utility of risk-benefit analysis for making
regulatory decisions (2-6) make a mockery of such analysis
on an individual basis.

The worker's need to know is thus substantial, but within a
limited framework. If we had perfect scientific knowledge of

risks and appropriate exposure levels, that need would be
limited to understanding the rationale of certain work practices or to assisting enforcement of protective regulations.
Without that knowledge – and we will be decades in acquiring
it – the need to know the extent of our knowledge, our uncertainty, and the facts of daily exposure is essential to
survival.

The extent of a need is always an ingredient in the formulation of legal rights, but is never sufficient in itself to
establish those rights. Direct political action, resulting
in legislation or regulation, can also establish such rights,
as has now occurred in the United States with the enactment
of OSHA regulations giving workers broad access to their own
medical records and to all plant exposure records. (7)

For purposes of this paper, however, I shall concentrate on
the underlying ethics and values, as expressed in American
constitutional and common law, which form the consensual
foundation for establishing an independent <u>right</u> to know
chemical identities and monitoring results in the workplace,
regardless of specific proof of need or political strength in
an individual workplace. It is hoped that this more general
discussion will have a measure of applicability on an international basis. The right to know, as discussed here, is
never a substitute for collective societal responsibility to
protect against unhealthful exposures by changing the workplace, but is rather a complementary individual right to
exercise personal judgement about vital life-affecting
matters.

The right to know and American Law

The right to obtain information necessary to make personal
decisions about health is not a concept newly created by
unions or the Occupational Safety and Health Administration.
Rather, American law has consistently upheld such a right,
based on profound national values of personal autonomy and

fairness. Where these values have been pitted against societal and individual interests in protecting trade secrets,
they have generally been judged more important and thus
preeminent.

First, American constitutional law, which preempts all other
laws of the country, protects "independence in making certain
kinds of important decisions." (8) This general right has
been applied at various times to protect freedom of choice
in marriage partners, procreation and abortion, child rear-
ing, and education. The corollary right to obtain sufficient
information to choose effectively has also received judicial
protection against interference by state statute. (9) More
recently, a federal Freedom of Information Act (10), the
national Privacy Protection Study Commission (11), and other
experts (12-13) have applied this right to obtaining one's
own medical and exposure records.

Second, American law of liability of "defective" products
has evolved in such a way that manufacturers have a number
of duties toward the ultimate users or consumers of their
products. At the outset, the manufacturer has a responsibility to design and make a safe product insofar as is
possible. He must test and inspect the product before
marketing, keep abreast of research by others, and otherwise
perform as an expert on his own product. (14) But our law
recognises that some products may be "unavoidably unsafe."
For those products the law requires that the maker communicate an effective warning and (if known) safe handling
instructions to the worker or consumer. (14) The warning
must be comprehensive: compliance with government labelling
requirements may be insufficient where more is known; or the
warning may have to be bilingual where the foreseeable users
speak only a non-English language. (15) Indeed, the absence
of an effective or adequate warning has formed the basis of
most personal injury actions filed by workers injured by
toxic substances. In the most dramatic of these incidents,
it has been shown that the asbestos industry kept secret from

its own and other employees for thirty years the true
hazards of asbestos. Even as late as 1966 its sole warning
was that inhalation "in excessive quantities over long
periods of time may be harmful," held by the courts to be
inadequate to encourage the wearing of respirators or
reduction of exposure. (14) In another case, the company
even hid X-ray results from its workers so that they would
continue to work and would not claim workers' compensation
benefits. (16)

The premise of these products liability rules is that tran-
sactional fairness demands that an entity with superior knowledge and resources should disclose unseen problems to an inexpert and unsuspecting user. The further premise is that
the manufacturer has the superior ability to research and
eliminate product hazards, plus the mechanism for spreading
those costs to the consuming public via higher prices.

A third area of American law providing a foundation for the
right to know is that which governs a physician's relationship to those he or she examines. In part because of the
substantial reliance placed upon medical advice, and in part
because of the physician's superior knowledge, the law
imposes a duty upon physicians to reveal health-threatening
conditions to all workers they examine or treat. This rule
is sometimes said to stem from the "Good Samaritan" rule that
one who undertakes to render services necessary for the
safety of another becomes subject to a duty to use reasonable
care in rendering such services. (17) Where the relationship
goes beyond a pre-employment physical, the obligation is also
said to stem from the physician-patient relationship (18), a
relationship of trust which obligates the doctor to reveal
all pertinent information to his patient. (19)

For many years, the physician was given the power to decide
what information would be in the patient's best interest to
know. But recently, perhaps due in part to the decline of
personal relationship between doctor and patient in a world

of medical specialisation, courts have held that they alone
will decide whether disclosure is sufficient, measured by
whatever information would be material to a patient's health
decisions.(20)

In an occupational context, company doctors have an even
higher duty. Specialists in a field have a legal duty to
know the latest discoveries. Where, as here, the specialists
have a Code of Ethical Conduct which requires them to know
the hazards of the workplace and to communicate those hazards
to the worker (21), the law will often treat the ethical duty
as a legal requirement. In at least one case, the physician's duty has significantly been extended to require notification of former patients regarding hazards discovered
after the relationship has terminated.(22)

These fundamental precepts of American law have given legiti-
macy and impetus to the movement to obtain a specific right
to know chemical identities, monitoring results, and the
contents of one's own medical records, resulting not only in
OSHA's standard granting such access, but also in specific
legislation in several states granting worker access to such
information. (7,23) The right of unions to such information,
as necessary for effective collective bargaining, is also
clear in theory, but is presently being challenged by
industry in pending cases, based on industry's fears that
valuable information could be disclosed to competitors.(24)

At the same time that the right to know has achieved legiti-
macy in American law, it has been increasingly challenged by
demands for confidentiality of certain information in order
to protect individual rights to privacy and industry investment in trade secrets. The right to privacy - "the right to
define one's circle of intimacy" (25) - applies principally
to the disclosure of highly personal information to persons
who might use it to stigmatise, ridicule, or otherwise mis-
treat the individual. It has no application to disclosing
the results of environmental monitoring, and little or no

application to the disclosure of biological monitoring results. An exception to this statement might be the disclosure of chromosomal aberration monitoring if the disclosure of such results could result in workplace ostracism or ridicule by fellow workers. For the most part, however, privacy concerns are not at issue in the disclosure of workplace monitoring results, and are more appropriate to a discussion of access to personal medical records.

The protection of trade secrets, rather than pitting one personal right against another, pits personal rights to self-preservation against corporate economic rights to protect valuable investments. Society protects trade secrets to encourage innovators to create new and better products for the benefit of us all.(26) A trade secret loses protection if it is not truly secret. If a company does not employ security measures to restrict its employees from knowing or divulging such secrets, or if the information could be acquired fairly easily by others, trade secret status is lost.(26,27)

Trade secret concerns applicable to the disclosure of workplace monitoring results are several. The initial claim is that employees or their representatives will disclose those results to industrial competitors. The second claim is that those results will provide competitors with (i) the identity of chemicals used in manufacturing, (ii) the identity of catalysts and intermediates used in manufacturing, (iii) the percentage of such chemicals in a mixture, and (iv) clues to secret manufactuuring processes. As a result, compromises have been suggested in which monitoring results would be summarised, chemical hazards but not chemical identities would be disclosed, or industry would exercise discretion to remove chemical names when deemed by industry to be irrelevant to the worker.

An analysis of these claims narrows the issues considerably. First and foremost, the claim of industrial espionage by workers seems more a figment of imagination than of fact. In

the U.S. OSHA hearings on its access standard, not one wit-
ness was able to give an example of such misdeeds.(28)
Workers who would sell to the highest bidder usually already
know far more valuable information about a company than would
be added by results from workplace monitoring. Contracts
requiring confidentiality are common in industry, and would
put the wrongdoer in legal jeopardy. The practical effect of
being discovered could be even worse - occupational ostracism
within sometimes tight-knit job markets. Workers also
usually have an interest in the success of their company,
especially where their workplace is organised and a competitor's may not be.

Second, the claim of trade secret protection for most chemical identities is spurious under American law. Analysis of
end product constituents by modern techniques is simple and
relatively inexpensive compared to other operating costs and
potential profit margins. Trade secret protection is therefore inappropriate.

This is not to say that there are no legitimate trade secret
concerns regarding disclosure of monitoring results. Recent
American statutes as well as the OSHA rule on access to monitoring results protect against disclosure of mixture composition and manufacturing processes, while mandating disclosure
of health and safety study information (including chemical
identities and exposure levels under the OSHA rule). (7, 29)
A more general discretion to provide only testing summaries,
on the other hand, would be broader than needed for trade
secret protection, while substantially limiting the ability
of individuals to understand their risks. More importantly,
under American law, unions have the right for collective
bargaining purposes to review the employer's testing protocols and, if necessary, conduct tests of their own. (30)
These collective rights, more important than those of the
individual in achieving practical changes in the workplace,
should not be restricted without substantial reason.

These decisions seek to accommodate competing interests, but do so with a presumption that trade secret protection must yield to the public interest when the two conflict. American constitutional and common law support this presumption in the few cases where the conflict has surfaced. Thus when manufacturers refused to list ingredients in food because of trade secret concerns, the U.S. Supreme Court responded:

> (I)t is too plain for argument that a manufacturer or vendor has no constitutional right to sell goods without giving to the purchaser fair information of what it is that is being sold. The right of a manufacturer to maintain secrecy as to his compounds and processes must be held subject to the right of the state, in the exercise of its police power and in promotion of fair dealings, to require that the nature of the product be fairly set forth.

Statutes specifically requiring disclosure of such information have uniformly been held to be valid. (32) Other cases have required disclosure of trade secrets in litigation where public health and safety interests are involved. (33) Indeed, one celebrated California case implies that industry must voluntarily and affirmatively disclose such secrets whenever a substantial threat to public health is involved, a decision in accord with a recent American statute requiring industry to report adverse effects of its products. (34) It therefore seems clear that the right to know exposure monitoring results must prevail over business rights to protect trade secrets.

Conclusions

Workplace monitoring is a valuable tool for research and enforcement purposes. The worker's right to know these results is solidly based in American laws recognising a right to independent decision-making on vital personal matters and

a right to be warned of hazards by those with superior knowledge. American labour law also recognises the union's right
to such information for purposes of collective action. Given
the scientific and regulatory uncertainty which currently
plague our efforts to control toxic hazards, the right to
know is an essential part of the right to self-preservation.
In the face of these rights and needs, legitimate trade
secret concerns are limited. Accommodating those concerns is
often possible, but concerns for enterprise profit cannot
achieve a higher priority than the protection of human
health. For as Bernardino Ramazzini stated over 250 years
ago, "Tis a sordid profit that's accompanied by the
destruction of Health." (35)

References

1.   Calabresi, G. The Cost of Accidents (1971). See
        also Slovic, et al., Cognitive Processes and Societal
        Risk Taking, UCLA School of Engineering and Applied
        Science, No. 7598, at 291 (1975).

2.   Green, The Risk-Benefit Calculus in Safety Determina-
        tions, 43 Geo. Wash. L. Rev. 791.

3.   Mishan, Evaluation of Life and Limb, 79 J. Pol. Econ.
        687 (1971).

4.   Zeckhauser, Procedures for Valuing Human Lives, 23
        Pub. Policy 419 (1975).

5.   Schelling, The Life You Save May Be Your Own, in s.
        Chase (ed).

6.   Nash, Future Generations and The Social Rate of
        Discount, 5 Environment and Planning 611 (1973).

7.   U.S. Department of Labor, Occupational Safety and
        Health Administration, Access to Employee Exposure
        and Medical Records, Final Rule, 45 FR No. 102,
        35212-35303 (May 23, 1980):29 C.F.R. Sec. 1910.20.

8.   Whalen v. Roe, 429 U.S. 589, 97 S.Ct. 869, 876
        (1971).*

9.   Carey v. Population Services International, 431 U.S.
        678, 687; 97S.Ct. 2010 (1977).

*Citations to American legal decisions are here referenced
in the form most acceptable to the legal profession.

10.   5 U.S.C. sec. 552.

11.   Privacy Protection Study Commission, Report: Personal
        Privacy in an Information Society 295-300 (1977).

12.   Westin, A., Computers, Health Records, and Citizen
        Rights,(National Bureau of Standards Monograph No.
        157, (1976) at 289-294.

13.   National Commission on the Confidentiality of Health
        Records, Dilemma, (1978).

14.   Borel v. Fibreboard Paper Prods. Corp. 493 F. 2d
        1076, 1089-1090 (5th Cir. 1973): See Generally
        Restatement of Torts, 2d, Sec. 402A.

15.   See, e.g., Rumsey v. Freeway Manor Minimax, 423
        S.W.2d 387 (Tex. App. 1968); Davis v. Wyeth Labs.,
        Inc., 399 F. 2d 121 (9th Cir. 1968); Hubbard-Hall
        Chemical Co. v. Silverman, 340 F.2d 402 (1st Cir.
        1965); Gall v. Union Ice Co., 108 Cal. App. 2d 303
        (1951).

16.   Johns-Manville v. Superior Court, 165 Cal. Rptr. 858
        (1980).

17.   Restatement of Torts, 2d, Sec. 323 (1965); See Union
        Carbide and Carbon Corp. v. Stapleton, 237 F.2d 229
        (6th Cir. 1956); Hoover v Williamson, 236 Md. 250,
        203 A.2d 861 (1964); Coffee v. McDonnel-Douglas, 8
        Cal.3d 551, 105 Cal.Rptr. 358 (1972); Wojcik v.
        Aluminium Company of America, 183 N.Y.S.2d 351
        (1959); and Jines v. General Electric Co., 303 F.2d
        76 (9th Cir. 1962).

18.   See, e.g., Betesh v. United States, 400 F. Supp. 238
        (D.C. Cir. 1974).

19.   See, e.g., Tabershaw, Whose "Agent" Is the Occupa-
        tional Physician, 30 Arch. Environ. Health 412
        (1975). Bundy, How Do We Assure That The Workers'
        Health Is The Occupational Physician's Primary
        Concern?, 18 J. Occup. Med. 671 (1976); Warshaw, The
        Malpractice Problem and the Occupational Physician,
        19 J. Occup. Med. 593 (1977); Whorton & Davis,
        Ethical Conduct and the Occupational Physician; 54
        Bull N.Y. Acad. of Med. 733 (1978).

20.   Cobbs v. Grant, 8 Cal. 3d 229, 242; 104 Cal. Rptr.
        505, 513; Canterbury v. Spence, 464 F. 2d 772 (D.C.
        Cir. 1972); Truman v. Thomas, 165 Cal. Rptr. 308
        (1980).

21.   See generally, Standard of Care Required of Medical
        Specialists, 21 A.L.R.3d 943; See American
        Occupational Medicine Association, Code of Ethical
        Conduct, Sec. 6, 8, 9 (1976).

22.   Tresemere v.   Barke, 150 Cal. Rptr. 384 (1978); com-
         pare John-Mansville v. Superior Court, 165 Cal. Rptr.
         858 (1980), supra.

23.   See, e.g.,   26 Maine Revised Stats., ch. 22 (1979);
         N.Y. Stats, ch. 551 (1980); Calif. Stats. ch. 874
         (1980).

24.   Colgate-Palmolive Co., Case No. 17-CA-8331, __ , NLRB
         __(March 27, 1979); Minnesota Mining and Manufactur-
         ing Co., Case Nos., 18-CA-5710-11, ___ NLRB ___
         (March 13, 1979); Borden Chemical, A Division of
         Borden, Inc., Case No. 32-CA-551, ___ NLRB ___ (April
         25, 1979).

25.   Briscoe v. Reader's Digest Association 4 Cal. 3d 529,
         534,93 Cal. Rptr. 866, 869 (1971).

26.   Kewannee Oil Co. v. Bicron Corp., 416 U.S. 470, 486-
         487; 94 S.Ct. 1879, 1888 (1974).

27.   4 Rest., Torts, sec. 757; see, e.g., Motorola, Inc.
         v. Fairchild Camera and Instrument Corp., 366 F.
         Supp. 1173 (D.Arz. 1973); Wilson Certified Foods,
         Inc. v. Fairbury Food Products, 370 F. Supp. 1080 (D.
         Neb. 1971) (insufficient protection of secret; no
         secrecy found); compare K-2 Ski Co. v. Head Ski Co.,
         Inc., 506 F.2d 471 (9th Cir. 1971); Telex Corp. v.
         IBM Corp., 376 F. Supp. 258 (N.D.Okla. 1973) (meas-
         ures ranging from modest to elaborate to protect
         secrets.

28.   See Reference 7, at p. 35238.

29.   See Section 14 of the Toxic Substances Control Act,
         15 U.S.C. sec. 2601, 2613; Section 10 of the Federal
         Insecticide, Fungicide, and Rodenticide Act, 7 U.S.C.
         sec. 136h.

30.   See, e.g., Fafnir Bearing Co. v. NLRB, 362 F.2d 716
         (2nd Cir. 1966).

31.   Corn Products Refining Co. v. Eddy, 249 U.S. 427,
         431-432 (1919). See also Savage v. Jones, 225 U.S.
         501, 32 S.Ct. 715. (1912) (animal feed); Plumley v.
         Massachusetts, 155 U.S. 461 (margarine); Patapsco
         Guano Co. v. Board of Agriculture, 171 U.S. 345
         (fertilizer); Id. at 431-432; National Fertilizer
         Ass'n v. Bradley, 301 U.S. 178 (1937).

32.   See, e.g., FCC v. Schreiber, 381 U.S. 279 (1965);
         Utah Fuel Co. v. National Bituminous Coal Comm'n, 306
         U.S. 56, 60-62 (1939).

33.   Uribe v. Howie, App., 96 Ca. Rpt. 493 (1977) (pest
         control reports); Carter Products, Inc. v. Eversharp,
         Inc., 360 F.2d 868 (7th Cir. 1966) (patent
         infringement); Wilson v. Superior Ct., 225 P. 881

(1924) (chemical composition of explosive); U.S. v. 48 Jars More or Less, 23 F.D.R. 192 (D.D.C. 1958) (FDA suit for seizure and condemnation of misbranded article); Cf. Jacobson v. Massachusetts, 197 U.S. 11 (1904) (compulsory vaccinations).

34. See Tarassoff v. Regents of University of California, 131 Cal. Rptr. 14 (1976) (psychiatrist must disclose confidential murder threat to potential victim); Toxic Substances Control Act, 15 U.S.C. sec. 2601.

35. Treatise on the Diseases of Tradesmen (1705).

MULTIDISCIPLINARY APPROACH TO PREVENTION AND HEALTH PROTECTION
BY MONITORING: ROLE OF INDIVIDUAL DISCIPLINES.   THE ROLE OF
TRADE UNIONS - I

A. MAZZOCCHI (USA)

Summary

*To date, ambient and biological monitoring programmes have had
the effect of removing or altering workers to conform to the
existing contaminated workplaces. Methodical monitoring programmes that meet particular requirements of an individual
work environment have not, as a general rule, been developed.
Instead, monitoring programmes, together with results derived,
have been seen by management as a device for removing the
victim from the job rather than dealing with the contaminant
itself. However, it has recently been ruled that where
monitoring data exist, workers should have access. However,
management still has the prerogative over who and where they
monitor. The paper suggests improvements to the present
arrangements.*

It is the view of a significant sector of the labour movement
that ambient and biological monitoring cannot be discussed
within its present context of corporate control. Ambient and
biological monitoring programmes to date have had the effect
of removing and/or altering workers to conform to the existing
contaminated workplaces. Biological monitoring programmes, in
many instances, are totally irrelevant simply because they do
not take into account the nature of the specific work
environment.

As a general rule, it has been our experience that there has
not been methodical industrial hygiene monitoring of work
environments and subsequent biological monitoring programmes
developed that meet the peculiar requisites of the individual
work environment.   In fact, in the oil industry where
there is specific collective bargaining language such as the
following:

> "Such research surveys shall include such measure-
> ments of exposure in the workplace, the results of
> which shall be submitted in writing to the Company,
> the International Union President and the Joint

Committee by the Research Consultant, and the
results will also relate the findings to
existing recognised standards.

The Company agrees to pay for appropriate
physical examinations and medical tests at a
frequency and extent necessary in light of
findings set forth in the Industrial Consultant's reports as may be determined by the
Joint Committee.

The Union agrees that each Research Report
shall be treated as privileged and confidential
and will be screened by the Company to prevent
disclosure of proprietory information or any
other disclosure not permitted by legal or
contractual obligations.

At a mutually established time, subsequent to
the receipt of such reports, the Joint Committee will meet for the purpose of reviewing such
reports and to determine whether corrective
measures are necessary in light of the Industrial Consultant's findings, and to determine
the means of implementing such corrective
measures."
>   (OCAW/Oil Industry
>   Health and Safety Clause)

our experience has been that regardless of the fact that the
industry acknowledges that industrial hygiene surveys should
precede the development of biological monitoring, the companies have moved unilaterally to structure medical surveillance programmes without the benefit of the industrial
hygiene survey being conducted.

Unilateralism in establishing biological monitoring programmes characterises the practice in the United States.
Management uses medical surveillance as a worker removal
device. It seeks to find out whether an employee has been
adversely impacted by virtue of his workplace exposures. If
an abnormality is discovered, the monitoring programme is not
used as a device to address the causative factors; instead it
removes the victim from the job rather than addressing the
contaminant itself.

Additionally, management has taken the position that ambient
and biological monitoring is strictly a management prero-

gative, and contrary to existing labour law, they need not discuss the design and implementation of these programmes.

In a now classic case, management was conducting blood tests on workers in a facility where styrene was made, and it was believed by the work force that the blood testing programme was attempting to discern damage possibly from benzene exposure. The union attempted to find out: (i) the nature of the blood test; (ii) the results of the blood testing; and (iii) notification to the worker of the results.

In this situation, management took the position that they need not disclose the nature of the tests or the results to either the bargaining agent or the worker himself. Subsequently, the Union filed for arbitration on the basis that we could not appropriately represent the employees unless the nature of the tests was disclosed and the results released so that we could address the cause of the damage, if indeed there was damage. The arbitrator ruled in favour of the Union, maintaining it could not carry out its duty of appropriate representation unless it understood the nature of the biological monitoring programme. Incidentally, this plant had an excess of leukaemia.

In another instance, ambient monitoring was never conducted in a dye facility where benzidine, a known bladder cancer inducer, was being used. Instead, a biological monitoring programme was instituted by the employer in which the employees were sent to a health institution nearby and were cystoscoped yearly and, in some instances, more than once a year. Bladder cancer was discovered among numerous employees. The employees were treated and sent back to the point of production without ever being told the nature of the surveillance programme, the results of the programme, nor were they ever told they were working with benzidine and the fact that it is a known bladder cancer inducer.

The cases cited are not aberrations; they are the general rule. I can relate in detail and at length any number of situations that are similar to the two described episodes.

Ambient monitoring programmes that have been instituted by management have not been effective means for exposed workers contaminated at the point of production. The results of ambient monitoring programmes are kept from workers and management has refused to disclose this data.

The Assistant Secretary of Labor, in a recently promulgated rule, will allow for access to those data where they exist. However, who monitors and where they monitor is still the prerogative of management. Physicians, industrial nurses and industrial hygienists are a captive profession. In order to liberate these scientists, it is our view that control is the key question. Who controls the monitors? We propose that these professionals be allowed to conduct their activities without restraints imposed upon them by either management or the workers' representative. Management should pay for the surveys as a cost of doing business, but the professionals should not be obligated to report the individual results of biological monitoring to either the Union or management. Management and the Union should receive only the aggregate data, which in the final analysis, is the only data necessary to make corrections in the work environment.

Industrial hygiene monitoring ought to be done after joint consultation between management and the Union, and the hygienist ought to be directed to monitor in a comprehensive fashion and on a systematic basis, and the results of the monitoring made known to all parties affected.

The system of funding a separate entity that would hire the professionals is not very difficult to develop, since health insurance and other welfare provisions in the collective bargaining agreement have, in many instances, been established just in this manner. Workplace biological monitoring

and ambient monitoring programmes in their present configuration are counter-productive and serve to perpetuate the
existing deteriorating work environment and its subsequent
impact on the workforce.

MULTIDISCIPLINARY APPROACH TO PREVENTION AND HEALTH PROTECTION
BY MONITORING: ROLE OF INDIVIDUAL DISCIPLINES. THE ROLE OF
THE TRADE UNIONS - II

P. SILON (BELGIUM)

Summary

*For the trade unions, one of the most important aims of a good
health and safety policy is to ensure that monitoring is no
longer necessary.   Such a state of affairs could be achieved
by removal or replacement of toxic agents, or by way of safe
technologies and working methods. It is felt that monitoring
can fulfil an alarm function, an intervention function, a
study and research function, and an inspection and evaluation
function. Although biological monitoring is acceptable under
certain conditions and even necessary in some cases, priority
should be given to ambient monitoring.*

*It is hoped that the Community will harmonize monitoring
methods and procedures and perhaps certify the quality of
laboratories that agree to a strict control of their monitoring results.*

The trade union view of the relationship between monitoring and health and safety policy

For the trade unions one of the most important aims of a good
health and safety policy is to ensure that monitoring is no
longer necessary: either by keeping toxic agents out of the
place of work as far as possible or by replacing agents of
high toxicity by agents of low toxicity or by keeping the
risks of exposure to the absolute miminum by using safe technologies and working methods.

The former require thorough research into the toxicity of substances before they come on the market and are used in the
production process, research performed under the direct or
indirect supervision of workers and government. The latter
means bringing pressure to bear on the industrial and commercial equipment market so that only safe articles come on to
the market.

Organisation of this type of health and safety policy requires more commitment and creativity than does a policy
which merely imposes ambient and biological monitoring plus a
number of limit values.

If, moreover, we refer to toxic substances only and not to
harmful substances or physical agents, we limit the scope of
the problem, which is perhaps not advisable. This does not
imply that the problem of monitoring is not important, since
as long as we do not have the basic elements of a good health
and safety policy, good ambient and biological monitoring is
of great importance to workers' health.

The functions of ambient and biological monitoring

The functions of monitoring can vary. It is our opinion that
its most important function in connection with preventive
values is the alarm function. In the case of physical monitoring this alarm function is fulfilled by direct indication
of:
    - a steep rise in the concentration
    - values far in excess of the limit suggesting an
      incident, leakage or radical change in working
      conditions.

The 'alarm' thus given makes it possible to take direct
action and remove the cause of the increase in concentration. Biological monitoring can under certain conditions
(see below) also act as an alarm system. Good functioning of
the alarm system requires a well-thought-out and suitable
monitoring method.

Another important function of monitoring is creation of the
possibility of good specific intervention. Continuous analysis of the monitoring results must provide a good picture
of ways in which exposure risks manifest themselves in the
undertaking. Physical and biological monitoring must also be
organised so as to provide useful indications about the

nature of risks and for creating healthier working conditions. The interpretation of monitoring results must thus
provide useful information for the purposes of specific and
effective health and safety measures, if monitoring is to
have real value for health and safety. In the case of biological monitoring in particular, the relationship between the
individual and his environment must be analysed thoroughly
before. monitoring can suggest measures to improve the environment. It is also necessary to adapt the frequency of
monitoring to health and safety requirements. In other words
biological monitoring must take place at intervals which
still make it possible to take preventive measures and undo
any harm or limit it to a strict minimum.

Monitoring also has a function as regards <u>study</u> and <u>research</u>
about the environment and the relationship between the environment and the individual. Without examining this function
more closely, it should be emphasised that the trade unions
do not accept the way these studies and research projects
often serve as an alibi and a reason for postponing urgent
technical health and safety measures in connection with
substances whose degree of toxicity is not known with any
great certainty.

Finally, monitoring fulfils an 'inspection and evaluation'
function. It enables the workers involved, their organisations, health and safety experts and the government to check
whether the imposed or agreed standards are complied with.
It also enables the persons involved to evaluate health and
safety policy and examine the effectiveness of the measures
taken.

In connection with the monitoring of limit values, it must
also be made clear that the trade unions do not accept that
<u>limit values</u> should be used in the sense of <u>acceptable
standards</u>; they are to be regarded as temporary guide values.
Various reasons for adopting this position include the facts
that:

- there is no clear-cut limit between harmful and
  non-harmful concentrations and for a number of
  substances, 'nil' concentration is the only
  absolute guarantee of safety;
- the worker is frequently exposed - at his place
  of work and outside it - to toxic substances
  and the cumulative effect is often difficult to
  assess;
- the working conditions under which exposure
  takes place often differ greatly;
- individual reactions to substances differ and
  limit values are based on the reaction of
  the average person.

Thus the trade unions urge that all technical means should be
used to reduce exposure as much as possible, and in some
cases eliminate it completely, not least because substances
are not only toxic but also cause discomfort.

Priority should be given to ambient monitoring

From the health and safety point of view the trade unions
give priority to ambient monitoring because all harmful exposure should be avoided and biological monitoring takes place
after the event....in other words when the damage has been
done.

Biological monitoring is also more stressful and less safe
for workers, less suitable for monitoring certain effects
and costly because of technical, measurement and interpretation problems. The trade unions have the impression that the
large amount of money spent on this would be better used for
research and measures to improve the environment.

Biological monitoring is, however, acceptable under certain
conditions and even necessary in some cases. It is for instance quite clear that biological monitoring is indispensable to the study of the relationship between the environ-

ment and the individual. Biological monitoring can also
fulfil an 'alarm' and 'intervention' function where toxic
substances are taken up by various routes (by inhalation,
through the skin, orally) or where the worker is exposed to
the same substances outside his place of work (traffic,
nutrition).

To sum up, it can be said that biological monitoring is
acceptable under certain conditions provided that:
- it complements ambient monitoring;
- it forms an integral part of health and safety
  policy as a whole;
- it takes place under decent conditions.

The role of workers and their representatives as regards monitoring

The trade unions require that workers and their representatives receive adequate and suitable information about toxic
agents and the monitoring of toxic agents by way of a procedure which ensures that:
- all workers have the right to inspect their
  medical records either direct or through their
  general practitioner;
- workers' representatives must always be able to
  check ambient monitoring and monitoring
  results;
- industrial confidentiality cannot be given as a
  reason for preventing workers' representatives
  from inspecting all toxicological data and
  monitoring results;
- the results of biological monitoring must be
  presented in a way that makes it as difficult
  as possible to know individual results.
The trade unions require that workers and their representatives should be vested with genuine influence over the whole
monitoring procedure and methods. This influence will ensure
that the monitoring results are representative, reliable and

as objective as possible. The workers' practical experience
and knowledge of the working environment are moreover an
indispensable aid to obtaining good monitoring results and to
their interpretation.

The trade unions urge that biological monitoring should take
place under the best possible conditions. Certain material
requirements should be met (good premises, sanitary installations, heating) and discretion guaranteed.

The trade unions are making every effort to provide information and training so that monitoring results may be accurately assessed and form an aid to the introduction of safety and
health measures. The trade unions are prepared to cooperate
with all serious efforts to improve the objectivity and
quality of monitoring. They therefore hope that the
Community will harmonise monitoring methods and procedures at
a high level of quality. In conclusion perhaps the European
Commission could also exercise greater influence on laboratories by certifying the quality of laboratories which agree
to a strict control of their monitoring results.

MULTIDISCIPLINARY APPROACH TO PREVENTION AND HEALTH PROTECTION
BY MONITORING: ROLE OF INDIVIDUAL DISCIPLINES. THE
INDUSTRIALIST: INDUSTRY'S VIEW OF MONITORING I.

G. BUNGE (BELGIUM)

Summary

*Laws and regulations have existed in the chemical industry
for over 100 years as have professional organisations to look
after the protection of workers against hazards. The aim has
always been the reliable prevention of hazards working within
objectives that have commitment from all levels in a company.
This paper discusses monitoring from the standpoint of regular updating as new analytical techniques emerge. It states
industry's position regarding cancer prevention programmes
now and in the future and makes proposals for the development
of a code of good monitoring practice. It concludes with a
request for a greater convergence between countries, and
between industry and authorities.*

Introduction

Chemistry touches everyone's life, everyday and the "work
place", concerns not only the approximate 2.3 million of
workers and employees in the 10,000 or so chemical enterprises
of West Europe but many more persons who come into contact
with chemicals in their daily work. Chemical substances and
compounds penetrate into many industrial installations. The
number of chemical products is on the increase; many chemicals
however are low volume products.

Our enterprises, in concert with authorities and workers, try
to ensure that chemical agents likely to be harmful to health
"should not be present at the wrong time in the wrong working
place, in the wrong amount". Contact with these agents should
be limited to amounts below a no effects level.

Since the beginning of the modern chemical industry, internal
safety and health of the workers and employees has played a
role in all companies. Laws and regulations exist; some of
them have done for more than 100 years. The interest of
society and public has increased over the years, especially

after World War II, with the great advance of science and
experience.

The documentation about the situation has improved and
measures for prevention are continuously updated. Apart from
medical services existing in the companies for a long time
already, the first professional organisations of employers
and employees to look after the protection of workers against
hazards were established in the 1880s (Alkali Inspectorate,
Institut de Securité Industrielle, Berufsgenossenschaft,
etc...).

Now, a hundred years later, we are going into a decade where
major initiatives are proposed by authorities, the public and
the unions, to improve health and safety at the work place.
Industry welcomes these initiatives.

The working environment of chemical workers is safer than
industry's average. We endeavour to keep and improve this
record devoting increasing amounts of investments to comply
with occupational safety and health standards. As a result
of improving control and monitoring, (when presenting
industry's view of monitoring, I refer, of course, mainly to
the chemical industry of West Europe) the incidence of acute
industrial occupational diseases is falling in some
countries.

Objectives and principles

I believe that there is no disagreement between the public
and people in industry in aiming for the reliable prevention
of hazards, whilst people work in industrial installations.
We know that there is no such a thing as zero risk but with
the available knowledge, according to the best state of
technology, a good management of prevention of risk is today
possible. This finds the support of industry.

Industry supports the objectives in the "Council Directive on
the protection of workers from harmful exposure to chemical

physical and biological agents at work". This framework
Directive will lead to other Directives where industry may
express a different opinion, for instance, in the area of
carcinogens.

Objectives should be:
- introduction of a systematic and balanced in-
  plant monitoring scheme;
- determination of priorities;
- agreement on definition of terms to achieve
  inter-comparison of methods;
- uniform understanding and interpretation
  between Government and industry;
- incorporation of these and other principles
  and details into companies' codes.

Industry is defined as "systematic labour for the creation
of value" or "habitual employment in useful work". In modern
language, one might add the concept of "under safe and
healthy conditions". Industry is but one part of society,
perhaps an important part, in the sense of contributing to
the standard of living, but above all, a part which should be
equal under law with that part of Society which is non-
industrial.

The responsibility of industry can only be discharged
properly if there is a clear apportionment of rights and
duties and a clear framework of law and regulation including
that part where industry's own responsibility and initiative
is recognised fully. Participation of industry in programmes
of Governments is needed because the experience of the
"frontier" is needed and self-initiation of measures to
improve safety and industrial hygiene should be encouraged.

Commitment to the objectives has to come from all levels in a
company, beginning with top management. This commitment must
be supported by understanding on behalf of the rest of
society (the legislator, the public, the mass-media) for the

particular problems industry is faced with. Only this understanding can create a participation of all in a safe working
environment. Over the years, national parliaments and
authorities have established many laws and regulations and
international institutions have contributed, as opinion
makers to legislation. This has led both within countries
(USA) or communities - the European Community (EC) - to some
overlapping, sometimes to contradictions and to a feeling of
insecurity vis-a-vis the law; this is a problem especially
for small enterprises. Another objective should also be a
contribution on an international basis, to clarification and
simplification.

Monitoring, tests, assessment

Following modern scientific methods industry has achieved
the lowering of limits of sensitivity and shortening of the
cycles of analyses. Detection can now be done on a ppb, or
even on a ppt range. Hence the element of uncertainty in
handling chemical products has been much reduced.

Hazards in chemical industrial installations appear as
solids, dust, liquid particles, gases, or vapours. Monitoring
in industry must adjust accordingly and make sure that each
technique considers sensitivity, accuracy, precision and
relevancy of tests.

The relative toxicological risk is classified according to
different grouping systems, either chemical or biological/
medical.   Obviously, the various forms of potential toxicity
such as: neuro- nephro- pulmonary- or other forms, must be
listed when establishing a full monitoring system.

Many companies have manuals for the monitoring system, establishing details of personal monitoring, area monitoring,
designation of workers, etc... These manuals should be
updated once per annum following the development of science,
or if new products are manufactured, or if the manufacturing
process changes.

Analytical   techniques keep improving and the challenge to
industry to define the safety measures in installations will
remain.   In the various countries of Europe, one observes
different approaches to testing and to monitoring. Apart
from the national approach, one also observes attitudes which
are purely scientific or sometimes influenced by political
institutions. This leads to a different appraisal of testing
and monitoring.   Industry will maintain that, with methods
existing today, it is possible to come nearer to the task of
real protection of workers and employees and to control
effectively occupational hazards.

The concept, the system and the terminology referring to
exposure limits are different in European countries. Also,
the accepted limit value is different in size and sometimes
in threshold.   The EEC is endeavouring to achieve harmonisation in this area but this is likely to be a long and
tedious exercise.   Industry would favour a reduction of the
differences but is aware that work practices are much
influenced by local and national authorities. The EEC has
succeeded in establishing a glossary of key terms and common
principles for the definition of exposure limit values.

Similar differences of classification concern biological
monitoring tests.   Further evaluation of biological trials
must be undertaken to contribute more to risk assessment,
which is essential for industry's appraisal and decision.

Though in the major part of chemical enterprises, medical
monitoring is following similar ways, in the laboratory testing or in clinical examination, the differences in physicians'
referral patterns make the interpretation of data uncertain.
Industry physicians working in the medical departments of
chemical enterprises try, however, to accept common criteria
to harmonize the principle lines of occupational health care.

Total "man monitoring" must then include the coordination of
analytical, biological and medical tests. The profile of the

chemical product will be established and will lead to the determination of the occupational risk.

I believe that more regular monitoring will come both on a voluntary and on a statutory basis. Authorities and industry should establish jointly the type and volume of monitoring needed, considering size, nature and site of a chemical plant. Final judgement of the results must take into consideration factors outside industry's fence, for instance: age, constitution of the employee, diet, smoking habits, etc... The records of personnel and monitoring data are the responsibility of local management and the medical department. Documentation is already or should be computerised. This facilitates full appraisal. It would be worthwhile also to endeavour to harmonize computer systems.

Carcinogens

Industry is in favour of a cancer prevention programme, providing the best possible protection. Monitoring and assessment are particularly difficult because it is doubtful that any method is sensitive enough for reliable detection of all carcinogens. Since there is no agreement yet on the cause of cancer (a single agent or a multi-stage development?) it is at present impossible to define precisely the attribution of cancer to occupational exposure. The estimates of the percentage of cancer cases relating to occupational factors are different. Industry is interested in clarifying further this question and favours a scientific approach based on factual epidemiological evidence.

The Occupational Safety and Health Administration (OSHA), the International Agency for Research into Cancer (IARC), the European Communities, the European Chemical Industry Ecology and Toxicology (ECETOC) and others have endeavoured to classify chemical carcinogens. The European chemical industry would favour the ECETOC definition, "a contribution to the strategy for the identification and control of

occupational carcinogens", but would also support the trial
to harmonize internationally this classification. Based on
short term tests, animal studies and epidemiological
findings, the carcinogenic potential must be established;
this will enable industry to control actual human exposure
under circumstances of an "acceptable quantified risk".

Guidance exists or comes in for industry from OSHA, the
International Labour Organization (ILO) and, in the near
future, from the EEC. At present, the criteria for definition of occupational carcinogens and consequently regulations
differ widely in the EEC Member-countries. European industry
would, therefore, favour the EEC guidance to come, both for
listing carcinogens and for generic policy. Industry should
be consulted in working out together with the authorities the
concept based upon which an EEC Directive would be established.

Industry is not in favour of a complete ban, though regulations of this kind exist already. Endorsement of legislation
is the prerogative of nations and if law or regulations concerning prohibition of production of certain chemicals are
not endorsed worldwide, the possibility of "exporting the
hazard" exists. Having said this, I would like to stress that
industry does not object to strict observance of stringent
regulations controlling occupational carcinogens.

Industry would also be in favour of a separation of the
evaluation of carcinogenicity and the establishment of law
and regulation. The evaluation must be arranged by a scientific advisory body, including scientists who speak on behalf
of industry, based on their experience in industrial installations. This advisory body should define the quantitative
risk assessment.

Epidemiology

These studies and findings - of great importance for industry
to present experience data to appraise hazards of occupational

origin - need an international clarification of their design
and conduct. The World Health Organisation (WHO) has provided guidelines which - as far as I know -have not been
accepted worldwide. Epidemiological data contribute to a
better risk assessment, for instance in the area of
carcinogenic chemicals. Industry is in favour of a closer
contact between independent or government epidemiologists and
industry's experts. I would like to suggest an international
panel of epidemiology with a mandate of WHO, EEC, ILO, OSHA
and perhaps some other authorities which would have a role in
this field. Industry would like to be represented on this
panel.

Good laboratory practice (GLP)

The principle of GLP was pioneered by the Food and Drug
Administration (FDA) with the aim of improving work and
results of laboratories. The European industry favours an
harmonization of the basic attitude vis-a-vis GLP and attempted by the Organisation for Economic Cooperation and Development (OECD). Accreditation, including inspection, is unavoidably bureaucratic because several groups of institutes
must find approval, regardless of different traditions of
mentalities. Industry sees however that a major divergence
of laboratory practices in different countries could create
problems. Industry must rely on laboratory findings, which
are comparable; these laboratory findings have, of course, an
influence on the appraisal of occupational risks in industrial installations. European Industry would favour the
proposals for GLP as worked out by ECETOC ("Good Laboratory
Practice").

Some thoughts on the present and the future

This seminar should contribute to a form of a globally
balanced interdependence of industrial countries regarding
occupational health. If, on the other hand, fragmentation
remains and the national policies concerning the safety and

health of workers remain very different, this would distort
the condition-parameters under which industry has to operate
in various parts of the world.

It is not possible to aim for total "harmonization" but it is
advisable to have as a task - both at Government level and in
industry - agreement on a uniformity of standards and interpretation of these and establishment of a systematic approach
to assessment. This could result in a code of Good Monitoring Practice.

The major part of organisations are able and, I think, also
willing to contribute to such a code as listed below:

United Nations and specialised agencies	World Health Organisation (WHO); International Agency for Research into Cancer (IARC); International Atomic Energy Authority (IAEA); International Standards Organisation (ISO); United Nations Environment Programme (UNEP).
European Communities	Directorates-General III V and XII of the Commission of the European Communities; the European Centre for Population Studies (ECPS).
Organisation for	Economic Cooperation and Development (OECD)
National authorities and institutions	Ministries of Health; Ministries of Labour; Works Councils; Berufsgenossenschaften; Inspectorates etc.
United States	Occupational Safety and Health Administration (OSHA); National Institute for Occupational Safety and Health (NIOSH); Health and Human Service (HHS); Environmental Protection Agency (EPA); National Cancer Institute (NCI); American

Conference of Governmental Industrial
Hygienists (ACGI); Food and Drug
Administration (FDA); Consumer Products
Safety Commission (CPSC).

Societies   International Union of Pure and Applied
Chemistry (IUPAC); toxicological societies;
Deutsche Forschungsgemeinschaft; Royal
Society of Chemistry (RSC); Chimie et
Ecologie; etc.

Industry   National associations; Conseil Européen des
related bodies   Fédérations de l'Industrie Chimique (CEFIC);
Association of Plastics Manufacturers in
Europe (APME); Ecological and Toxicological
Association of the Dyestuffs Manufacturing
Industry (ETAD); Groupement International
des Associations Nationales Fabricants
Produits Agrochimiques (GIFAP); Chemical
Manufacturers Association (CMA); American
Industrial Health Council (AIHC); Chemical
Industries Institute of Toxicology (CIIT);
European Chemical Industry Ecology and
Toxicology Centre (ECETOC); MEDICHEM;
Japanese Ecology and Toxicology Centre
(JETOC).

Other bodies   International Commission for Protection
against Environmental Mutagens and
Carcinogens (ICPEMC); International Social
Security Association (ISSA); International
Archive of Occupational Health (IAOH); data
banks etc.

Good science provides good credibility. Scientific progress
ought to find support from all; the chemical industry has a
good record here. Interaction between industry, research
institutes and universities must be encouraged. Science must

prepare the ground - and industry must contribute reliable data - for legislation and decision on occupational health, which in the end is political. In order to discharge the responsibility, the scientific arm of Government and the scientific part of industry must have more educated staff and sufficient funds. Thus, the uncertainty is reduced and certainty enables us to do a proper appraisal and go for the right political decision.

Risk must be and can be controlled; total elimination, or zero-risk or the total ban of production - excepting rare cases - has on the one hand the virtue of simplicity but society appreciates the wealth-creating function of industry and favours a balanced approach, weighing risk against benefit.

More convergence should be supported in the area of classification of carcinogens, perhaps under the leadership of IARC acting as opinion-maker. It is likely that the number of substances for which carcinogenic properties are suspected, will increase and it is highly desirable that all tumour-related questions (potency, human or animal carcinogenicity, benign or malignant tumours etc.) are thoroughly studied and appraised. This is, of course, already going on and the number of research publications is legion. Nevertheless, the lack of internationally accepted expert opinion leads some-times to an absolutist approach to law and regulation and industry would take exception to this approach.

I favour naturally an exchange of experience; whether a pooling of monitoring data is internationally feasible remains to be seen; the range of measurement techniques is rather wide. Also, the confidentiality of data, e.g. medical data or industrial property has to be respected.

A programme of toxico-vigilance has been proposed and the implementation of present and future monitoring in industry is already a good part of this programme. Any thorough

toxicologist, however, would have to recommend extension of
this toxico-vigilance to all parts of the workers life. This
seems difficult to realise.

Very many managers - chemists, doctors, engineers, physicists
- work in industry for the common goal we discuss here today.
Often, enterprises voluntarily comply with work practices to
improve the control of risk ahead of regulation. This should
be encouraged by Government and the public alike. CEFIC,
through its committees and working parties, is a catalyst and
helps to work towards common European standards. We hope to
contribute to the good balance sheet of health which - in the
sense of a social audit - the chemical industry is working
for and caring for.

Some examples of convergence or divergence in the international field are given below:

Convergence	Divergence
Industrial lay-out.	Climate, site, local mentality
Industrial technology.	National standards.
Exposure limit objectives.	Exposure limit systems.
Objectives of law and regulation	Interpretation and implementa-tion of law.
Generic policy (e.g. carcinogens)	Listing, classification, criteria.
Objectives of industrial hygiene	Industrial hygiene standards
Common procedure for exchange of information, international "reference centre".	Information available but spread over many scientific journals, national registers publications.

Let us endeavour to achieve more convergence both between
countries or between industry and authorities.

Documents

D.F.G. - Maximale Arbeitsplatzkonzentrationen.   1979

DUPONT - Occupational Health and Safety.   1980

ECETOC - Good Laboratory Practice.   1979

ECETOC - A contribution to the Strategy for the Indenti-
          fication and Control of Occupational Carcinogens1980

EGAN   - Analytical Testing Procedure. A critical Review.1980

BUNDESRAT
        - 2 Novelle zur Verordnung uber Gefahrliche
          Arbeitstoffe.   1980

ESSO   - Benzene Monitoring Programme.

OSHA   - Generic Rules on Identification, Classification
          and Limitation of Toxic Substances representing
          a potential cancer risk at work place.   1980

KING   - Man Monitoring in Occupational Medicine.   1980

THIESS - Prevention and Control of Occupational Cancer -
          MEDICHEM.   1980

HUME   - Monitoring Airborne Hazards.   1980

EC   - Council Directive on the Protection of Workers
          From Harmful Exposure to Chemical, Physical and
          Biological Agents at the Work Place.   1980

EPA   - TSCA Cancer Hazards Working Rule - List of
          Carcinogens.

EEC   - Comparative Analysis of the principle and appli-
          cation of control limits in the Member States of
          the European Community.   1979

ENVIRONMENT DATA SERVICES
        - The EEC's Health and Safety Programme for the
          1980s.   1980

OECD   - Facing the Future.   1979

EEC   - Discussion document on Occupational Carcinogens.1979

SMEETS - Tests and Notification of chemical Substances in
          current legislation.   1979

CEFIC   - Position papers and Committees' conclusions.

MULTIDISCIPLINARY APPROACH TO PREVENTION AND HEALTH PROTECTION
BY MONITORING: ROLE OF INDIVIDUAL DISCIPLINES. THE
INDUSTRIALIST: INDUSTRY'S VIEW OF MONITORING II.

J.M. HOCHSTRASSER (USA)

Summary

Industrial hygiene monitoring is used more extensively by
industry industrial hygienists than by counterparts in labour
and government. Monitoring is used in all phases of an industrial hygiene programme (recognition, evaluation and control)
and plays an important part in the development of new sampling
and analytical procedures. Very little information is
presently available regarding formal logical approaches to
monitoring. However, the approach used by the Occupational
Safety and Health Administration (OSHA) in recently issued
occupational health standards can, with minor modifications,
be adopted for use by industry as a formal approach to all
industrial hygiene monitoring.

Introduction

Monitoring of employee exposure to potential occupational
health hazards must be the basis for every viable industrial
hygiene programme. Monitoring is essential to all three major
phases of any industrial hygiene programme, those phases being
recognition, evaluation and control. The monitoring of chemical and physical agents, in the workplace, provides qualitative and quantitative information relative to an employee's
present exposure, possible previous exposure, potential future
exposure and is essential to the decision-making process if
corrective action is indicated. Monitoring data must be used
to implement effective administrative and engineering controls, including such engineering controls as may be necessary
to prevent a workplace problem from becoming an environmental
problem.

An industry overview

Industry's approach to the technical aspects of industrial
hygiene monitoring should not differ significantly from the
approaches of labour unions and government regulatory

agencies, at least where monitoring programmes are administered and managed by competent industrial hygienists.
Usually, when differences do arise, they are administrative
in nature and can be attributed to the limitations of time
and opportunity placed on the industrial hygienist. In this
regard, the industry industrial hygienist usually occupies
the advantageous position of having direct access to study
and evaluate each potential exposure. While the industry
industrial hygienist might be restricted with regard to time
and opportunity, the restrictions are less than those placed
on labour and government representatives. Therefore, the
industry industrial hygienist has the advantage of opportunity to monitor a given situation as frequently as
necessary to obtain as much data as may be required to reach
definitive conclusions in the decision-making process. It
should be mentioned that all three sectors are restricted by
lack of sufficient qualified personnel.

Industrial hygienists from labour and government must, of
necessity, base judgement decisions on very limited data.
Where an overexposure condition is indicated from interpretation of the monitoring data collected from a given
situation, recommendations for corrective action can differ
significantly. Industry, labour and government industrial
hygienists can each have different opinions regarding the
need for, and type of, corrective action to be taken. In
this aspect, differences of opinion can be due to differences
in education, training and/or experience or they could be
attributed to philosophical differences, such as technical
feasibility versus economic feasibility. Unfortunately, the
existing adversary relationship of industry, labour and
government often prevails when these differences exist and
the decision-making process is surrendered to the legal
system. The final result can be, and often is, counter
productive to the basic purpose of the monitoring process;
that being to ensure that each employee has a work environment that is not detrimental to his or her health and wellbeing.

It is important to recognise that the quality and success of any industry industrial hygiene programme depends on the quality of the monitoring data, the ability of the data interpreter to properly analyse the data and to make recommendations where indicated. However, no industrial hygiene programme can be successful if recommendations are not implemented and necessary corrective actions are not taken. Since industry industrial hygienists usually occupy staff positions their contributions to the implementation processes may be severely limited. The industrial hygienist's ability to positively impact the implementation process depends on many factors, including technical expertise, credibility, upper management support, delegated authority, ability to deal effectively with interpersonal relationships, including adversary staff/staff and line/staff relationships and a constant awareness of his or her moral obligations, such as those stated in the Code of Ethics, adopted by the American Academy of Industrial Hygiene; in other words, dedication to the profession.

Monitoring basics

The basic principles of monitoring are set by the state-of-art and are independent of the sector, industry, labour or government, which applies the principles. However, the different sectors may choose to apply different principles of monitoring depending on the ultimate purpose of the monitoring. For instance, it is rare that labour or government will use qualitative monitoring techniques to determine employee exposure. Industry frequently uses qualitative techniques to identify the presence of chemical substances which may not be regulated but might pose a threat to an employee's health.

It is beyond the scope of this presentation to discuss the technical aspects of monitoring. However, some of industry's application of monitoring principles will be discussed.

Qualitative vs. quantitative monitoring

The industry industrial hygienist uses qualitative monitoring techniques, in the "recognition" phase of a survey, to iden-tify the presence of potential occupational health hazards. The technique could involve taking a charcoal tube grab sample for mass spectroscopy analysis, a filter grab sample to identify fibres or particulate, or possibly the use of an explosimeter to ensure the absence of explosive concentra-tions of volatile chemicals. Bulk samples of the materials might also be collected to aid in identifying the proper quantitative monitoring method.

Quantitative monitoring techniques are used, in the "evaluation" and "control" phases of a survey, to evaluate the severity of a potential occupational health hazard and, where an overexposure is indicated, to identify a method of control. Quantitative techniques are necessary to demon-strate compliance with government regulations, to obtain data for comparison with biological monitoring data and to evaluate the effectiveness of engineering controls.

Both qualitative and quantitative monitoring must be employed in the development of sampling and analytical methods to identify potential occupational health hazards.

Personal vs. area monitoring

Personal monitoring is used to evaluate an individual em-ployee's exposure to an occupational health hazard. Quantita-tive methods are employed and the data can be used to define the exposure of other employees performing similar tasks, provided the differences between employees' exposures can be shown to be statistically insignificant.

Area monitoring is generally of a quantitative type and used to evaluate process emissions for purposes of designing and evaluating engineering controls. Area monitoring data can

also be used to predict personal employee exposures when
accurate time and motion data are available. This application of area monitoring is especially useful when a suitable personal monitoring technique is not available.

Personal and area monitoring can employ qualitative techniques but are usually quantitative in nature. The results
of personal and area monitoring are also used as previously
discussed under Qualitative vs. Quantitative.

Monitoring methods

The monitoring methods employed are usually those which have
been defined by recognised authoritative sources such as the
Occupational Safety and Health Administration (OSHA), the
National Institute for Occupational Safety and Health (NIOSH)
or the American Society for Testing Materials (ASTM). Whenever possible, the most sensitive methods are used. But,
when a monitoring method for a potential occupational health
hazard does not exist, a development programme must be
implemented.

Frequency of monitoring

Wherever possible, the frequency of monitoring should never
be less than that defined as minimal by OSHA. The actual
frequency of monitoring must be based on the industrial
hygienist's determination of whether or not employees are
overexposed, whether or not the potential for employee over-
exposure exists and many other aspects. The industrial hygienist must be capable of applying knowledge, experience
and common sense in determining monitoring frequency, number
of employees to monitor and in determining the number and
locations of area monitors. The application of statistical
monitoring methods may not be applicable in the constantly
varying industrial environment. The industry industrial
hygienist is constantly faced with unusual exposure situations which may elude a well-defined statistical monitoring
programme.

Wipe samples

The use of wipe samples as an occupational health hazard monitoring technique is increasing. It has been used for years as a technique to determine contamination in the nuclear and pharmaceutical industries. It is now providing the industrial hygienist with a technique to evaluate degree of contamination where carcinogens and systemic poisons are used. This is a valid method for auditing the effectiveness of housekeeping procedures and confinement of contamination, especially where the contaminant may be transported from the workplace into the outside environment via clothing and equipment.

Monitoring problems

As previously mentioned, the major differences between industry, labour and government monitoring are the limitations placed on labour and government by opportunity, and on all three sectors by time and the availability of qualified staff. In recognising these limitations, it would be well advised for all three sectors to develop a reference monitoring programme so that all data derived from such a programme could be used to its optimum effectiveness.

At the present time, the most widely publicised formal monitoring programmes are those included in occupational health standards developed and issued by OSHA. Segments of monitoring programmes, such as recommended statistical programmes, are available from NIOSH. However, no formal logical approaches to the collection or effective and exhaustive use of monitoring data presently exist.

Attempts to formalise monitoring programmes in industry increase as industrial hygiene staffs increase. However, these programmes are seldom implemented with forethought and planning. They are usually a progressive outgrowth of monitoring in a "firefighting" mode. Very often formal monitoring programmes, which have been developed by qualified industrial hygienists, including those developed in accordance with OSHA standards, are turned over to plant personnel for implementation. Such programmes have a tendency to deteriorate in time, even when they are closely audited by qualified industrial hygienists.

There has been a recent increase in the availability of information on statistical approaches to monitoring. Properly implemented and supported by reliable data bases, statistical programmes can be effective tools for monitoring programmes. However, failure of the user to understand the significance of all aspects of a statistical programme could result in the failure of the monitoring programme. The fact that the user has taken courses in statistical methods does not guarantee that he or she is capable of implementing a valid programme.

A logical approach to monitoring

At the present time, the only readily-available, logical approaches to industrial hygiene monitoring are published in OSHA Occupational Health Standards. The OSHA logic can be used as the basis for development of all monitoring programmes. With minor modifications, the OSHA approach to monitoring could be applied to any potential occupational exposure situation. However, the OSHA approach to monitoring logic should be considered minimal.

OSHA monitoring logic begins with an "initial" determination. The results of that determination dictate the future direction and magnitude of the monitoring programme. The results also dictate what additional steps must be taken to protect the employee, such as implementation of housekeeping procedures, biological monitoring and personal protective equipment. An industry adaptation of the OSHA Lead Standard monitoring logic is shown in Figure 1. Additional requirements keyed to the monitoring logic are summarised in Table 1. It

should be recognised that Figure 1 and Table 1 are an
adaptation of OSHA monitoring logic. One major observable
difference is that the logic presented in Figure 1 requires,
as a minimum, annual monitoring of an employee's exposure.
OSHA does not require annual monitoring when an exposure is
less than the "action level".

Conclusions

The industry industrial hygienist uses monitoring more extensively than his or her counterparts in labour and industry.
The industry industrial hygienist must be confident that the
monitoring results are representative of the actual workplace
conditions in order to make qualified judgements regarding
the relative hazard. to the employee and what types of controls (if any) are necessary to protect the employee in the
short and long terms. One approach to ensuring that monitoring and corrective actions are adequate is to apply the
monitoring logic as defined in OSHA Occupational Health
Standards. By accepting the OSHA monitoring logic as a minimal requirement, the logic can be modified to apply effectively to any circumstances in industry where an employee may
be exposed to a potential occupational health hazard.

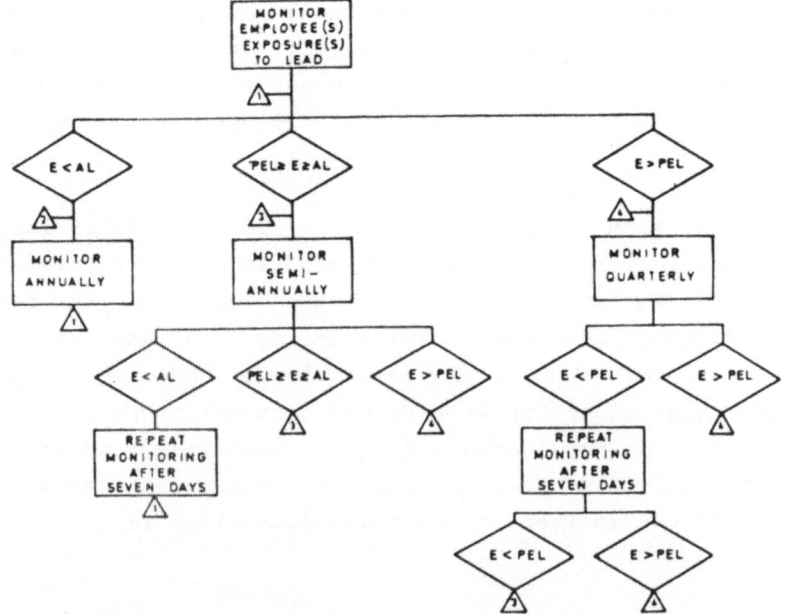

Figure 1. Monitoring logic occupational exposure to lead

Table 1. Occupational Health Programme - Lead Exposure
(Keyed to Monitoring Logic)*

Monitoring Results	Requirements
E < AL (Exposure Less than Action Level) (1 through 9)	1. Recordkeeping 2. Inform employees of monitoring results 3. Employee training 4. Respiratory Protection programme 5. Protective clothing & equipment 6. Housekeeping 7. Hygiene facilities & practices 8. Control equipment monitoring 9. Administrative controls audit
PEL ≤ E ≤ AL (Exposure greater than or equal to AL but less than or equal to Permissible Exposure Limit) (1 through 11)	10. Medical surveillance 11. Medical removal
E > PEL (Exposure greater than PEL) (1 through 15)	12. Engineering controls 13. Work practices controls 14. Written compliance programme 15. Warning signs

* Derived from OSHA Lead Standard (29 CFR 1910.1025)
Federal Register Vol. 43, No. 220, November 14, 1978,
pp. 53007-53014

References

1. U.S. Department of Labor - Occupational Safety and Health
Administration. Occupational Exposure To Lead; Federal
Register, Vol. 43 No. 220 - Tuesday, November 14, 1978;
pp. 52952-53014.

2. U.S. Department of Health, Education and Welfare; National
Institute of Occupational Safety and Health.
Occupational Exposure Sampling Strategy Manual; (DHEW-
NIOSH Publication No. 77-173); 148 pp.

3. Ibid. Handbook of Statistical Tests for Evaluating
Employee Exposure to Air Contaminants. (DHEW-NIOSH
Publication No. 75-147); 207 pp.

DISCUSSION - MULTIDISCIPLINARY APPROACH TO PREVENTION AND
HEALTH PROTECTION BY MONITORING

A. M. THIESS   From the outset it must be stated that our
subject occupies a central function in the list of duties of
any modern industrial society, and is thus of great importance for plant physicians, occupational medicine personnel,
industrial hygienists and epidemiologists.

We are presently occupied with preventing industrial damage
to health by means of the close medical supervision of
employees. With the continually improving methods of
analysis it has become possible to measure concentrations of
substances at the place of work in terms of ppb and ppt.
Although this undoubtedly represents real progress, it must
be stressed that interpretation of such data is the responsibility of the expert, as uncritical publications or non-
representative test results can cause uncertainties.

Effective cooperation between plant physicians, occupational
medicine personnel, industrial hygienists and epidemiologists
is essential not only for immediately recognizing the onset
of occupational illnesses but also for preventing these.

All the papers on this subject underline this importance. To
introduce the discussion let me make a few comments on the
various aspects.

1.   The Hygienist: Ambient monitoring - where - when -
and how?

To my knowledge, industrial hygienists are to be found only
in the United Kingdom and the Netherlands, and, within
Germany, at our BASF Works, in addition to the USA. In other
EEC countries, including the Federal Republic of Germany, the
duties of the industrial hygienist are performed by plant
safety personnel who are graduate chemists, engineers and

biologists who do excellent work in their particular fields of activity. Ambient monitoring at the workplace is a key element in any industrial hygiene programme. Although the monitoring is carried out by the industrial hygiene or industrial safety group, other members of the occupational health team as well as the personnel division join in sponsoring the work and utilizing the data.

Where should monitoring be carried out?

Ambient monitoring is necessary at all workplace areas where an exposed person's health could be impaired. It is important that workers should be informed about MAC levels and peak concentrations because they, too, are or should be responsible for supervising and undertaking routine or special monitoring.

Exact monitoring based on a special plan is necessary for medical case studies in establishing a casual relationship between occupational disease and exposure, and for epidemiological, engineering and analytical studies. A new concern for the hygienist, moreover, is the protection of the environment outside the works, as pointed out by Heuse.

When should monitoring be carried out?

Burgess has given a clear answer. The National Institute for Occupational Safety and Health (USA) has recommended the employee exposure determination and measurement strategy for OSHA regulatory requirements: The event that initiates repeat sampling in this plan is an exposure greater than the Action Level (TWA) which is nominally one-half the OSHA Permissible Exposure Limit.

How should monitoring be carried out?

The experience gained in the last two decades has led to major developments in monitoring methods and apparatus. Sometimes the identification of a single chemical species or family is very difficult, but the evaluation of exposure especially to carcinogenic substances during a long period of work, should, whenever possible, be recorded.

<u>Concerning   the recording and storage of monitoring data</u>, it
should be mentioned that under the "Arbeitsstoffverordnung"
in the Federal Republic of Germany of 01.10.1980, and the
protective measures stipulated by the "Employers' Liability
Insurance" for handling carcinogenic substances, regular
measures have to be taken and the data has to be stored for
60 years.*

Although it is considered vital for such hard data to be
recorded, it would be too difficult to establish a "Health
Protection Card" on which all data such as details of all
accidents, illnesses, aggravation bonuses, absence from work,
sport accidents, smoking and drinking habits, etc. are
entered. Maintaining such a "card" would entail enormous
difficulties and, for example, when a person changes jobs,
could have a negative rather than a positive effect. The
Federal German government and plant physicians in the German
chemical industry have opposed such a card, as have the
representatives of the CEFIC Health Protection Committee.

2.The Nurse: Role in the health team

The role of the occupational nurse changes according to the
number of other specialists employed in the medical team.
Where the nurse is the only health practitioner, he or she is
likely to undertake a wider variety of duties. Generally
speaking it can be said that, without specialist training in
occupational health, the nurse will simply try to use his or
her hospital experience. However, the nurse who works as the
sole health practitioner (small plants) must also be able to
advise the management on different tasks, especially in the
area of prevention. Appropriate basic education and additional knowledge and skills in the wide field of occupational
medicine are therefore necessary. The identification,

*   UVV   "SchutzmaBnahmen   beim   Umgang mit cancerogenen
Substanzen".

medicine are therefore necessary. The identification, monitoring and control of health and safety hazards in the work place environment and in the private sector constitutes primary prevention. Rahjes has pointed out that biological monitoring is a facet of secondary prevention and both are very important aspects of comprehensive programmes in disease and injury prevention in worker populations.

Appropriately trained nurses - and in this field we still have a lot to do in the USA and EEC - should - according to Radwanski and Rahjes - be able to perform all the many duties listed in their papers.

According to my experience it seems that the nurse in the USA has a broader education than the nurse in Europe. We doctors, politicians and employer and employee representatives, should all make every effort to develop opportunities for upgrading and enhancing their school education and providing further training in occupational medicine.

3 The Physician: Assessment of workers' exposure; ethics and reliability of biological monitoring

The plant physician must act in an advisory capacity to the employer and employees. He has freedom of choice in making decisions and giving instructions concerning the assessment of a worker's exposure in line with his duties, and is responsible only to his own conscience as a physician. The success or otherwise of his activities is governed not only by the physician's personality but also by whether he enjoys the confidence of the plant management and the employees, and how he can motivate such people as the industrial hygienist, the nurse and the epidemiologist.

The ethics and reliability of biological monitoring is a broad problem. Parmeggiani (ILO) referred in his paper to the legal status of biological monitoring in the different ILO Conventions and Recommendations (136, 139, 144, 147, 148, 156, 177). These Recommendations are not ratifiable instruments; they nevertheless serve as a guide when the corresponding conventions are being implemented and national legislation drawn up. An important aspect of these recommendations is the idea of incorporating biological monitoring into any statutory preventive and routine medical examination of workers.

Parmeggiani stated that biological monitoring can therefore be compared to biomedical research as described in the World Health Organization's Helsinki Declaration and appears therefore to be quite ethical under the clauses of the Helsinki Declaration, with which I agree and which cover:

- Information and appropriate explanations to the individual.
- Respect for an individual right to safeguard his integrity.
- The examination methods should not affect his physical wellbeing.
- Priorities between different parameters should be set up, etc.

Parmeggiani and Roberts have also raised a number of other problems which should be discussed here, for example:
- The role of management.
- Consent of workers.
- Confidentiality of results of medical examinations and studies.

Biological monitoring can act as an alarm system or alarm function, and can be thought of, as Roberts pointed out, in narrow or broad terms and the need for biological monitoring varies from worker to worker, from work-site to work-site, and it is an immense challenge to "recognize the situations in which biological monitoring are indicated".

4. The Epidemiologist Value of monitoring
Peters clearly stated that the epidemiological studies which

provide the most useful information for occupational health purposes are those in which the same attention is paid to the dose or exposure as to the response or outcome element. A single individual is not capable on his own of conducting a useful study and therefore multiple disciplines are required.

In considering the relationships between exposure and health effects he gave examples about
- acute exposure vs. acute effects (CO and SO_2)
- acute exposure vs. chronic effects (SO_2, cotton dust and TDI)
- chronic exposure vs. chronic effects (formaldehyde, TDI dermatitis and benzene) (the greatest challenge for the epidemiologist)
- chronic exposure vs. acute effects (benzene)

The epidemiologist also sees the value of monitoring in:
- Strict definition of cohorts
- Listing of chemical substances
- Cooperating with the other experts in a team by determining or selecting the investigation parameters for a study.

In the case of data collation we all agree that epidemiological data should be collated and evaluated on an international basis. Pooling of data is advisable where small groups ae involved.

Conclusions

In all the presentations, the role of the individual disciplines of
- hygienist
- nurse
- physician, and
- epidemiolgist have emphasized that successful health welfare and protection of the employee can be

practised only where there is good teamwork between all the experts involved. In addition, it is important to have scientific ability, personality, and, particularly, confidence in the team and the employer, and the employee should have confidence in the work which has to be done.

From my point of view, whenever possible - but this is not always reasonable (see aromatic amines) - priority should be given first to ambient monitoring, and then to biological monitoring.

Both can act as an alarm system and both should be considered very seriously. Both are steps towards ensuring that workers are not placed at risk. Both must be coupled with critical evaluation and interpretation. Both are very important aspects of comprehensive programmes in disease and injury prevention in worker populations.

It is important not to lose too much time in discussing which should have priority - ambient or biological monitoring, and to pay more attention to the supervision of our employees to whom we feel responsible. For this task both ambient and biological monitoring are important.

M. DROZ I have gained the impression that some of the participants look on biological monitoring as the exclusive domain of the occupational physician. I do not support this point of view. The industrial hygienist has an independent role to play in biological monitoring. Biological monitoring may be divided into two parts, depending on the objectives envisaged:-

- assessment of the dose
- assessment of the effects

The industrial hygienist is responsible for the former and the occupational physician for the latter. This approach has been applied successfully in our institute in Switzerland.

R. L. ZIELHUIS It has been shown that for valid ambient monitoring, biological monitoring and health effects monitoring often sophisticated tests, and not only simple tests, have to be carried out. There is a need for:-

- sophisticated tests and measurement strategies
- sophisticated equipment
- highly trained laboratory staff
- highly trained occupational health staff

My question is: what are the consequences of this for

- organization of occupational health services
- training of staff
- levels of regulating and controlling authorities, e.g. labour inspectorate
- national and international directives and regulations?

E. P. RADFORD The problem I see in occupational health is that the industrial nurse, or the occupational physician does not have adequate authority to carry out the necessary monitoring of exposures or evaluation of health effects. All too often the professional does not have access to top management, or even to a plant manager. For this reason, applying the techniques being discussed in the symposium will be unlikely until this authority becomes better developed.

D. M. RADWANSKI Employers need to be told what they need. Specialist training helps to give authority.

A. MUNN I cannot accept that the physician in industry has no authority. He generally achieves the authority that his skill and expertise and personality deserve.

Certainly in 30 years in the Chemical Industry I have had no difficulty in gaining access to top management. Perhaps I do not have the authority to spend 5 million dollars to remedy a hazardous situation, but I do have the authority to disclose the problem to top management, to discuss it, to make recommendations for action, as well as the opportunity to discuss such matters with both employees and regulatory authorities.

L. DE BOER On the "authority" of the occupational physician I agree with Dr Munn. In Europe most of the occupational physicians have easy access to management and mostly report to top management. I know, however, that in the USA managers have a stronger voice than occupational physicians.

W. J. HUNTER There are approximately 100 million workers in the Community, of which the majority are employed in small industries with an average of 15 workers per plant. Assuming that a single occupational physician can look after 2,500 people, the requirements for occupational physicians would total about 40,000 in the Community. Since resources do not allow such numbers of physicians to be made available, it means that greater emphasis must be placed on the development of the "health team" concept and more responsibility delegated to the occupational health nurse and the industrial hygienist.

N. J. ROBERTS Members of the health team must indeed have access to policy setting management. Many do have such access already. Where it is not available, the awareness of its importance must be brought successfully to the attention of management. Much can be done by educational efforts. Where this cannot be done with reasonable success, it may have to be regulation-driven by general duty type requirements.

M. RAHJES   All attempts to assure that we have the ability to
influence   management   are   not useful unless we can gain the
confidence and cooperation of workers.

G. KAZANTZIS   With   regard   to   retrospective   studies, the
epidemiologist   is   hampered   not   only by a lack of exposure
data   but   also by an inability to identify the population at
risk.   Medical records are often inadequate for such studies
as   they may have been initiated some time after the start of
the   hazardous   process   being   investigated,   or they may be
selective.   Personnel   records often provide a more suitable
data-base both   for   exposed   and   control workers. However
while   personnel records in some of the larger companies have
now   been   computerized   or   microfilmed, they are frequently
destroyed   after   a   minimal period on the grounds that space
for   storage   is not available. I would like to propose that
personnel records adequate for identification purposes should
be   retained throughout the Community and that this should be
made a legal requirement in the shortest possible time.

J. P. TASSIGNON   On the one hand it was mentioned that the
number   of   physicians,   hygienists, nurses, epidemiologists,
etc.,   is   insufficient.   On the other hand it has been said
that   the   threshold values tend to be progressively reduced.
The   result   is that the number of employees who must undergo
medical   surveillance   and   the   number   of   firms which must
monitor   exposure   levels increase at the same time. Unfortunately   capacity   -- in terms of personnel, equipment, methods
of   analysis   and   data storage - is by no means expanding at
the   same   rate.   Should   we   not   consider - with a view to
eliminating this bottleneck - legal exemptions, especially in
Europe, both as regards environmental and medical monitoring,
in   plants   in which risk of exposure is low? Should not the
"action   level"   concept (as defined by OSHA) be applied on a
general   scale?   This   would exempt plants considered clean,
from   very   burdensome   monitoring and enable us to focus our

occupational health and industrial hygiene resources on real priorities.

S. EPSTEIN   Does Roberts recognize the fundamental problem of conflict-of-interest in occupational physicians and other health professionals employed by management? There appears to be a well documented basis for suspicions on health and safety data generated and interpreted by professionals with direct and indirect economic interests in such data.

N. J. ROBERTS   The problem of conflict of interest interfering with the work of health professionals paid by employers has been raised repeatedly. In my judgement and experience it is more theoretical than real. Probably not a single employed professional in this room has ever been asked to compromise his or her professional integrity. There is no greater problem than a lawyer, accountant, engineer or other professional would have, nor than would be experienced by a university professor seeking tenure or advancement.

J. LEWALTER   The importance of biological monitoring and the role of the occupational physician in interpreting the findings have been generally recognized. Why is there a reluctance to recognize that the time and effort involved can only lead to real health protection provided job applicants fulfil certain health and hygiene conditions e.g. non-smoker, non-alcoholic, no hypertension, etc.? The value of epidemiological studies is enhanced by biological monitoring which focuses on specific working substances. Why should responsibility for biomonitoring be spread out among various assistants rather than left to appropriately trained occupational physicians? Surely the problems of epidemiological studies show clearly that such studies can only be carried out by suitably qualified assistants under the supervision of an occupational physician?

L. DE BOER With regard to the "independency" of the occupational doctors, a "natural" development will meet the difficulties: small companies cannot have their own occupational health service and have to use "inter-industry health services" which serve several industries. They are "managed" by representatives of employers and employees though medically directed by a doctor. In Holland there are already many of these regional services which cover almost all geographical regions. In fact this is the only answer to the needs of small industries and takes away the image of the doctor "being employed by the employer".

K. ROBOCK Evans, Lardeux, Fallentin and Bell have presented their personal and specific experiences, gained by the engineer and the analytical chemist in the field of technical prevention and health protection.

By example of coal conversion into gas and oil, Evans has very clearly described how it can be managed from the development of a process in the laboratory up to the commercial process, to reduce

- workers' exposure to potentially toxic products and the
- emission of such products into the ambient air to protect the general population.

This has been effected by
- modifying processes in such a way that generating of toxic products or by-products will be reduced or eliminated,
- developing and implementing appropriate control technologies,
- monitoring, so that hazardous concentrations will be detected in time,
- instituting appropriate protective measures for possibly occuring emergency situations.

While the first two items generally depict the basic preventive objectives for all problems displayed in this session, the four active measures indicate the feasibility of controlled handling of substances hazardous to health. This results in the first question which has to be discussed. Can we accept a controlled handling of toxic substances in our economic and social value system secured by utmost reduction of their concentration or shall we demand the zero-risk (nil concentration for toxic substances)?

From the technician's viewpoint, Lardeux entered into the same problems, however, added the necessities
- of special training courses dealing with occupational medicine and industrial hygiene aspects,
- to provide the knowledge on risk-problems,
- to exercise measurement and analysis,
- to provide instructions for protective measures,
- of team-work with occupational physicians, toxicologists, technical management, analysts and employees:
"Safety cannot be an individual, separate discipline. One person cannot be responsible for all and everything, everybody has to feel responsible!"

From Lardeux's contribution the following important questions have to be raised for discussion. What could be done to institute a uniform international, inter-disciplinary system in providing training and information on risk-problems? What could be done to standardize measurements of toxic substaces regarding sampling strategy and evaluation on an international basis? How could international training courses be performed on protective measures?

Fallentin especially concerned himself with the questions of sampling, measuring methods, and accuracy and precision of measurements and methods. He concerned himself particularly with the where, when, how and what of measurement; and with how to analyze and how to evaluate.

Thus he dealt with the very important problems of measuring
methods and, above all, measuring strategy which have to be
coordinated and standardized internationally. This had been
pointed out before, as for example for epidemiological
investigations, an international standardisation will be
essential.

By means of specific examples Bell, too, described these
problems and how standards are established in the USA on the
basis of measurements. He drew the attention to the fact
that the analyst is always confronted with new measuring
methods.

This results in the last question for discussion. Is it
imperative to always follow the latest development in measuring techniques or should a defined measuring method be maintained for longer periods in order to grant the feasibility
of testing and comparing the findings of occupational physicians and hygienists gained internationally?

Finally, I should like to stress the point that the physicist
should be always consulted in all questions regarding
accuracy and precision of measurements when defining the
concentration of toxic substances at workplaces and in the
environment and also when implementing protective measures.
In the discussion of these five questions within the scope of
this session, recommendations may be obtained and agreement
reached for the future.

M. S. BARAM I believe that of the four underlying issues I
cited at the outset of the meeting - educational inadequacy,
professional independence, cost consideration in health risk
decisions of government, and the new era of biological
monitoring, the first two have been dealt with. But neither
the cost consideration or cost-benefit issue, nor biological
monitoring have been fully discussed. Let us now try to
focus our discussion on these two.

With regard to biological monitoring, we have to be candid. It poses possible cost savings and more precise health effects information, but it could also work to the detriment of the worker.

Will industry use biological monitoring for restrictive screening of new employees, phasing out workers who show early stages of illness, for cheaper, polluted workplaces and personal protective devices so that workers will be faced with new stresses to avoid risk in a work environment of increasing risk?

How will government deal with biological monitoring? There is presently great difficulty in the USA and other countries to promulgate standards which will reduce risk.

Will this task be easier or even more complicated if new standards will be set not on the basis of air quality but on the different types of workers – men, women, old, young, big, small, etc.?

Finally what are the implications for workers? There will be the unpleasantries of blood testing and the like. In addition there will be problems arising from the use of workers for experimentations, which nominally will be for their benefit. But on the other hand if, as in the USA, the worker has a legal right or access to his own medical records and testing, the biological monitoring results offer a powerful set of evidence of a self-incriminating nature and can be used by workers filing claims against negligent employers.

P. SILON "Cost-benefit analysis" and "optimum safety" approaches are not acceptable as a basis for prevention. Health detriment cannot be expressed in money terms. In view of the limited resources available for prevention the effi-cacy of the various methods must be closely scrutinized so that more rational use can be made of the resources.

S. EPSTEIN One presentation made repeated references to "spurious safety factors" and "occupational standards 100 or 1000 times more than necessary". This is contrary to the established record which shows small or even negative safety factors for occupational in contrast to environmental standards.

L. LAVE No-one wishes to return to the period of extremely high risk when workers had a short life expectancy. Today the risks to workers are small, almost always smaller than the risks they assume in going to work or in their leisure activities. It is with this range of extremely small risks that it is necessary to weigh costs and risks.

Certainly there have been cases of bad data or analysis by companies and industry. We need to be more careful of the science and economics in order to get data required for more intelligent decisions.

Anyone advocating zero risk or total safety is, to be charitable, someone who has not thought through the consequences of this goal. Zero risk is incompatible with an industrial society. We can have high standards of living and acceptable risks, but not zero risk.

Cost effectiveness can be thought of as a moral issue or as a tool for helping workers attain a desirable compromise between risk and standard of living. The lives lost are statistical ones - the one additional cancer over the 101 predicted - where the individual can never be identified. The Marxian notion that control cost comes from profits is nonsense for the USA. Increased costs must result in higher prices or perhaps the closing of a company or industry. We must carefully weigh the costs and consequences of our actions.

P. B. MEYER Cost-benefit analysis, given the present state
of the art, is only one of a number of factors to be taken
into consideration when decisions are being made in the
safety and health field. Moreover the new law on working
conditions gives employees in the Netherlands an ample say in
decisions relating to safety and health.

D. GOMPERTZ We should consider the two types of error found
in both ambient and biological monitoring. One type comes
from sampling and the other source of error is analytical
error. We know that air sampling data is lognormally distributed and that errors are related to this distribution.
NIOSH has produced elegant guidelines for estimating compliance whilst taking into account this type of sampling
error distribution. In many cases the error of analysis is
much less than the error of sampling. This is also true for
biological monitoring. The main concern here is to take
account of the pharmacokinetics of the material being studied. Frequently we can measure the material with adequate
accuracy and precision but we are measuring it at the wrong
time or in the incorrect body compartment or fluid. When we
define a sampling strategy we must consider the relative
sampling and analysis errors associated with ambient and
biological monitoring and select the method which gives the
most accurate estimate of risk to the individual worker.

A. BERLIN Bell mentioned the use of wipe samples in
connection with benzidine in addition to air sampling.

In view of the insufficiency of air monitoring alone to
assess ambient exposure of workers to some chemicals, how
should we supplement quantitatively air monitoring data?
Should we quantify wipe sampling and determination of the
toxic agents on the skin surface to assess working methods
and protective measures?

Using such an approach, with biological monitoring, we could further maximize the protection of the worker's health.

L. MIKSCHE For protection of the workers' health we do need several approaches. Air monitoring will provide us with information on the possible level of exposure to dangerous agents. Biological monitoring, however, is the only way to gain information on the amount of a substance that a person has incorporated. Clinical examination by a physician will provide information on the health status of the worker. Information on the importance of personal hygiene at the workplace can help workers to prevent additional uptake of chemicals via contamination. All these approached together can help in the task of preventing health risks at the workplace.

P. WEINER Economists concentrate on costs and benefits to society as a whole. If we were indeed at a low level of risk, economists could usefully tell us the cost-effectiveness of any specific method for protection. In judging whether risks are acceptable, we must ask "acceptable to whom"? Economists ignore distributional questions, assuming that
- such questions are political and
- costs are the same no matter whom they are imposed upon.

This failure of economists to address distributional questions has led workers and consumers to regulatory laws as their only means of obtaining equal bargaining power and of imposing costs on industry, which has both the ability and, with these costs, the stimulus to conduct the research necessary to reduce hazards. Without such liability, taking lives may be more cost-effective then saving them.

"Zero risk" is a straw man raised by economists to indicate the need to consider costs. Both the risks and the benefits are largely indeterminate, and latency factors coupled with severe disease ensure the need to take action based on incomplete data. Economists should concentrate their energies on economic solutions to the distributional issues if they would have us abandon regulatory solutions.

L. DE BOER Silon remarked on the unacceptability of cost/benefit analysis in safety and health. This is psychologically understandable. When a safety committee in my company was discussing the high mortality (20 deaths) by accidents and decided to try to bring this down, the technical people insisted upon setting a "target of 10 deaths" for next year. As a doctor I could only accept "to try harder to get as close to zero as possible". The effort may be the same, the result also, but please formulate it better and more acceptably.

The vinyl chloride industry in Europe, immediately after the hazard was known, brought down exposure to reasonable safe levels (before there was legislation).

M. CORN The focus on economics of our field can also be viewed as a measure of our professional success. We are now spending large sums; over 10^9 have been spent by OSHA and NIOSH in the USA since 1971. It is estimated that the private sector has spent $10-30 \times 10^9$ to implement the Act. Those allocating funds seek better justification for expenses in our field versus those to be spent in other fields of health. In the face of these challenges we should seek to develop better measures of our ambient and biological monitoring. How are they to improve health?

One measure I suggested some years ago is the "workers removed from risk". When AM and BM indicate x workers have been removed from risk by lowering their exposures below a suitably adopted standard, we should tally this number. If

the risk was permitted to exist at the former high level of
exposure, disease would ensue. Thus one measure of performance could be "workers removed from toxic chemical exposure
risk" on an annual basis.

Members of the seminar are asked to develop further candi-
dates for measures.

M. S. BARAM Doctor and lawyer have a value system and a
professional responsibility to maximize the interest and the
health of the individual. Corn and Lave represent the recent
economic and engineering system approaches to the problem of
making decisions on health risk prevention, approaches which
focus on a larger "national interest" concern. Epstein, de
Boer and I, come from a humanistic perspective to this issue"
Lave and Corn from a quantitative, technical approach. This
is a major debate in the United States, and we seek to reduce
risk in a time of economic limits. I am sure the same issue
is important in Europe except that it is not openly dealt
with.

R. I. HIGGINS I would like to correct the Chairman's impression, which may be shared by others attending this Seminar,
that biological monitoring of industrial workers is a 'new
technological development'. In fact it preceded personal
breathing zone monitoring, as we now understand it, by four
decades or more. Chloride Group Ltd which currently employs
several thousand lead workers in 35 different countries, has
been using biological monitoring for over half a century as
an integral part of its occupational health service and
environmental control system. The experience we have accumulated over this period has shown that many persons who view
biological monitoring as something new, frequently have much
more trouble with the philosophy and theory than we have had
with the practice. It is a commonplace experience for
successful practice to precede intellectually satisfying

theory and there is no need to labour the analogy. If a procedure has been found to be effective in practice, the sensible person will go ahead and use it - until such time as something better comes along. To qualify as 'better' a proposed alternative must be either more efficient or more effective and, preferably, both.

The twin concepts of efficiency and effectiveness lead me to take up and develop the points made by Berlin and Gompertz concerning the relative usefulness of biological and air monitoring and the random and bias errors associated with sampling and analysis. To do so I start from the point that the purpose of any assessment or monitoring of a toxic agent at the workplace is to help achieve and maintain a satisfactory degree of control of that toxic agent. Now control is a word which falls so easily from the lips of many of us that we rarely pause to consider its meaning. It means "the detection and correction of a deviation from some operating standard". It is immediately clear from this that monitoring is only one of the three essential elements of any CONTROL SYSTEM. It is the DETECTOR element. The other two elements are the corrector or REGULATOR and the OPERATING STANDARD. It is readily apparent that a fundamental requirement for consistency or stability of performance of a control system is that the signal from the detector element which is fed back to actuate the regulator should be as free as possible from confusing and misleading noise, i.e. it should have the smallest practicable statistical variance. Thus when seeking to compare the relative value of biological and ambient monitoring as detector elements in a control system we can define the problem as follows:-
"What is the relative cost of obtaining equally precise (consistent) information from biological and ambient monitoring?"

Straightforward application of standard statistical theory then reduces the problem to a calculation of the relative number of the two measures which is necessary to achieve the same (normalised) variance.

Thus:-

Operating cost of the biological monitoring detector

Operating cost of the ambient monitoring detector

$=$ (normalised variance x cost) for a single biological measure

(normalised   variance x cost) for a single ambient measure

We have applied this criterion to a group of 80 workers engaged   on   the same job in a lead-acid battery factory where we
have found that the geometric standard deviation of the blood
lead   measure   is   1.20 and that of the personal (1 hour) air
lead   measure 2.0.   The costs of each measure are about equal
at approximately £6.   The cost ratio defined above calculates
out therefore at about 0.069.   An alternative way of expressing   the same underlying relationship is to say that it would
require   14 one hour lead in air tests to give information as
precise   as   one blood lead test.   This means that to monitor
this   group   of   workers   by   biological testing (every three
months)   costs   about   £500   each time it is done.   To obtain
equally   precise   information   by   lead in air sampling would
cost   no   less than.£7,200.   The difference in these costs is
very   far   from   trivial.   It   demonstrates that, for these
workers,   biological   monitoring is by far the more efficient
measure   of   the   interaction   between   the   worker   and his
environment from the standpoint of both statistical precision
and cost-effectiveness.

If   we   extend   this   treatment   to embrace the TOTAL CONTROL
SYSTEM   we   note   that   any   money spent unnecessarily on the
detector   element   represents   so much less available for the
all   important   corrector   or   regulator.   The   substantial
difference   in   the   monitoring   costs derived above provides
persuasive   evidence   of   the markedly superior efficiency or
cost-effectiveness   which can be achieved by a control system
based   on   a   biological   monitoring   rather   than an ambient

detector element. But the finding is not unique to this particular group of lead workers. A variance ratio in the region of 0.07 for the biological and ambient measures described above is, in fact a common finding in a well controlled lead works. It is for this simple and compelling reason that the lead industry bases its ambient control systems on biological monitoring and, until such time as the variance of the lead in air measure can be reduced dramatically, will continue to do so.

The major component of the random error variance in the lead in air measure is caused by minute to minute and day to day variation in the true airborne concentrations to which the worker is exposed. In practice, measuring errors in the air sampling instrument and subsequent analytical errors make a very minor contribution to the total variance of the lead in air measure and there is very little to be gained by fussing with them. This finding seems to be found everywhere it is looked for regardless of worker, process, industry or airborne substance. The general experience can be summarised succinctly by saying that the concentration of airborne substances generated by work activity and measured in the personal breathing zone of a worker will generally be lognormally distributed with a GSD in the range of 1.5 - 2.5. This observation sets some illuminating limits on the random error variance or precision which we can expect from a detector element based on SINGLE personal breathing zone measurements. For example, variations ranging from 4 to 1 up to 20 to 1 will commonly be found in an individual's breathing zone measurements even though there has been no REAL change in the activity. We can, of course, reduce the variance and improve the precision of the signal if we combine (integrate) several results. We must be careful that we do not integrate so many results that we suppress the variance below that which truly occurs in the relevant biological compartment of the worker. It turns out that this places an acceptable upper limit on the integration period of about one biological half-life in the relevant body compart-

ment for serial measurements. For simultaneous measurements
made across a group of workers the number which can be safely
combined is most conveniently obtained from an empirical
determination of the variance ratio of the biological and
ambient measures in the manner already explained.

An important but remarkably simple conclusion can be drawn
from all this. If the biological half-life of the airborne
substances is less than a working shift, single personal
breathing zone measurements will normally provide a detector
element for the control system which is as precise as that
based on single biological measurements. The choice will
then be made largely on the basis of cost and convenience.
If the biological half-life exceeds a working shift, single
biological measurements will always have the intrinsic
capability of providing a more precise detector than single
personal breathing zone measurements. Whether this capability is realised in practice will depend largely on the
analytical errors associated with each methodology.

The precision of monitoring the exposure of cadmium workers
is a topic of current interest. Since the biological half-
life is some orders of magnitude greater than a working
shift, biological monitoring clearly has the potential to
give the more precise measure. To decide how precise the
biological measure for cadmium must be for this potential to
be realised we can appeal to the experience gained by monitoring lead exposure in the lead industry. In this case an
analytical precision corresponding to a coefficient of variation of 0.1 (or less) has formed a basis for an effective and
efficient control system when applied to GROUPS of workers.
This provides a sound basis for selecting it as the criterion
to be satisfied by an efficient biological measure for
cadmium. To allow meaningful transfer of experience from one
works to another concerning the adequacy of control and the
health of results achieved in relation to LEVEL of exposure,
bias errors in the analytical measure have also to be taken
into account.

Any attempt to use the current quality of biological measures for cadmium as instruments for dogmatically asserting the health status of an individual, with all that this implies, or for enforcing national Regulations, would at worst be scientifically dishonest and at best be grossly inefficient because of the size of the confidence limits which would necessarily be involved. In the case of cadmium the uncertainties of measurement of the biological parameters are compounded by equally great uncertainties regarding their significance to the worker's health particularly if we try to infer this through an intermediate correlate of physiological effect. The statistical variance in the overall equation becomes so great that it mocks any pretence to cost effective utilisation of resources for the protection of the worker's health, if we attempt to protect it in this way.

It seems that until both the precision of the biological measures and our knowledge of their health importance can be improved we are more or less forced into making the best use we can of cadmium in air measurements as the principal detector element in our ambient control systems. This is the approach which we have adopted in Chloride Group Ltd and for this purpose we have recently developed a "group sampling frame" methodology which is an elaboration of the approach described earlier in the Seminar by Corn.

S. EPSTEIN An emphasis on the alleged high costs of regulation is consistent with the emerging trend to use economic arguments to limit regulation. However, while there is no reasonable objection to considering economic questions, there is substantive objection to the use of inexpert or biased economics.

One presentation ignored the high delayed costs of failure to regulate the lack of full information on hazards to exposed workers; the difficulty in monitoring the costs of failure to regulate; the improved industrial efficiency induced by regulating; the growth of the antipollution industry, and the established track record of industrial exaggeration of the costs of regulation.

Furthermore I am unaware of any data that would substantiate claims of "spurious safety factors" and "occupational standards 100 to 1000 times more than necessary".

J. M. HOCHSTRASSER I would like to clarify some of the points mentioned by Epstein. First, the original cost estimates submitted by industry for control of vinyl chloride monomer were submitted for a "lowest detectable level" not for control to a TWA of 1.0 ppm. Also industry does not presently control at the 1.0 ppm level. We in industry still experience VCM exposures in the 1 - 3 ppm range which when averaged with other exposure data result in an overall worker profile of less than 1.0 ppm.

L. LAVE Corn is correct that public health people are being taken seriously. Previously we could afford moral judgements but now must confront reality.

Weiner mentioned the never-never land of economic theory. Current regulation has not fared well; I am seeking a way of making the regulations work better. Economists think that saving lives is different from compensating survivors.

Epstein asked for examples - benzene, and photochemical oxidants are cases, although the political nature of the process has prevented these from going as far as the agencies would have desired.

J. M. EVANS I have heard a great deal over the past few years of zero risk or zero emission. It sounds good! It is a goal which is admirable, but on a practical engineering basis I do not believe it is possible. Zero risk or zero emission by definition is 100% of the time; this does NOT happen in the practical world.

Secondly such improvements will cost money. What are we willing to pay in terms of inflation and negative productivity.

Thirdly, is nil concentration of substances in the workplace really zero risk? I suggest that the health worker and the physician must tell us what values are zero risk rather than the simple approach of "zero concentration will obviously be zero risk". For the practical engineer this is impossible.

There is a reasonable level to which we must remove contaminants from the workplace. But what is reasonable? Certainly not the lowest detectable concentration. Control technology can help attain a reasonable risk.

I suggest that our economic and social value system is not ready for zero emission. If new developments show that older methods are in error, then the new should be implemented quickly. If the improvement in accuracy is small, look at the cost-effectiveness.

R. L. ZIELHUIS Kliesch is a representative of the German authorities and has criticized biological monitoring on a large number of grounds. The fact that a method has been abused (e.g. in sport) is never a valid ground for rejecting a good method. His views contradict these of other representatives of the Federal German Labour Ministry. Moreover, the DGF intends to publish biological tolerance values for working substances in the MAK list in 1981. Have official views changed in the past few weeks?

A number of participants at this seminar are members of a "captive profession", in that they are the captives of an incorrect and confusing definition of biological monitoring, although a better definition was drawn up by the CEC-WHO-EPA three years ago. The negative comments on biological monitoring are liable to unjustly discredit a method which is of essential importance in the prevention of disease.

G. KLIESCH Both biological monitoring and ambient monitoring have proved their worth in the context of occupational health care. However, one should be aware of their limitations, so as to obviate unnecessary conflicts at the workplace. Thus: no change of viewpoint on the part of the specialists.

The work done by the DFG on biological threshold values is valuable and essential. Whether an official list will be prepared on the basis of this work is a matter to be discussed.

A. J. LEBRUN When discussing cost/benefit one should be sure to use the same terms of reference in the numerator and the denominator. Too many people are saying the workers pay the cost (measuring in health damage), the company or the share-holders reap the benefits (in dollars). That is a dangerous sophism. Carbon tetrachloride under certain conditions is a carcinogenic agent in man. It also is the main raw material for manufacturing refrigerant gases. The benefits of refrigeration in the field of nutrition alone are immeasurable. Food does not spoil anymore. Therefore more of it, of better quality, is available at lower cost to more people. Food can travel long distances and feed starving people. Carbon tetracholoride is also used as a preservative for grain, wheat and other foodstuff stored in silos and therefore increases world reserves. How do you enter those elements in a simple cost/benefit ratio? It is indeed a very complex equation that would mix dollars and human suffering. That is a societal decision in which neither the economical profit (and cost) nor the human benefit (and cost) should be neglected. The question of the ethical behaviour of physicians in management has been brought into discussion twice. We all know about corrupt union leaders, unscrupulous lawyers and politicians, even dishonest scientists. That does not mean that whole professions and all members are discredited. Physicians are not different. Some are unethical; most are honest people, morally and intellectually, and doing a good job.

I am not sure that having the physician operating from an "independent" organization would change anything. Indeed, a rotten apple will still be a rotten apple regardless of the basket. And honest people do not need a "gimmick" to discharge their professional responsibility.

R. E. YODAIKEN Cost-benefit analysis cannot be measured in the way suggested. There is no question that most people in industry are not primarily concerned whether the worker has been informed of existing hazards or not. I would also like to agree with Lebrun on another issue. While Weiner gave an exemplary paper, I take issue with him in respect to a statement in his paper, namely that the physician's "power" was given to him by society. In fact the relationship with the patient is special, embedded in history and long-standing societal mores. If this relationship has deteriorated, the deterioration has been aided and abetted by over enthusiastic and sometimes unscrupulous lawyers. There is no question that some physicians are "bad" but doctors nevertheless as a profession have been active in improving the environment; from the disaster at Minemata, through the vinyl chloride angiosarcoma tragedy both of which were brought to light by physicians.

S. EPSTEIN The issue which requires resolution is whether there is a fundamental conflict of interest built into the relationship between occupational physicians and other health professionals and the industry that employs them. Can such conflicts be resolved by employment of health professionals by joint management-labour health and safety committees?

A. BERLIN As regards the right to positive information and the right to participation, it should be remembered that a Community law has existed in this field since 27 November 1980, when the Council Directive on the protection of workers against hazards caused by exposure to chemical, physical and biological agents at the workplace entered into effect.

When this Directive has been implemented by the Member States, the workers will have a right to obtain information on hazards due to chemical agents; they will have access to the results of ambient and biological measurements and to the results whenever these limits have been exceeded. The workers' representatives at the workplace will have a "right of observation", be in a position to check the application of the limits and the implementation of monitoring systems.

As regards medical confidentiality, how can this be adhered to when there is an obligation to remove a worker from his workplace when over-exposure is established and at the same time an obligation to inform the employer of the reasons for the request to remove the worker? Should results of measurements of biological indicators of exposure be considered as medical data?

P. WEINER Doctors used to withhold information regarding risks of operations or jobs at their discretion, e.g. if the patient was too "stupid" to understand them or if the doctor thought that the information wouldn't change minds. Injured patients had no recourse but to ask courts to order that such information be routinely disclosed. I think most doctors would agree with this.

I do not mean to imply that all physicians are unscrupulous. The participants in this conference are certainly exemplary. But the contract physicians who serve most small plants (and thus most workers) are less likely to know workplace hazards and are more subject to pressure from management. We must recognize that these problems exist. Even in large corporations, there is an ethical question - not necessarily answers - where an admittedly needed and cost-minimized action is recommended but rejected by management. We must all consider answers to these questions in the future, lest the courts decide them for us.

J. LEVY   As a trade unionist I was glad to hear said that - in contrast to what an economist claimed this morning - the workers are concerned not only with pay but also with working conditions, health and safety, a fact pointed out in several contributions.

However, I would like to put a question to Morin: what influence and power does the occupational health inspector have when the occupational physician shows insufficient proof of his independence vis-à-vis his employer in cases when the employer is not willing to inform employees?

B. MORIN   Is it not true that occupational health inspectors have been employed in Germany for 100 years (and not just 7 years)?

G. KLIESCH   This is something I did not deny. In Germany a large body of occupational health inspectors was established well before the adoption of a legal obligation to employ occupational physicians.

B. MORIN   What is the relationship between the occupational health inspector and the occupational physician who does not respect his own independence vis-à-vis his employer?

J. LEVY The occupational health inspector cannot himself impose penalties - he can only inform and persuade the occupational physician and submit an opinion to the factory inspector when the latter requests him to do so.

E. P. RADFORD Monitoring has been discussed on the assumption that results can be compared with some limit in the form of "acceptable" values. There has been no discussion of how these limits will be agreed upon.

The EEC this year issued exposure limits for ionizing radiation based on the International Commission on Radiological Protection recommendations. The ICRP is held out as a model of how scientific data can be evaluated for Regulatory purposes.

It is a bad model. The IRCP is self-appointed responsible only to the International Congress of Radiology, a user of radiation, and operates in such a way that membership is markedly biased toward members of the Government laboratories or agencies with a stake in nuclear development. I believe the standards adopted are not defensible on scientific grounds.

L. LAVE My earlier comment was directed to what scientists attempt to build into standards. The standard setting process generally stops this from occurring in occupational standards.

Epstein said that no one advocated zero risk as a goal and that I had knocked down a straw man. Yet I have heard zero risk advocated during the whole conference. Obviously I didn't knock down the straw man. Zero risk is impossible to obtain and a pernicious goal. It will hurt worker health not help it. But if we cannot rely on zero risk as a goal, we must find methods of trading risks against benefits. Biological monitoring has no role in defining zero risk; it does, in a more intelligent framework, trade risks against benefits.

M. STEINER   In connection with the emission of lead or cadmium dust at the workplace; how are wipe samples collected and do they reveal anything significant?

What would be the significance of the measurements if one dealt with the emission of large particulates which settle on the ground rapidly and may not show in air samples collected in an operative worker's breathing zone?

J. M. HOCHSTRASSER   Wipe test samples are taken in facilities such as showers, clean change rooms and lunch rooms where there is a danger of ingestion or transport of the material from the workplace to the home environment.

Where high dusting operations are encountered, wipe tests are of little significance except where the conditions indicated above are encountered.

The collection method for wipe samples has been documented by OSHA and involves using a wetted personal sampling filter wiped over a specific (sized) area.

L DE BOER   In answer to Dr Berlin on the difficulty of disclosing the information to management if a man has to be taken off work: there is no difficulty, provided the procedure is known both individually and collectively (works council, union), that the possibility exists that based upon the result of biological monitoring, someone may have to be taken off his work (often a legal requirement). The actual value does not need to be disclosed to management.

G. E. BETTINGER The use of biological monitoring in conjunction with ambient air monitoring, as well as a coordinated effort by plant and corporate management has resulted in the reduction of worker exposure to one toxic substance by a factor in excess of 500 fold. This shows that, in practical terms, biological monitoring can result in very positive steps to improve worker safety. Continued monitoring can only result in continued reductions and this is one aspect of biological monitoring that needs increased emphasis. I speak of regular, weekly monitoring such as with urinary metabolite programmes. The biological monitoring that has been focused on, is a problem of much less frequency, such as quarterly or semi-annual sampling. That is more surveillance than monitoring, and could not have led to the level of reduction I spoke about.

A. MUNN One of the more infuriating habits of trade unionists is that they are frequently right for the wrong reasons. Although I disagreed with many points made by Silon, I am in full agreement with his summing up which I commend to you:

"Biological monitoring is acceptable provided that:

-   it complements ambient monitoring
-   it forms an integral part of health and safety
    policy as a whole
-   it takes place under decent conditions"

He further added on the role of the worker: "The worker's practical experience and knowledge of the working environment are an indispensable aid to obtaining good monitoring results" and I hope that every participant appreciates the wisdom of this comment.

When Bunge spoke, he may have given the impression that the European chemical industry would like to have a generic standard for carcinogen regulation. Insofar as I can speak for the industry, I assure you that the reverse is the case. I would like to make some constructive suggestions. Let us have harmonization in Europe, not simply of regulations about monitoring, but about enforcement of these regulations. Let us have less emphasis on "medical examination", and more monitoring, whether ambient or biological. Let the regulators encourage better record-keeping to facilitate epidemiology, and let us know greater recognition in Continental Europe of the important role played by the professional industrial hygienist.

J. T WILSON In view of the inference made from his remarks, I should like to ask Hochstrasser if environmental and biological monitoring records are combined and used in making decisions about environmental conditions?

J. M. HOCHSTRASSER The industrial hygiene and occupational health monitoring records are kept separately. Access to industrial hygiene records is different from access to medical records. However, the close physical proximity of the industrial hygiene manager and occupational physician provides for direct exchange of data.

A. JEAMMAUD With reference to the pertinent point raised by Dr Berlin on medical confidentiality between occupational physician and employer, I would like to point out that a provision was introduced some years ago into the French Labour Code which makes it incumbent on the employer to take into consideration the occupational physician's opinions on

the employee's state of health. If a factory doctor informs
the employer that a certain employee cannot remain at his
present workplace, the doctor is not obliged to provide the
exact health details on which he has based this opinion, so
as to ensure that medical confidentiality is respected. If
no other workplace is available, the employer may dismiss the
employee. The latter has no possibility of having this
dismissal judged as "unfair", as the employer can claim that
he did not have to request details from the physician in
order to determine whether dismissal was called for. Thus
medical confidentiality is first exercised by the physician
vis-à-vis the employer and then by the employer vis-à-vis the
employee. This explains its ambivalence.

The Directive of 27 November 1980 seems very interesting.
However, I wonder whether it will bring about any changes in
French law. I fear that certain governments may once again
take refuge behind the argument based on the principle of
"pre-established harmony", although this approach has been
condemned by the Court of Justice of the Communities. I also
wonder to what extent its strict application in national law
will eliminate existing difficulties stemming from the conflict between the right to information, which has gradually
been recognized, and obligations of medical confidentiality
and professional secrecy.

On a more general level, I would like to point out how difficult it is to draw up appropriate legal formulae and I would
like to warn against thinking that the law can provide a
definite solution to these problems. Indeed any precise
confirmation of a prerogative aimed at benefiting workers
means in effect limiting this prerogative or prerogatives
which may be claimed by others. As regards the right of the
worker to obtain information on the results of examinations
and analyses carried out such an approach might be used to
justify refusing any information (out of respect for privacy)
to other workers equally concerned by the toxic substances
which have affected the worker who has been examined.

STANDARDISATION, GOOD LABORATORY PRACTICE AND QUALITY CONTROL:
EXCHANGE OF INFORMATION AND INTERNATIONAL COOPERATION I

J. BERKY, R. HART AND B. GOUGH (USA)

Summary

*In this paper there are presented some of the Good Laboratory
Practice (GLP) concepts of the Food and Drug Administration
(FDA) and the Environmental Protection Agency (EPA) and there
are suggested some changes or extensions of the GLP in terms
of test system interface, automated information systems,
worker safety, waste disposal and in the area of inspector
training. Whereas the member countries of OECD and the CEC
have provisionally accepted the GLP Principles - at least for
review and comment, there are still opportunities for regulatory interchange which can only enhance economic cooperation.
International standardisation of quality controls applied to
test guidelines and test systems, Principles of Good Laboratory Practices and in the mechanisms of compliance can lead
to removal of restrictions on data acceptance, reductions in
testing - cost and volume - and the acceleration of scientific data and its understanding from the laboratory to the
world market place.*

Introduction

The principles of international Good Laboratory Practices
(GLPs) as considered for "provisional acceptance" by member
countries of the Organisation for Economic Cooperation and
Development (OECD) are awaiting final review and revision
by the Expert Group on GLPs (lead country: USA). Certain
issues evaluated by the Expert Group include the interfacing
of OECD Test Guidelines with the OECD/GLP Principles and
development of "GLP specific protocols". Currently, two of
the United States regulatory agencies, the Food and Drug
Administration (FDA) and Environmental Protection Agency
(EPA), use GLP regulations or standards for all non-clinical
laboratory studies in support of safety investigations on
drugs, food additives, biologics, radiation emitting devices,
and medical devices, as well as a variety of industrial
chemicals falling under the Toxic Substances Control Act. In
the United States, separate regulatory approaches cover
clinical investigations and manufacturing processes, including FDA's regulations on Good Manufacturing Practices.

In the area of toxicity testing and toxicology research, many aspects of laboratory operations fall under the general concept of GLP principles but are currently excluded because of their association with basic research, methods development/validation and toxicokinetics. The OECD definition of Good Laboratory Practice emphasises the organisational and planning processes of laboratory studies, how they are performed, monitored, recorded and reported (1). The stated purpose of the OECD GLP is to promote the validity and quality of test data. Since these are goals that must be common to all scientific studies, the question of whether or not GLPs should be expanded to include every type of test system covered under the proposed Test Guidelines, at least to a modified form for each specific testing protocol, must be decided. In order for such decisions to have any meaning and not interfere with trade, international cooperation and standardisation in quality control, quality assurance and compliance must first be achieved and implemented using the resources and techniques presently available.

Evolution in the Good Laboratory Practice concept

In order to ensure a reduction in restrictive trade barriers between nations and the potential duplication of costly testing procedures, we must immediately standardise methodologies to assure international acceptance of test data, and develop an international reference archive, standardised method of training of GLP inspectors and an international toxicological data management and information service. This service will also, in addition to storing data, evaluate data and project relationships of compounds to one another relative to their toxicological effects. Fragments of all these systems presently exist and should be used to expedite implementation and reduce costs. In concurrence with this, the FDA GLP regulations in the USA do not address the "science" of toxicity testing but are restricted to the process by which studies are organised, coordinated, documented and reported.

This is reasonable, since at most universities and at least some federal and industrial research facilities, the use of internal and external peer review accomplishes the evaluation of the proposed "science". In the USA, the GLP regulations were proposed technical concepts derived by a combination of bench scientists, laboratory managers and regulatory scientists within government and subsequently peer reviewed by the regulated industries, scientific societies and representatives of academia to assure rational execution and data management. They were broad in scope, had applications to many fields within toxicology, were process-orientated and were restricted to safety testing of items submitted for government regulatory review. While affecting the process of science, the GLPs were not initially aimed at standardisation of protocols or test guidelines. Nor did the GLPs propose to impact on worker safety or the problems of waste disposal resulting from the safety evaluations and the efficacy/ functionality testing required of new drugs or of industrial chemicals having both positive economic value and a potential for some level of toxicity during manufacture, purification, distribution or use.

The purpose underlying the development of GLPs in regulatory agencies in the USA was for "upgrading the processing of data". The impetus for its development was the occurrence of specific instances of faulty testing, particularly long-term animal toxicology experimentation. The principal types of testing of concern in the USA to the FDA included:

- Acute Toxicity Studies
* oral, dermal, inhalation
* LD_{50} and LC_{50}s

- Subchronic Toxicity Studies
* oral, dermal, inhalation (90-day)
* neurotoxicity
* teratogenicity

- Mutagenicity and Carcinogenicity Studies
* short term vs. long term
* in vitro vs. in vivo

- Toxicokinetics

- Chronic Studies
* oral, dermal, inhalation (12 months)
* general toxicity
* carcinogenicity (18 - 30 months)
* combined chronic toxicity
and carcinogenicity studies

While the GLP principles span many areas of chemical testing, four areas are of special interest to OECD:

- definition of physicochemical properties;
- studies evaluating chemical fate in the environment;
- ecological investigations evaluating effects on the environment; and,
- evaluation of human health effects: toxicity testing/toxicological studies.

Both the GLPs promulgated in the USA by the FDA (2) and the proposed rules of the EPA on GLP standards in the USA for health effects (3) deal with minimal characterisation of test substances, and both refer to standardisation and/or calibration of equipment used in the generation, measurement and assessment of data, and in the control of environmental conditions affecting test situations.

The OECD Good Laboratory Practice concepts presented at the High Level Meeting of the Chemicals Group (Paris, May 19 - 21, 1980) focused on the three key elements of the GLP concept: (a) test guidelines, (b) principles of Good Laboratory Practices and (c) compliance, and included coverage of:

- organisational matters: test facility, managerial responsibilities, investigators, and an internal review system;
- technical aspects of studies: their performance, test data control, reporting and record keeping; and,
- certain areas dealing with test systems - particularly with respect to long-term animal tests in toxicology.

Since all existing GLPs agree on these broad, general approaches and this very nonspecificity has encouraged international acceptance, it is now an appropriate time to initiate discussion on how implementation might best be achieved and additional areas of collaboration added to the present programme.

Standardisation of innovations in GLPs; quality assurance, compliance

Five aspects inherent in any good laboratory practice which may aid in standardisation and implementation of Good Laboratory Practices and in achieving international acceptance of these principles may be discussed. These include:
(a) development of an international reference library for chemical standardisation, (b) the incorporation of automated research support systems into the overall toxicology laboratory operation - including the quality assurance function, (c) the inclusion of those aspects of laboratory practices which are directly relevant to worker safety and wellbeing within the GLP scope and particularly in toxicity testing, (d) the inclusion of practices dealing with laboratory waste disposal of toxic materials resulting from toxicological experimentation - not just the chemical residues, but feed, bedding, animal waste, contaminated test systems, etc. - and (e) a concept of training in bioresearch monitoring for inspectors and auditors of toxicological testing in areas of both health and ecological effects of industrial chemicals, biologicals, drugs and food additives.

It is at this point that details of standardised methodologies and the OECD Test Guidelines have the potential for
interface with international GLPs. GLP requirements for test
article characterisation lend themselves to standardised mass
spectrometric methods for determination of compound identity,
for HPLC or GC procedures for purity and for those methods
used to ascertain stability of chemicals incorporated into
carriers or mixtures. The utilisation of internationally
accepted methodologies (4) and the OECD Test Guidelines, when
interfaced with international GLP Principles, remains a goal
of prime importance to both toxicologists and the industrial
sector. Previously, unless we knew just how a drug, a
chemical, a food additive had been characterised, we tended
to reassay, i.e. to start the entire toxicity testing procedure over again - in our own laboratory, in each of our
countries. However, a recent meeting of an OECD Expert Group
committee dealing with the interface between GLPs and specific test guidelines concluded that there was no overlap or
conflict, and that GLPs should not in themselves detail
"protocol specific" tests. These decisions are current,
opportune and point toward international GLP acceptance and
implementation. However, for uniformity of record keeping,
development of effective communication and efficient implementation, an international archive linked by computer to
central points in each participating nation should be established with an oversight function being delegated to a committee composed of representatives of interested nations.
Such an archive should contain reference samples of all
compounds tested, copies of all chemical characterisation
data on each compound, reference to the site of experimental
study and summary of the results of such tests and be in
accord with trade secret requirements and needs.

Automated information systems

Information systems developed in the USA within the FDA, and
utilised at its NCTR, include data collection, data storage
and reporting and data retrieval and audit [(5) and (6)].

Starting with a protocol analysis, details of experimental design are defined in terms of animal cage and rack configuration, treatment codes, allocation and sacrifice dates, operator identification, experiment and location identifications, plus those aspects of the experiment plan calling for direct computer input of analytical data. Current systems include a Breeding Information System, Experiment Information System, and a Post Experiment Information System. Together these three systems cover details of breeding colony management, productivity, diagnostic surveillance, environmental monitoring, health observations of the test species, food consumption, weight change, gross and microscopic pathology observations and clinical chemistry on the test system. Sub systems of these sections deal with microbiological quality assurance of test species and chemical surveillance of diet.

We are currently developing computer-assisted systems for diet preparations and overall system tracking, the chemical characterisation of test articles, data summary systems for experiment reporting and quality control. We are attempting to place as much of the data review and auditing by the quality assurance unit (QAU) on-line and, available through query language processors, as is possible. Rather than inundate the QAU with the multitude of data obtainable through automated data recording systems, we are attempting to devise key "exceptions" -reports on, e.g.: missing animals, missing organs, checks on action dates - sacrifice schedules, animal organs processed in pathology vs. those called for in the protocol, results of quality control procedures and so on.

An automated QA information system, with its own system of quality control checks, will allow a more thorough review of studies underway and represents those innovations to the GLP so necessary in these days of increased testing. It should also accelerate development of international data review procedures. Where quality assurance activities can augment laboratory quality controls using professionals with expertise in these areas (7), a very real opportunity exists for achieving international quality assurance standards.

Laboratory worker safety in the GLPs

Another point of interest to member countries of OECD and CEC, but not expressed in any detail in the existing GLPs, is the detailing of safe working practices to protect scientists and science support personnel. In the USA, these are covered in extensive detail with Department of Labor OSHA rules and standards. However, a significant opportunity to incorporate some details of safe carcinogen handling into GLP Principles does present itself. In a recent presentation to the American Society for Quality Control, Carl Morris of the EPA (8) cited an IARC document on laboratory worker safety entitled "A Manual on the Safety of Handling Carcinogens in the Laboratory" with specific reference to GLPs under Section 4 of the U.S. Toxic Substances Control Act (9). At NCTR, as at many large testing and research laboratories in the USA, we have developed specific guidelines for laboratory and facility operations safety with emphasis on the toxicity testing procedures underway in our establishment. These guidelines include both national (OSHA/NIOSH) and specific agency (NCI, NIEHS) concepts, as well as our own ideas resulting from eight years of multidisciplinary toxicology testing and research. As a part of this programme, special safety guidelines are developed for each new chemical/protocol introduced at NCTR and specifics for good safety practices are spelled out for all personnel involved. The approach has been to formulate these guidelines in a format usable for technicians and caretaker personnel, yet containing key data for the scientist investigators, as well. These have been well received and represent the type of guideline which the international community is constantly addressing and the exchange of which could be extremely useful.

Incorporation of a limited, but concise, segment of a safe carcinogen handling procedure into the international GLP could provide a measure of discipline for worker safety, without overextending the basic intent of such principles.

Similarly, in the support of a U.S. National Toxicology Program, we have developed a substantial number of Executive Summaries of potential test chemicals which must eventually be considered for some testing phase in the United States and in member countries to test protocols or experiment plans and, in many cases, provide the first step in assessing the testing rationale, e.g.: the application of specific Test Guidelines - as defined by OECD.

Waste disposal and the GLP concept

The proliferation of national regulations relating to industrial waste disposal is known and appreciated by all. The application of rules and standards to testing and research laboratories engaged in toxicity studies has lagged because of the relatively small amounts of test materials ordinarily used. However, modern toxicology facilities have expanded to include extensive diet preparation and animal holding areas capable of supporting many simultaneous studies in a variety of species. These, _in toto_, can generate tons of disposable materials and animal carcasses as well as toxic chemical and solvent residues requiring regulatory compliance in their disposal. A list of toxic chemicals compiled by EPA (10) may be utilised by the Agency to require specific reporting requirements and use limitations of 1 kg/month by testing laboratories. Such restrictions could well affect testing laboratories where several long-term tests on a given substance could exceed these proposed standards. Again, laboratories in the USA have developed guidelines (11) which not only address the safety of all workers potentially exposed to such substances, but define and recommend methods of disposal of laboratory quantities of carcinogens, radio-nuclides, solvents and contaminated materials generated in the day-to-day functioning of the modern toxicology laboratory. These, in turn have as their basis the regulations imposed by the

United States Environmental Protection Agency, the Occupational Safety and Health Administration and the Nuclear
Regulatory Commission.

If these sections in the international GLPs are to be expanded, with emphasis on monitoring test integrity, they should
be addressed by the appropriate Expert Group of the OECD and
sufficient details be provided on collection, storage, decontamination, transportation and methods of disposal of laboratory toxic waste. In 1981, the NCTR will have available an
advanced design, high temperature pilot-scale incinerator
(2500°C.) to begin a series of studies with the EPA on
destruction of selected industrial chemicals and, hopefully
will be able to contribute to guidelines for such activities.

International training: BioResearch monitoring

A final aspect of GLPs and their implementation which may be
considered in terms of standardisation is that aspect of compliance dealing with training of inspectors. The rationale
derives from a need for coordinating and harmonising the
inspectional approach to toxicological investigations of
products destined for potential world-wide marketing. If we
can agree on the Testing Guidelines and their methods of
selection, and the principles for Good Laboratory Practices
during the application of test systems, then we have a real
opportunity for compliance at international levels. The
standardisation of QC and QA action, the development of a
universally accepted GLP, the acceptance of uniform Test
Guidelines will result in:
- mutual acceptance of data;
- reductions in trade barriers;
- reduction in the accelerating costs of health and ecological effects testing, and
- more effective utilisation of test facilities and
  scientific manpower.

The Expert Group on GLPs recently met in Washington and drafted policies on comparable enforcement programmes for GLPs which may facilitate mutual acceptance of test data. It was recommended that member nations should promulgate enforceable GLPs and compliance efforts must include inspection systems to be effective. A committee of that group further recommended that national inspection systems should include both data audits and GLP compliance inspections.

The development of uniform inspectional procedures for laboratories hinges on the development of training programmes for inspectors or "scientific auditors" which are acceptable to the OECD and CEC member nations. Eventually, systems of accreditation and/or inspection of toxicology laboratories and their certification will be a fact, and their development is a matter for immediate concern. At present, we can best address compliance-inspectional techniques, how inspections can best serve the scientific and industrial community engaged in health and ecological testing and attempt to provide a framework for quality control, research quality assurance of toxicity testing and the conduct of studies under international GLPs.

Compliance actions under GLP standards in the USA have been largely accomplished through the use of inspections conducted by FDA personnel and according to the FDA's Compliance Manual (12). This compliance guidance manual provides inspectional details for: chemical contaminants, (EPA), food additives, biologics, human drugs, animal drugs and for investigational device exemption monitoring. While the compliance concept for U.S. GLP regulations was being developed, the practical problem of inspecting some 200 regulated laboratories had to be met.

The FDA's approach to this challenge was to assign to the FDA/EPA toxicology research centre, NCTR, the mission of developing courses in biological monitoring for the agencies' enforcement units. During the past 5 years, we have conduc-

ted 16 BioResearch Monitoring Courses for FDA and EPA investigators, compliance officers and supervisory consumer protection officers, with a total of over 500 attendees. We
have taken the approach that once the inspectors, usually
graduates in biology, chemistry, microbiology, or related
fields of science, have had some field inspectional experience in foods, drugs, etc. and several years' exposure to
regulatory aspects, they require specialised training in
toxicology studies and in "GLP surveillance" inspections.
The former has been provided by the scientific staff at NCTR
and includes overviews of most toxicology disciplines and
their involvement in GLPs. Equal time is provided for work
sessions on FDA/EPA regulatory aspects and inspectional
techniques, actual case reviews and problem solving. But the
key to inspector training has always been the actual conduct
of an inspection of one of NCTR's ongoing studies, with
direct involvement of the inspectors with study personnel,
study documents and the actual data. Inspectors have been
able to delve into problems of the scientists, assure GLPs
and the adherance to them, and are able to develop their
reporting skills by participation in the exercise.

In line with this concept of international compliance, FDA is
currently developing a proposed "Inspectional Procedures
Manual" for presentation, via the GLP Expert Group, to the
OECD for discussion and review in 1981.

It would be opportune to consider the simultaneous development of an International GLP Compliance Training concept for
review by OECD member groups at the same time. We recommend
for the consideration of the CEC, and the OECD, the
development of a system for international training in
compliance.

References

1. OECD, High Level Meeting, Environment Committee, Principles of Good Laboratory Practice, April 11, 1980.

2. Federal Register 43 (247), DHEW, FDA, Nonclinical Laboratory Studies, Good Laboratory Practice Regulations, 60013-60020, Dec. 22, 1978.

3. Federal Register 44 (145), EPA, Proposed Health Effects Test Standards for Toxic Substances Control Act Test Rules and Proposed Good Laboratory Practice Standards for Health Effects, 44054-44093, July 26, 1979.

4. Quality Assurance Practices for Health Laboratories, ed: S.L. Inhorn, American Public Health Association, Washington D.C., 1978.

5. Konvicka, A.J., et.al., Effect of Good Laboratory Practice (GLP) on Design of Automated Research Supports Systems; Drug Information Journal, 75-78; June, 1977.

6. Taylor, D.W. and C.L. Johnson. Data Systems Support for a Large, Long-Term Carcinogenicity (ED_{01}) Study; Journal of Environmental Pathology and Toxicology, 3:221-230, 1979.

7. Marash, S.A. Organisation and Reporting Chain (GLPs), Clinical Toxicology, 15:613-626, 1979.

8. Morris, C. Quality Assurance Aspects of the Toxic Substances Control Act, American Society for Quality Control, Cincinnati, Ohio, October 21, 1980.

9. U.S. Toxic Substances Control Act (TSCA) (Pub. L. 94-469, 15 U.S.C. 2601, et.seq.)

10. Federal Register 45 (98) EPA, Hazardous Waste Management Systems: Identification and Listing, 33084-33133, May 19, 1980; and 33136-33137 - Proposal to Modify 40 CFR, Part 261, Hazardous Waste Lists.

11. U.S. FDA/EPA National Center for Toxicological Research, Laboratory and Environmental Safety Manual, October 1980.

12. U.S. Food and Drug Administration, Compliance Program Guidance Manual, Chapter 48 - Human Drugs: BioResearch Monitoring, Good Laboratory Practice Program (Nonclinical Laboratories), September 30, 1979.

STANDARDISATION, GOOD LABORATORY PRACTICE AND QUALITY CONTROL:
EXCHANGE OF INFORMATION AND INTERNATIONAL COOPERATION II

S. CRISP AND H. EGAN (UK)

Summary

*Good laboratory practice embraces both standardisation and
quality control. It is applicable to all aspects of laboratory operations and to all types of laboratories. The concept
of GLP is still evolving and this paper reviews current developments in thinking on the subject. There is interest in GLP
at the international level in the Organisation for Economic
Cooperation and Development (OECD) and there has been a significant stimulus from action at Community level. The paper
reviews developments in several countries and discusses problems associated with the exchange of information between
groups and between countries.*

Introduction

In the general sense, good laboratory practice is a system
of laboratory conduct designed to ensure experimental results
which are reliable, reproducible, accurate, free from bias
and differing from the true value to within a known, limited
and acceptable extent. In practice it embraces both standardisation and quality control, the latter being a system
designed to monitor the parameters characteristic of good
laboratory practice and to enable corrective action to be
taken where necessary. Such systems have developed in many
circumstances, in individual laboratories or in those associated through industrial, commercial or simply professional
association both locally or nationally and internationally
over the past century; and, more particularly, the past 20
years. They apply to all aspects of laboratory operations; and
to all types of laboratories.

Both standardisation and quality control are part of Good
Laboratory Practice (GLP), which may therefore be taken as
the main focus of this paper. The concept of GLP is still
evolving. It is appropriate to review current developments
and by so doing to encourage the various views towards an

internationally accepted consensus. The scope of GLP depends on the viewpoint taken. The Royal Institute of Chemistry (now the Royal Society of Chemistry) in Britain, for example, is concerned with the professional aspects of chemistry and its published Code of Practice (1) is concerned with laboratory hazards, safety and legal responsibilities. This is one aspect of the broader concept of GLP as developed by industry and government in organisations such as ECETOC (2) and OECD (3).

Discussion

The OECD definition of GLP relates to the organisational process and the conditions under which laboratory studies are planned, performed, monitored, recorded, and reported. The term embraces all those factors that contribute to sound and valid scientific studies or test procedures and which ensure the quality of test data. Major factors considered include training and experience, facilities and equipment, conditions and handling of test systems, test substances and safety, management and personnel responsibilities, record keeping and retrieval, reporting and quality assurance procedures. At present it has been possible to do little more than to lay down useful guidelines and objectives. Individual codes are required for specific types of laboratories e.g. radiochemistry, physical testing and animal experiments. A more comprehensive approach to GLP is through the detailed specification of testing protocol. This has been criticised by ECETOC as embracing the whole field of standardisation of methods. Although vitally important to GLP, specification of methods tend to make the documentation unmanageably large.

The main purpose of GLP is to ensure the quality and integrity of test data. In order to realise this objective, due regard to current skill is necessary. The scientific fraternity would resist the imposition of an arbitrary system such as one that may result from committee deliberations. Wherever practicable, differences in national laboratory organisation and management practices should be accommodated, otherwise unnecessary work is created and valuable data lost. The text of any code should be unambiguous without restricting scientific initiative, experience, expertise and judgement. Laboratory practices have to allow for the dynamic interplay of science, technology and politics to permit future re-organisation and harmonisation with other groups. GLP should be sufficiently broad to cover all types of testing including physical and chemical properties and health effects.

The current interest in GLP has received a significant stimulus from the requirement in the sixth Amendment to the 1967 EC Directive on classification, packaging and labelling of dangerous substances. The advantages of an accepted GLP code are considerable: test data is acceptable internationally, with the elimination of multiple testing and of non-tariff barriers to trade. The safety aspects are of benefit to laboratory staff and, in the case of the assessment of chemicals, man and his environment is better protected.

OECD is in process of formulating a scheme to assess the toxicity of chemicals in which GLP are to be followed and in 1979 a survey of the position in various countries was conducted. The Federal German Republic included GLP in a draft Bill regulating chemicals (4); the Netherlands had regulations on food and pesticides which incorporated regulations on how to perform tests in line with the OECD principles of GLP and they were preparing a law on non-regulated chemicals; in UK the Health and Safety Executive was preparing a code for the sixth amendment to the EC Directive and the Home Office was revising legislation on the care of experimental animals; and in Switzerland discussions on GLP were taking place between government and industry: Denmark and France, although having no specific codes, favoured an international system. Outside Europe, the USA had GLP backed by the force of law for non-clinical studies administered by FDA (5) and EPA (6) had proposed GLP for testing health effects and were considering GLP for testing pesticides, chemical fate and ecotoxicological effects.

Registration schemes for Test Houses operate in Australia (National Association of Testing Authorities), New Zealand, (the Testing Laboratory Registration Authorities) and the USA (National Voluntary Laboratory Accreditation Program), and were under consideration in Canada. In 1979 the National Physical Laboratory in the UK published proposals for a voluntary scheme of accreditation of Test Houses. (7)

An important element of GLP is the standardisation of methods. This is particularly well illustrated in the field of analytical chemistry, itself widely used in monitoring ambient conditions in the workplace and often used as the best practical substitute for a direct measure of biological quality and so in effect as a means of biological monitoring also.

The standardisation of analytical methods is normally regarded as one of the first objectives when developing good laboratory practice, although this will not always be immediately attainable when methodology is still in the course of development. It may also be difficult to achieve when the more sophisticated of the modern analytical techniques, calling for a high degree of involvement of advanced instrumentation such as mass spectrometry or nuclear magnetic resonance, are concerned. There are two main approaches to standardisation, the collaborative study and the cooperative study; but there is no uniformity of approach to either of these. A collaborative study can be defined as 'an inter-laboratory experiment designed to estimate the characteristics of an analytical method'. In it, a sample or samples, are distributed to all of the participants together with a detailed statement of the experimental procedure to be followed. In a co-operative study the samples are again distributed but the choice of method is left to the individual analyst. One of the fundamental principles of the collaborative study is that the prescribed method should be followed in all circumstances. The study is intended to check the method, not the analyst: indeed, a standard method can be regarded as one that is selected for the ability of different analysts using it to obtain harmonious results which sufficiently represent the value.

There has been a strong interest in the development of internationally acceptable standard methods and many international organisations have developed highly organised systems for the establishment of collaboratively studied methods and the publication of these and considerable headway has been made in the adoption of the format of ISO Guide 18 for the standard presentation of an analytical method. But there are also divergencies and some unintended duplication, and a need to reconcile or harmonise such methods and to direct new efforts towards unifying the approach of international organisations.

In most of the cases where an organisation develops analytical methods on a collaborative basis, there is a well-developed framework for the evaluation of results and for the acceptance of the methods. This is well illustrated by the AOAC, whose Methods Book and manual on "Statistical Techniques for Collaborative Tests" by W.J. Youden and E.H. Steiner (1975) are perhaps the best known examples. These set out considerations relating to the number of participants in a collaborative study, the number of replicate analyses and the statistical treatment of the results obtained. But it is sometimes necessaary to 'settle for less'. The International Agency for Research on Cancer for example is currently producing a manual of selected analytical methods for nitrosamines, vinyl chloride and polynuclear aromatic hydrocarbons: for some of these, no full collaborative analytical studies exist and a start has to be made on the best methods available as judged by more limited criteria. But even where collaborative studies have been done and published, except in some limited areas there is at present no systematic co-ordination between the various bodies and there is no simple means by which others needing new methods can ascertain whether those already available will meet their needs. There are no agreed procedures for the comparison of two (or more) methods, each of which has individually been studied (perhaps internationally) on a collaborative basis. This can be very frustrating, since the members of one group may in these circumstances see no reason why all of the reagents, conditions and apparatus for its established method should be abandoned in favour of that of another group.

In order to test the reliability of an analytical method it is necessary first to identify and agree upon the parameters which characterise the method. In order to test the reliability of an analytical method, three things are necessary. Firstly, the parameters which characterise an analytical method need to be identified and agreed. Secondly, definitions of the parameters selected need to be established and agreed, so that the methods for quantifying each of them can also be agreed and understood. Finally, the values of the various parameters, or the limits between which the values should lie, for the acceptance of a method, or for agreement that two (or more) methods can be regarded as equivalent, need to be established. The parameters concerned are such features as accuracy, precision, repeatability, reproducibility, sensitivity, selectivity, specificity and limit of detection, range of applicability and (perhaps) practicability.

This is where the problem begins, since there are no universally agreed definitions of these parameters and certainly no internationally agreed framework on which to base the acceptance or comparison of methods, whether these are established by a full collaborative professional backing or not. The whole question of the harmonisation of collaborative analytical studies is being considered by the International Union of Pure and Applied Chemistry, (IUPAC). Four analytical parameters have been selected for further consideration: accuracy, limit of detection, sensitivity and precision (reproducibility).   Definitions for each of these, based on some of the existing IUPAC definitions and the Statistical Vocabulary of the International Organisation for Standardisation (ISO) are being considered, as follows:

accuracy: the   closeness   of agreement between the   true value and the mean results obtained   by applying the experimental procedure a very large number of times.

limit of   the   smallest   concentration   (or detection: amount) of substance which can be reported   with a specified degree of uncertainty   by a definite, complete analytical procedure.

sensitivity: the change in measured value resulting   from   a concentration change of one unit.

precision   the   closeness   of agreement between (or repro-   the results obtained by applying the ducibility): experimental procedure several times under   prescribed   conditions   in an interlaboratory collaborative study.

The standardisation of chemical analytical methods spans many decades and embraces a vast body of experience and expertise. By   contrast   the   field of toxicology is in a state of flux. There   is   no general agreement on what tests should be done. Procedures   for LD_{50} are   well   established   but tests to assess   ecotoxic   and   mutagenic   effects   of   chemicals, for example,   are   more   difficult to establish.   Many such tests have   been   proposed but the problem is to select those which give   meaningful results without excessive demands on laboratory resources.

An essential adjunct to any code of Good Laboratory Practice, even   using standard methods, is a system of quality control. Quality   control   begins   with   the   recruitment   and initial training   of   personnel   of suitable intellectual ability and

practical skill. It is also important that expertise within
any laboratory is maintained as staff changes occur. Staff
should be issued with clear written instructions and, as far
as possible, understand the principles of the tests being
done. In the case of some tests, for example, the monitoring
of manufacturing processes, there are statistical procedures
of evaluating quality control. One way of checking quality
of work is by the duplicate testing of sample both within and
between laboratories. Alternatively a laboratory can assess
its methods by use of standard reference methods. In some
countries there are registered Test Houses to assure quality
and ISO have published a guideline on the assessment of such
laboratories. (8) In the proposed UK scheme of accreditation of Test Houses, membership would be open to any laboratory which satisfies a regular assessment procedure. The
scheme is intended initially for engineering testing.
Ideally, GLP backed up by a sound scheme of quality control
would provide reliable data of use to scientists, environmen-
talists, government officials and traders.

Two general problems are associated with the exchange of
information, the volume of data and confidentiality. Thus,
it is estimated that the sixth amendment to the 1967 EC
Directive will generate between 20,000 and 30,000 items of
data within the EC. As far as confidentiality is concerned
two types of information can be distinguished, that which may
not be required to assess toxicity and that which would
damage a company's competitive positon if disclosed. Information is often required by law in connection with exports and
it would be advantageous if international uniformity could be
achieved as to what data are needed. As far as chemicals and
chemical products are concerned, (only) data to ensure the
protection of man and his environment should be required,
based on the minimum necessary. There are problems both
between and within countries in relation to the exchange of
information. Some governments restrict the exchange of
information and concepts of what constitutes commercially
confidential information differs. Others require the dis-

closure of information, claims by industry for confidentiality being denied. Public disclosure of information can lead
to misunderstanding if technical data is subsequently used
selectively (or even deliberately misinterpreted) by the
popular press or pressure groups. The problems of the volume
of data, uniformity of official requirements and confidentiality have to be faced realistically. These matters are
being studied by OECD in its efforts to encourage the exchange of reliable data to facilitate international trade.

The widespread concern about the effect of chemicals on man
in the workplace and the general environment has stimulated
much interest in the testing of the toxic effects of chemicals. This has strong implications for international trade
and cooperation on the harmonisation and use of information
is essential, otherwise a chaotic situation may develop beset
by non-tariff trade barriers. The first requirement is an
internationally agreed set of pre-marketing data for new
chemicals for the assessment of toxicity. This is quite
possible in a group such as the EC and the work already done
by OECD represents an important achievement on a wider international scale.

GLP, internationally accepted, is a key factor in the international exchange of information. Confidence in another
nation's data avoids the delays and expense of multiple testing. OECD have substantially incorporated the ECETOC proposed general principles of GLP, which have thus gained wide
acceptance. Two aspects of GLP should be recognised in this
context: those affecting the scientific integrity of data and
those concerned with personnel matters such as safety. The
organisation of the latter is best dealt with by individual
countries by codes of practice, guidelines or laws developed
by government, industry, the professions and the trade
unions. The scientific quality of data is assured by the use
of standard methods, standard reference materials and the
specification of equipment performance. International
organisations such as ISO and IUPAC play an important part in

formulating standard methods. A greater and more widespread
commitment to such organisations should be encouraged. Publication in the scientific literature contributes to the process of standardisation and much valuable documentation
exists in the form of official guidelines. There is a need
to bring this information together. There is also some duplication of effort in producing methods. For example,
several organisations are developing analytical methods for
substances such as asbestos, lead and vinyl chloride: and
international organisations such as ISO, UIPAC and the
International Agency for Research on Cancer can play a
valuable role in these circumstances.

Conclusions

In conclusion the need for exchange of technical information
and international cooperation is the result of the transition into a post-industrial era, the environmental impact of
technology and the dominance of economics in world politics.
Scientists can respond to this challenge by organising their
resources in order to define high standards of laboratory
practice. There is already much scientific capital on which
to draw and there is the potential to meet new problems more
effectively than in the past.

References

1. Code of Practice for Chemical Laboratories, (1976) Royal
   Institute of Chemistry, London.

2. Good Laboratory Practice, (1979) Monograph No 1, European
   Chemical Industry Ecology and Toxicology Centre,
   Brussels.

3. Draft Good Laboratory Practice 79. 17, 3rd Review, 7th
   November 1979, Organisation for Economic Cooperation and
   Development, Environment Directorate ENV/CHEM/MC/79.5
   Annex III.

4. Entwurf eines Gesetzes zum Schutz vor gefährlichen Stoffen -Chemikaliengesetz, Bundesrats Drucksache 330/79.

5. Federal Register (1978) <u>43</u> 60013 - 60020.

6. Federal Register (1979) <u>41</u> 27362 - 27375.

7. Department of Industry, National Physical Laboratory, (1979) The Accreditation of Test Houses. Proposal for a Voluntary National Scheme. A Consultative Paper.

8. ISO Guide 25 - 1978 (E), Guidelines for Assessing the Technical Competence of Testing Laboratories: International Organisation for Standardisation, Geneva.

EDUCATION OF THE WORKER/MANAGEMENT AND THOSE INVOLVED IN THE
MULTIDISCIPLINARY APPROACH - I

C. FALLING (DENMARK)

Summary

*In Denmark there is a long-standing tradition of compulsory
working environment training. Under the Working Environment
Act there is a requirement that 'necessary' training is provided. This is achieved in a basic training course which is
described in the paper. In addition further training courses
are being planned; among these are courses for people doing
work which can involve special risks for themselves or
others. One such course, concerned with dangerous substances
and materials, is also described.*

Introduction

There are so many different types of working environment
training courses in Community countries that it would not be
possible for me, in a short time, to give a comparative
summary of them all. This paper therefore concentrates on a
detailed description of the Danish training system with
special reference to the training of workers, particularly of
safety representatives.

It is generally true to say, as regards working environment
training courses in the EEC, that employers in Community
countries are obliged by law to ensure that employees receive
the necessary instruction/information required to enable them
to carry out their duties in safety. There are, however,
differing interpretations from country to country as to the
meaning of 'necessary'. In the United Kingdom, for example,
the interpretation is influenced by various factors, one of
them being economic considerations.

One significant feature which distinguishes working environment training courses in the other Community countries from
those in Denmark is that the former are based on the workplace. In the other Community countries, safety representa-

tives have no general training courses such as exist in
Denmark, but it is possible to some extent to have such
training at individual work places. This is so, for example,
in Germany, where enterprises with 10 -20,000 employees have
their own training departments. Another point worth noting
is that in Germany it is often customary to provide instruction on the working environment as a part of vocational
training. Generally speaking, working environment training
courses in Community countries are often provided by the
trade union movement and sometimes by trade organisations.

Denmark differs from the other Community countries in having
a long-standing tradition of compulsory working environment
training. In the EEC countries a safety organisation is
provided in undertakings above a certain size but the powers
and duties of such safety organisations vary from country to
country.

Denmark has allocated a very important role to its safety
organisation, giving it wide-ranging powers and duties, these
duties being a matter of statutory obligation. In order to
ensure that the safety organisation can cope with its
responsibilities we have organised a compulsory training
system which does not have its counterpart anywhere else in
the Community.

Training

The Working Environment Fund is responsible for the training
of the members of the safety organisations, the statutory
compulsory training referred to as Section 9 training (this
being a reference to Section 9 of the Working Environment
Act), which stipulates that the 'necessary' training must be
provided. It has been agreed between both sides of industry
that the 'necessary' training can be provided in a 32-hour
course and they have also decided the content of the course.
Such courses are organised by the Danish Employers'
Confederation, the Danish TUC in its National School and the

Working Environment Fund, either as external evening courses at various centres throughout the country or as internal courses in undertakings and in local and central government offices.

A feature of the Danish training system is that no distinction is made between workplaces traditionally considered dangerous and other workplaces such as offices and shops. The guiding principle is that all members of the safety organisation should have the same basic training for their duties, on the grounds that, in offices for example, new types of working environment problems have come to the fore in recent years. I am thinking here of new equipment such as data display terminals, cash check-outs in supermarkets and many other such developments which have a significant influence on the individual employee's working environment.

In principle, all members of the safety organisation receive the same training but they have, however, been divided into three groups. The main components in the three basic types of training are the same but there are slight variations of emphasis.

Courses have been organised for three main sectors: there is one for the building and construction industry, another for shop and administrative workers and there is also a general course which covers most of manufacturing industry.

As stated above, the Working Environment Fund is the body responsible for Section 9 training. A survey carried out by the Fund shows that there are at present in the Danish work force 130,000 representatives of the safety organisation, which means that, out of a total Danish work force of 2.5 million, 130,000 have taken or will take the compulsory basic training course. It is the duty of the employer to ensure that the members of the safety organisation, safety representatives and supervisors attend such a course and the Labour Inspection Service has to check that they do so. The safety representatives must first complete the compulsory training course before they can be officially recognised as members of the safety organisation. The survey carried out by the Fund showed that about 67,000 people in general manufacturing industry would be taking the general course, about 14,000 would take the building and construction industry course and about 48,000 the course for shop and administrative workers. About two-thirds of the 130,000 have already completed the course and the remainder will do so within the next year.

There will be a steady turnover of safety representatives since they are elected for a period of two years, so, even when the 'training bulge' of 130,000 levels out, there will still be a need for the compulsory training course.

The Section 9 basic training course consists of a number of modules. The modules for the general training course are as follows.

Module One aims to provide instruction in the basic elements of the relevant legislation including its scope and structure and the liabilities, duties and sanctions deriving from it. It should enable participants in the course to identify the duties and responsibilities of the different parties.

Module two deals with the basic elements of health and safety work in the undertakings. The participants learn how safety work is organised, what duties are involved and what facilities are available.

Module three deals with health and safety planning at the workplace, the principles to be applied in examining work-places and work processes with special reference to the prevention of occupational accidents and exposure to toxic substances, and internal and external accident statistics including reporting of vocational accidents and cases of exposure to toxic substances.

Module four is concerned with certain topics: internal transport, the safety group's day-to-day work in its own department, routine inspections, personal protective devices, safety instruction.

Module five aims to provide participants with the knowledge required to deal with problems that can arise in a physico-chemical working environment. This module deals with light-ing and temperature, draughts, dust, smoke, gases/fumes and noise, and includes the showing of a set of slides on work processes illustrating health and environmental problems in an undertaking. These slides provide the basis for discussion and for group tasks in the course of which the participants are asked to consider how the safety group can help solve problems associated with various substances and materials, i.e. they consider ways in which they can contribute to solving actual working problems arising from substances and materials. The instruction does not deal with substances as such but is directed rather at the analysis and solution of problem situations.

(In this module the participants have to answer a number of questions, one of which is concerned solely with substances and materials. The aim of the exercise is to familiarise the participants with the regulations concerning classification, packaging and labelling with particular emphasis on the need to show on the label the substance's coding according to the toxic substances list, the supplier's name and address, its toxicity rating and symbol, details of the hazards and safety directions. In this module it is also impressed on partici-pants that the safety committee can request information from e.g. the supplier, who must supply clear instructions (in Danish) on the use and transport and of the substances in question and any necessary safety measures (respiratory equipment etc.). It is also stressed that it is the supplier's duty to determine whether the substance can be used without giving rise to any toxicity hazard and he must be able to give adequate information on any of its component

elements which might endanger health; also that the employer
is required by Section 21 of the Working Environment Act to
have tests carried out if the situation calls for it. Thus,
in this module the members of the safety organisation are
instructed in the most important basic regulations concerning
the labelling etc. required for substances before they are
admitted to the workplace and they are also informed of their
right to have substances analysed).

Module six of the Section 9 training allows the participants
to correlate the information on the working environment provided in the previous modules and they are also made familiar
with the planning process whereby the safety group can introduce changes within a department.

Special modules seven and eight provide instruction on substances and materials but are concerned with specific
branches of industry to a greater degree than the other
modules. They provide the participants with information on
permissible limits of exposure, how substances can affect
health, how best to provide protection against harmful
substances, and in this module stress is laid on the
principle, enshrined in Danish legislation, that a dangerous
substance must, as far as possible, be replaced by one less
dangerous.

This basic information on the use of and work involving
dangerous substances and chemicals is thus at present given
to 5.2% of the total work force in Denmark, i.e. the 130,000
members of safety organisations in Danish workplaces. We in
Denmark can therefore feel quite sure that persons in such
workplaces engaged on work with dangerous substances and
chemicals can rely on a safety organisation which has had
basic instruction in the problems involved.

I should like to make it clear at this point that my own
personal opinion is that this basic instruction does not go
far enough where dangerous substances and chemicals are

concerned and we in the Working Environment Fund are therefore busy planning courses which provide a more detailed
insight into such problems. However, attendance at these
courses is not compulsory and, in my view, the fact that the
basic Section 9 training courses are compulsory is of prime
importance for labour market training, especially with regard
to the working environment and the safety and health of the
individual worker; I think it would be dangerous to leave too
much to personal initiative and good intentions. Before I
say something about further training courses which we in the
Working Environment Fund are planning, I should like to
mention a new working environment training course which we
have organised in Denmark, a compulsory course which deals
with a specific type of product.

Section 41 of the Working Environment Act empowers the
Minister of Labour to lay down rules providing that work
which may involve substantial risks of accident or disease
may be carried out only by persons who have been specially
trained, have passed a test or are above a certain age. The
Minister of Labour used these powers in Labour Inspection
Service Notification No 486 of 5 October 1978 relating to
polyurethane and epoxy-products and like substances and
materials with similar properties hazardous to health.

In Section 7 (1) of the Notification it is laid down that the
employer must ensure that work with such substances is
carried out only by persons who have followed a special
course of training designed by labour market organisations
and approved by the Labour Inspection Service. This is not
the first time that the Minister of Labour has used his
powers to prescribe a special course of training for persons
doing work which can involve special risks for themselves or
others - such a requirement was previously imposed in the
case of cranemen and drivers of fork-lift trucks - but it is
the first time the Minister has prescribed a special course
of training for persons working with dangerous substances and
materials. Although work with polyurethane and epoxy-

products does involve a special hazard, it is on the face
of it surprising that a training course was required only
for a very limited group of substances which is far from
covering all the dangerous substances and materials used in
industry today. However, the uses to which polyurethane and
epoxy-products are put are in many ways different from those
of other products since, although the substances, or some of
them, have been known and used for many years, there has been
a considerable increase in their production and they have
been more extensively used in a large number of trades where
they have taken the place of traditional materials and
methods.   Since the working processes in which the products
are used are often of a simple nature and the work is often
done at mobile workplaces by persons with no specific training in the relevant methods or products, it is necessary to
provide safety training in the use of those products.

During drafting work in 1978, agreement was reached on the
content of the Notification including Section 7 (1) which
deals with the type of training to be provided. But there
was naturally a number of problems concerning the form which
the training course should take, its content and its
organisation.

In addition there were some questions about the teaching
methods to be employed and it was also necessary to ensure
that a more or less uniform type of course could be made
available throughout Denmark.

It took a long time to deal with these questions and it was
not until April 1980 that the course could be started in
Denmark's Special Vocational Schools.

The fact that the courses are held in these schools means
that all those who work with the substances in question have
reasonable training opportunities, that the instructors hold
satisfactory recognised qualifications, that the necessary
facilities are provided and that the course, which lasts two

days, is recognised as a labour market training course and consequently no tuition fees are payable and any loss of wages is refunded.

When the course was first started the schools received about 7,000 applications. In August 1980 about 2,000 had completed the course and it is hoped that by the end of the year the waiting lists will have been cleared. It is evident that the products concerned have many more uses and involve many more people than was first supposed. It is therefore not possible at present to assess how great the demand for the courses really is. A cautious estimate is that approximately 15,000 persons work with polyurethane and epoxy-products and therefore need to attend training courses. It is not possible either to estimate what the demand for the course will be from workers newly allocated to work with these substances since this will depend both on the future development in their use and the degree of job rotation.

In the longer term it is intended to incorporate the training course in the relevant basic training for different trades and in specialist or further training courses but also to keep it as a special separate course.

Briefly, the course consists of the following: an introduction dealing with the background to the Notification on the products, the contents of the Notification and its scope. One section will familiarise participants with the use and composition of the products, classification, labelling, warning signs, instructions for use, inspection measurements and health hazards. Another section is devoted to personal protection and deals also with personal hygiene, facilities for personal hygiene, workplace design and isolation of the working area. The course also provides information on procedures in the event of accident and injury, product handling including storage, air pollution etc. Instruction is also given in work processes both in manufacturing industry and in the building and construction industry. A comprehensive manual has been prepared for the course. The two types of compulsory training I have described are intended for the safety organisation - i.e. for the employees' safety representative and for the supervisor in the safety group - and for the workers. In addition there has recently been established a compulsory training course intended solely for employers which is usually referred to as AMAL. It is a 20-hour course which deals with the position of the employer vis-a-vis the working environment. A total of about 50,000 employers are to take this compulsory training course which is concerned mainly with statutory responsibilities and obligations and to a lesser extent with specific problems of the working environment such as those associated with substances and materials.

Since it is recognised that the compulsory training courses do not give those working with dangerous substances and chemicals adequate specialist knowledge and since these substances and chemicals are being used more and more extensively in Danish industry the Working Environment Fund is, as already mentioned, preparing a course dealing specifically with this topic.

We are at present trying out a course which aims to give participants a general knowledge of the physico-chemical factors encountered in the working environment. It is designed to answer the needs of the participants and to enable them to deal with situations which arise in connection with their work. The course provides an introduction to the subject, involves group activities and practical exercises and also includes visits to workplaces.

Participants are given detailed instruction in the problems of a physico-chemical working environment and are shown how to take readings for the purposes of vocational hygiene and how to use measuring apparatus etc. There are also visits to workplaces where the participants are able to make their own measurements of various factors affecting the working

environment after which they prepare a report based on those
measurements. Finally, there is a discussion of the measurements and of the conclusion which may be drawn from them.
Since the course is still only at an experimental stage it is
not possible to say how great the demand for such a course
would be. Work is at present being done on another course
dealing solely with chemical factors in the working environment but its content has not yet been decided in detail.

We know that there is among workers a feeling of great uncertainty about work involving the use of chemical substances
and materials, a feeling which is not reduced but rather
intensified as new reports appear on the effects of materials
used in work processes. The interest shown in research into
the use of dangerous substances and materials is very great,
as is the need for such research. In Denmark, research in
this area is encouraged but it has to be admitted that the
resources we can call on for such research are quite inadequate. In the brief period during which resources have been
made available for research the total amount allocated has
been about Dkr 12 million, a third of which was spent on
research into the effect on workers of chemical substances
used in industry. Before funds were made available we made
sure that the results of this research will be seen in such
things as practical advice and instructions which can be
incorporated in the teaching materials for the optional and
compulsory training course. The compulsory training of the
members of the safety organisation is at present being
reviewed and this presents us with an opportunity to ensure
that information given to participants in the courses is up-
to-date.

However, this is not the only use to which the research
results can be put. It is the duty of the Working Environment Fund to disseminate information on matters concerning
the working environment. One method by which this is done is
the publication of brochures, which in recent years have been
devoted to a large extent to problems associated with

dangerous substances. The results of the research could be included in such material and would thus quickly reach a wide circle of users. In Denmark as in the other Community countries information on and training in the use of chemical substances is of interest not only to public bodies. Trade unions and trade organisations in different branches of industry provide special courses and chemical undertakings, for example, organise training for their staff when any special knowledge is required.

I have concentrated on the Danish training system because it is uniform and compulsory and because it ensures that all safety representatives have some knowledge of the problems of the working environment. Whether that knowledge, as regards the use of dangerous substances and materials, is adequate in all workplaces in Denmark is very much open to question. Yet in Denmark as in the other countries of the EEC there is a statutory duty on employers to ensure that employees are adequately instructed and informed about safety. The fact that an employer's safety representatives have attended a Section 9 training course does not mean that he has fulfilled his obligation in the matter. He must himself provide any further instruction that may be necessary.

Other Practices

It is relevant to note here that German legislation requires an employer not merely to give instructions to workers engaged in work with dangerous substances but to ensure personally that they are given training. Such training must be provided regularly and not less than once a year.

In Germany a considerable effort is made to provide guidance on the use of dangerous substances in industry. Thus the Bundesanstalt fur Arbeits-schutz und Unfallsforschung in Dortmund provides comprehensive working environment instruction manuals for vocational training purpose and the institution also, as part of the further training facilities in undertakings, organises special courses in the use of dangerous substances. It also helps with internal training in the undertakings which aims to ensure that safety representatives can see to it that all necessary precautions are observed during work with dangerous substances.

It is not possible here to describe the facilities for working environment and training provided in all the countries of the EEC, but a comprehensive report entitled 'Training and the organisation of work', has been produced by the 'European foundation for the improvement of living and working conditions' in Dublin.

EDUCATION OF THE WORKER/MANAGEMENT AND THOSE INVOLVED IN THE
MULTIDISCIPLINARY APPROACH - II

N. NELSON (USA)

Summary

*Industry serves two chief objectives: one is that it produces
a product that is useful to society and the other that it
provides a satisfying productive activity for the worker.
The production process has as its main objectives maximum
quality and quantity of product consistent with an optimum
quality of life for the worker. This paper discusses how the
above sets of objectives may be approached by way of a programme of education and training. It examines the varying
educational procedures required and analyses the relative
roles of groups by way of a matrix of function against
performer.*

Introduction

The objective of industry and technology is a product, not
the process. However, central to the produce is the worker
who is the key-figure in the process and the product. On the
other hand, the process as it involves the worker can be
regarded as an important social objective in itself. Thus,
we can see that industry as it has evolved in society serves
two chief objectives. One is to produce a product that is
useful to society, and the other is to provide a satisfying
productive activity for the worker.

The evolution from the days when the hunter and gatherer
supplied his own and his family's needs within a relatively
short distance of his particular location, often on his day
of need, to the present extremely elaborate and complicated
social endeavour has been a long path. At the present time,
the social machinery erected around the industrial process
is extremely involved and often fragile and vulnerable to
misuse and misdirection; it involves a large cast. Figure 1,
attempts to illustrate, in very much simplified form, some of
the players (but only a fraction) in this extremely complicated set of endeavours.

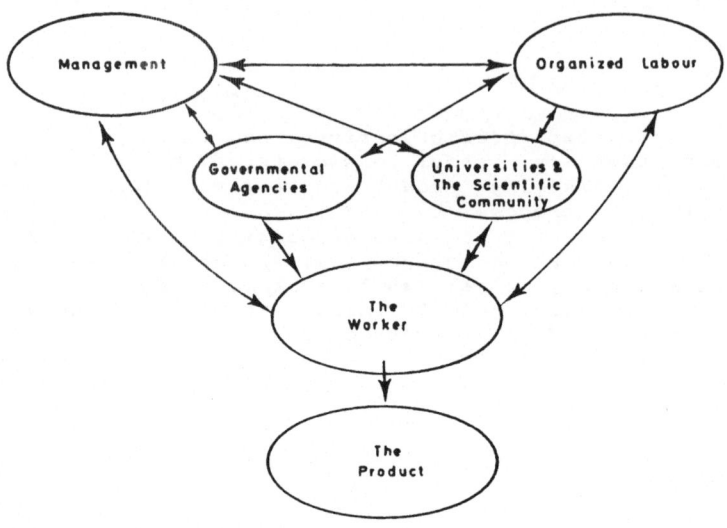

Figure 1.   The production process

The worker is deliberately placed in the central role as one
who carries out the process, which leads to the other vital
component, the product.   Management and labour are colla-
borators in planning and overseeing the production process,
and in safeguarding the interests of the worker. Amongst the
many additional players in this social activity, there are
only two groups, illustrated here, governmental agencies and
the community of science and universities. There are obviously many others involved in these activities, but for the
purposes of this presentation, these are concentrated on.

The salient objectives in the production process are the
maximum quality and quantity of a product consistent with the
optimum worker quality of life. These two objectives call
for good health, fair pay, a fair product price, the need
maximise worker interest and to minimise tedium. Said
another way the work should include more than assurance of

good health and fair pay; it should also recognise that pride
of person as well as intellectual and emotional satisfaction
are legitimate objectives. The minimisation of purely repetitive activities and the satisfaction of participating in
the crafting of quality products should be part of these
objectives.

Let us now concentrate on the health of the worker as the
component of the process of production of first interest to
those gathered here. Clearly, the two major partners,
management and labour, have self-interest in assuring good
health to the worker. From the management standpoint it has
been demonstrated again and again that the most profitable
business is the one that does not produce its product at the
expense of the worker's health. On the other hand, labour
itself, as the collective voice of the worker, has, as its
two major objectives, assurance of the good health of the
worker and of a fair return for the day's work.

In the centre is the worker himself and his legitimate desire
to maintain his good health and that of his family. In addition, he has a right to expect a contribution to a preventive
approach to health maintenance, to aid in anticipating and
avoiding incipient disease or injury. The role of the
industrial medical department has never been wholly clear on
this, but it is generally agreed that a cooperative role in
preventive medicine with the other parts of the health
delivery enterprise can legitimately be expected from an
occupational medicine programme.

Table 1 lists potential participants in optimising good
health.

Table 1. The participants in optimising good health

Worker	Engineer
Foreman	Governmental Administrator
Manager	Inspector
Union Official	Lawyer
Physician	Epidemiologist
Nurse	Analytical Chemist
Industrial Hygienist	Economist
Safety Expert	Computer Specialist
Industrial Toxicologist	Basic Scientist

The first four in the left-hand column, the worker, the foreman, the manager, and the union official, are all related to the production process itself as well as to maintenance of good health. The others play a variety of roles. The classical four major professional groups include the occupational physician, the occupational nurse, the occupational hygienist, and the safety expert. The others play their specialised roles from time-to-time depending on need. Clearly, with a cast of participants of such size and diversity, something more than a casual approach to mutual understanding and education is required. This means that some degree of planned instruction is required. Although an individual commitment is an indispensable ingredient, a mutual understanding of responsibilities is required to assure an effective team approach to the provision of good health services. This will normally involve a composite of formal training aimed at an understanding of each other's tasks and needs. Associated with such training should be a continuing examination of the adequacy of the current programme and a search for means of improvement. Regardless of the specifics of the programme aimed at these objectives, a most important ingredient is good sense and an understanding of the interplay of mutual responsibilities.

The components of training are divided into two categories; those having to do with technical understanding of occupa-

ational disease and injury on the one hand, and, on the
other, a mutual grasp of the responsibilities and rights of
the various constituencies who are involved in the health of
the worker.

Under the technical aspects, we are first concerned with
occupational disease and injury, the sources of the disease,
the types and gravity, the means for diagnosis and treatment
and for determining prognosis; traumatic injury is also a
highly technical field. Although occupational disease is
primarily the speciality of the physician, all the persons
involved should have some understanding of occupational disease, its sources, its treatment, and its prognosis, including elements of toxicology and the mode of action of chemical
and physical agents. This understanding should include the
worker at a level appropriate to his interests and to his
level of technical education. Similarly, although the detection and measurement of environmental agents is the province
of the industrial hygienist and analytical chemist, nevertheless, each member of the team needs to have a comprehension
of what the procedures are, their limitations, and their
capabilities. Control generally becomes the responsibility
of the engineering profession, but here also there is a
legitimate need for management, labour officials, and the
worker to have a grasp of some of the terminology and some of
the principles (e.g., containment, substitution) which govern
the control of occupational hazards.

Equally important with the technical aspects of occupational
disease and injury is the need to grasp and understand the
responsibilities and rights of the various constituencies
involved in this interlocking and complex set of activities.
Some of the major players are: management, labour organisations, the worker, governmental agencies. Obviously, there
are others, but it is imperative for these four components to
have a grasp of how interrelationships are established and
what the mutual responsibilities and rights are. Clearly,
the level of detail will vary depending on the particular

responsibilities of these collaborating units. Thus, both management and labour need to have within their organisations persons familiar in minute detail with the legal statutes governing the operation of a plant. The workers should have as a minimum a general comprehension of this. All should have a clear understanding of the ethical issues involved. Thus, we have a mixture of those whose knowledge must be of a detailed professional nature along with partners whose knowledge need not be so detailed, but who should have an understanding of the guiding principles and issues. Accordingly, all participants need to have some training and understanding of each of these components ranging from detailed to general.

The varying participation of professionals and non-professionals is illustrated in Table 2.

Table 2. Who does what

Performer

Function

Function											
Normal Health Care & Surveillance	A	P	-	A	A	-	-	A	A	P	N
Normal Environmental Surveillance	A	P	A	A	A	P	P	P	A	A	N
Special Medical or Toxicological Assistance	P	A	-	A	A	-	-	A	P	A	P
Require Reporting	P	P	A	A	A	P	P	P	-	-	-
Legal Issues	P	A		P	A	P	P	P	A	A	A
Education: Worker	A	P	A	A	P	P	P	P	A	A	A
Inspector	A	A	A	A	A	P	P	P	A	A	P
Professionals	-	-	-	-	-	-	-	-	P	A	P

A = Assists or Advises
P = Primary or Major Performer
N = As Needed & Available
* = Where Applicable

The major objective of the Table is simply to illustrate that each performer is likely to have some role in most of the functions which health maintenance in industry requires. Indeed, it will be noted that it is suggested that there is a place for each of the performers in education of the worker. The Table implies that in this multidisciplinary area there must be a high degree of crossover instruction and communication.

Just as a degree of detail varies depending on the responsibilities of the various participants, so the educational procedures used will vary depending on whether detailed professional understanding is required or whether only a general grasp of the principles and goals is the objective sought. Thus, in Table 3,

Table 3. Kinds of training

Formal Degree Programmes (or components thereof)
      Physicians, undergraduate, postgraduate, residency Nurses
      Industrial Hygienists
      Toxicologists
      Epidemiologists
      Safety Experts
      Plant and Process Managers
      Control Engineers
      Occupational Health Administrators (e.g., MPH)
Certificate Training
      Inspectors
      Aids to Nurses, Industrial Hygienists, Safety Experts
      Laboratory Technicians
Short Courses
      Workers and all participants
Conferences and Workshops
      All participants
On-the-Job
      All participants

one can understand that formal degree programmes at a university level of training will be required for the physician,
for nurses, for industrial hygienists, for toxicologists, for
epidemiologists, for safety experts, for plant process
managers, for control engineers, for occupational health
administrators, and for lawyers. A less intensive course of
formal training akin to what we in our country would describe
as certificate training may be adequate for most inspectors,
for aids to nurses, to industrial hygienists, to safety
experts, and for laboratory technicians. Short courses,
conferences, workshops, and seminars are effective means of
training in all of these activities and, indeed, they are the
procedures of choice for the joint training of multidisciplinary groups. Whether such training is formalised in short
courses or takes form in conferences and workshops, there
should be always adequate opportunity for free participation
in discussion and questions. On-the-job training is the
ultimate polish for each participant in these endeavours.
Clearly, those once trained in highly specific technical
topics will need refresher courses from time to time, and updating in their understanding of the technical issues as
science and knowledge progress. I would like to elaborate
slightly in respect to the training of occupational
physicians. For those physicians going into the full-time
practice of occupational medicine, there are at this time,
for all practical purposes, three types of training. One is
the formal residency programme normally taking a minimum of
three years; this is unquestionably the most desirable
approach. However, even though the production of trained
occupational physicians by this means has increased
substantially and will increase still more, it is quite
certain that it will never meet the full requirements of
those entering the full-time practice of occupational
medicine. Presently, such programmes are producing some 40
graduates per year. Even if this were to double, a most
optimistic expectation, this is probably less than one-
quarter of the annual entry into the full-time practice of
occupational medicine; most physicians enter by moving
laterally from another speciality or from general practice.

Such physicians have two options; one, to learn on the job, the other, to do as best they can with the limited availability of short course training presently available in universities in the United States. It would seem to me that this is a very logical place for a systematic development of a series of modules aimed at accelerating the grasp of the purely technical aspects of occupational medicine so that these individuals will be able to become effective more rapidly and to master fields not likely to be effectively learned on the job.

Although the highly professional training will remain the responsibility of the universities to a major extent, other kinds of training will require the participation of management, of governmental agencies, of the labour unions, and other components of the industrial enterprise as well. Although optimists always hope for an atmosphere of confidence in the good intentions of others, there is no substitute for a free and open exchange of ideas as a basis for solid, mutual confidence and respect. In addition, a grasp of some of the technical aspects of worker health programmes as well as the specifics of legal rights and responsibilities is a very wholesome base on which to establish a sense of mutual understanding and reassurance as to the competence and good faith of the other participants in worker health activities. Thus, a deliberate programme of training, including conferences and workshops with open discussions, is imperative if the worker health effort is to operate in a smooth and effective manner with a minimum of mutual suspicion.

DISCUSSION ON STANDARDIZATION, GOOD LABORATORY PRACTICE,
QUALITY CONTROL AND EDUCATION

L. DE BOER The papers of the previous sessions dealt mainly
with the basic philosophies, techniques and procedures of
ambient and biological monitoring (with many examples related
to specific compounds) and with the role of the various
disciplines in it. From that it became clear, that whatever
the reservations and ethical restrictions, Biological Monitoring and Health Surveillance (indeed two different things)
play and will continue to play an important role in the care
of the health of the workers (provided it is incorporated in
a total programme of preventive occupational health care).
For even if the situation is, or seems to be, safe, constant
vigilance is needed because failures can always occur and
production processes will no doubt change continuously.

It also became clear that there is no sense in establishing
standards if, at the same time, requirements are not established in regard to techniques, protocols and strategies of
monitoring these.   But even if this is all agreed and fixed
there is still an important key issue: the quality of the
analytical tests and the proper education of all involved.

The session dealing with Good Laboratory Practice was very
essential.   In his paper Hart mentioned the OECD activities
in this field, the purpose of which is to promote the validity and quality of test data. He described the developments
in this field in the USA, the purpose of which was originally
"upgrading the processing of data", using the resources and
techniques presently available.   The 3 key elements of the
OECD proposals are: test guidelines, principles of GLP and
compliance. Elements like setting up of an international
reference library, fixing requirements in regard to safe
working practices in laboratories and the handling of laboratory waste disposal (which can become quite a problem) as
well as the development of inspectional procedures for
laboratories were discussed in his paper. Interaction with

occupational health is necessary. Crisp, in his paper referred also to the EEC directive and the OECD effort and discussed in a more general way the problem of Good Laboratory Practices. Collaborative studies as well as cooperative studies are made, in which respect the method and the analyst are checked, leading to standardised methods, giving harmonious reproducible results. Of course he had to point to difficulties, not only technically but also principal ones, like the field of application and the decision on parameters to be considered in regard to acceptance of a method as a universal method (accuracy, limit of detection, sensitivity, precision, etc.). Anyhow the OECD guidelines do not aim at completely uniform test protocols. Further international efforts in this field are certainly needed, preferably led by well known international organisations like ISO, IUPAC, IARC, etc.

Another key issue of this session (also touched in previous sessions) is the proper education of all involved in safe working conditions and practices. This means not only proper training and qualification of the members of the various experts (industrial hygienist, occupational physician, safety officer, industrial nurse, chemical engineer etc.) but also, as outlined in Nelson's paper, a proper understanding by all of them of the work of the others. In other words there should be a good sense and an understanding of the interplay of mutual responsibilities. They should have a comprehension of each others' procedures, capabilities, limitations, ethical aspects etc. This needs special attention in the specific training of these professionals as well as in the training of those who need a basic understanding in this field, which in fact is everybody working in the relevant industry. The paper of Falling dealt with such a mass-educational effort in Denmark, which is unique because of its scale and because it is uniform and compulsory. All representatives from industry dealing with safety (usually serving for two years as such) have to attend this course, in agreement run by employers and employees. 130,000 persons are involved

every two years. A training course especially for foreign
labour is being planned. In addition special courses are
arranged dealing with the hazards of specific compounds,
compulsory for all those handling these compounds (like
polyurethanes, epoxides), which covers another 15,000
persons.

In addition a compulsory training course is organised for
employers, mainly dealing with statutory responsibilities and
obligations. Altogether these two papers confirmed the
philosophy from the other sessions: safety cannot be an
individual separate responsibility. Everybody should feel
responsible and should have the necessary basic knowledge
leading also to mutual confidence.

Berlin, trying to get the discussion on the track,
stressed that our object should be good monitoring practice.
Biological monitoring, if done, must be of high quality and
must lead to the same or at least easily comparable results,
otherwise it loses its meaning and the confidence of those
involved.

For regulatory reasons and for use in epidemiology there must
be harmonisation and a certain amount of standardisation.
But as anyhow within industry some BM has to be done, good
practice should not limit its application. In the general
discussion most agreed to the necessity to have standardisation wherever possible and practicable. Some felt however
that it was sufficient to check the quality of the work, not
the method: if the quality of the work is good any method
will do. Reference methods may be needed, not standard
methods. It was stressed that standardisation should not
only apply to the analytical methods but also to the sampling
techniques and procedures. There was less general agreement
in regard to international reference laboratories and inspection systems, though there will no doubt be some on a national basis. Safety of laboratory workers should also be taken
into consideration, preferably incorporated in a proper
occupational health programme.

On education several delegates reported about national or
industry activities in this field. All agreed to the high
importance of proper education and information of all
involved in safety and health, workers as well as managements. All disciplines can and should play a role in this
training, especially also industrial nurses. Instruction
and training in teamwork is essential in this field. For the
training of workers in the small scattered industries in
Denmark a mobile unit is used. It was stressed that proper
education has sucess only when it is in the "language" and
within the possibilities of understanding of the trainees
(e.g. the workers). This applies especially to foreign
workers which need special courses.

In regard to the training of the professionals in the team it
was concluded that the required qualifications depend on the
type of monitoring and thus of the roles of the various
disciplines in it based upon that profile. Anyhow it was
clear that much more has to be done in regard to proper
education of management as well as workers and in regard to
more and better qualified professionals (like occupational
doctors, nurses, hygienists.) Proper education of journalists in this field was also considered important to guarantee better information of public and thus of the workers.

Training facilities for the various professionals of which
there is still a shortage (occupational doctors, industrial
nurses, hygienists) should be promoted, perhaps after proper
reassessment of their respective roles. But whatever their
specific aims, in this training emphasis must also be laid
upon the principles and practice of teamwork, based upon good
understanding of each others capabilities, limitations,
ethical aspects etc.

In regard to the required qualifications of the members of
the team dealing with monitoring, it was concluded that this
depended on the type of monitoring programme and thus the
required roles of the various disciplines, for which thus a
profile could be made.

Apart from this specialistic training of the professionals, everybody working in relevant industries should receive basic education and certainly the workers delegates in the field of safety. Education is equally important for managers. In fact apart from the special courses safety and health should be an item on all kinds of courses.

The training should be adapted to the possibilities of under-standing of the trainees and this applies especially to foreign workers for which special courses should be arranged in their own language.

Altogether the papers as well as the discussion confirmed the philosophy from the other sessions. Safety cannot be a separate individual responsibility of the professionals. Everybody should feel responsible and should have the necessary basic knowledge, which will also lead to a better mutual understanding.

J. M. EVANS One of the large areas of concern of this meeting has been biological monitoring (BM) vs ambient monitoring (AM) and BM + AM. It has been suggested that BM or AM or BM + AM may be used to aid in the development of safe-health workplaces. It occurs to me that, at least in the USA, BM will not be accepted by all workers. I have run into this too often. It also seems to me that without full cooperation by all workers in the workplace, it is difficult, if not impossible, to define what the workplace contains. AM will do this!

While AM does give variable results (due not necessarily to the sampling technique or analytical technique itself), BM, will give far more variable results. BM, it seems, is most useful for monitoring the individual. These data in the aggregate may be useful in determining that regulatory levels in the workplace are in fact satisfactory or that something has been left out in the industrial hygiene programme.

In short I feel that <u>AM</u> must be used as the main or primary means of monitoring in the workplace; BM to monitor the worker himself but not to be <u>substituted</u> in <u>any way for AM</u>.

The second thing we heard was zero risk/zero emission. As an engineer I feel that zero emission is impossible. However, from my limited experience in occupational health, I am not certain that zero risk = zero emission, except perhaps in the field of radiation.

Thirdly: may I suggest that the seminar recommend that the regulatory agencies in the several nations represented here extend their efforts from regulation/inspection/enforcement to education? Education might be specific to the individual workplace and might be required where violations are found. I suggest that this could be far more effective in reducing workplace health hazards than monetary fines alone. Education would include management/bio-management/workers/worker representatives, etc.

Lastly: may I second the recommendation made from the floor that efforts be made to standardize sampling. If the sample is not taken correctly, nothing done down-stream will help.

<u>D. GOMPERTZ</u> I would like to challenge the concept of standardized methods for use in biological monitoring as proposed by two speakers earlier. I will do this by giving some examples of possible alternative approaches to analytical problems. The first example is the measurement of albumin; should this be by immunological or by dye-binding methods? Methylene bisorthochloroaniline (MOCA) is measured in urine by both gas chromatography and by high performance liquid chromatography (hplc). With the gas chromatographic approach, should one use an electron capture detector or a gas chromatography mass spectrometry system with single ion monitoring?

If one uses hplc, is an ultra violet or an electrometric method better? In the case of metals, say lead or cadmium, what choices should be made between atomic absorption (flame and flame-less) and indirectly coupled plasma emission? In the field of enzymology (say for cholinesterase determination) the choice is between an end-point of kinetic assay, and with other areas the choices include gas-chromatography and EMIT assay methods.

The choice of method frequently depends on the range of instrumentation in the governmental, hospital, university, industrial or contract laboratory. We should use quality control programmes to identify method bias; and if there is no method bias then any method with adequate precision performance is acceptable. Our experience with lead and cadmium quality control programmes is that it is laboratory size, throughput and experience that matters, not the choice of the method.

K. PEKARI The need for quality control is obvious, but there are no available control systems that would cover in the field for a laboratory performing accepted analyses in biological monitoring.

We in Finland have been happy enough to take part as outsiders in an inter-laboratory survey arranged by CEC in the metal field, but there has not been available any programme for organic compounds of occupational interest in biological samples. We started with eleven Nordic laboratories an interlaboratory comparison programme.

So far we have had two rounds of measuring mandelic acid in urine and also two rounds of urine samples containing penta - and tetrachlorophenol.

We have had a trial run to extend the programme through the Commission of European Communities to those laboratories interested in biological monitoring. The increased number of laboratories brought into the system make statistical analysis more reliable and sufficient.

I have a feeling that more co-operation all over the world would be needed to provide more reliability to toxicology analyses.

J. BARNARD   I would like to make a comment about the education of the worker. We have heard about the education of employee representatives specialists in the workplace. In some of the countries represented here there are considerable numbers of nurses employed in workplace for the occupational health care of workers; some may be working within a team of several occupational health specialists. In Britain and the United States, specific training is available for occupational health nurses. In Britain health education is particularly emphasized in training courses and includes the learning of specific educational techniques. I would like to suggest that in future consideration should be given to using nurses far more in the general health education of individual workers, or groups of workers.

Since they are frequently in day to day contact with many employees when treating them, providing care or counselling, perhaps visiting them in the workplace, they have an excellent opportunity to educate them, this may be an informal approach and include not only advice and information about the hazards to their health of the products or processes with which they work, but also personal hygiene. When relevant they may also be made to explain the purpose of personal biological monitoring.

Providing they have the consent of management or have discussed the subject with their medical colleagues nurses could also give more formal sessions on general aspects of health care and the prevention of ill health. However, the

nurse will be that much more effective, of course, if she has
been able to undertake some form of additional training herself, to equip her with the appropriate knowledge, as well as
teaching communication skills.

W. F. SUNDERMAN Expanding upon Crisp's discussion of
international efforts to establish reference methods for
analytical techniques and to promote collaborative harmonization programmes, I draw attention to the role of the IUPAC
Commission on Toxicology. This Commission is undertaking
programmes to establish reference methods and harmonization
schemes in the sphere of biological monitoring of occupationally related xenobiotics. A reference method for analysis
of serum and urine has already been developed by the Commission's Nickel Subcommittee; similar methods are now being
formulated by the Cadmium and Aluminium Subcommittees. These
efforts involve intensive collaborative work by scientists
from all of the industrialized nations. To date the breadth
and scope of these IUPAC efforts has been limited by the
paucity of funds available to IUPAC. The Commission of the
European Communities should consider supporting the expansion
of the international programme under IUPAC administration.

I emphasize the desirability of reference methods of
establishing accuracy, that can be used to evaluate the
performance of routine methods, and concur that standard
methods for routine use are neither necessary nor desirable.
Each laboratory should be free to select its routine method
for biological monitoring, provided that satisfactory
accuracy, precision, detection limits, and sensitivity are
documented by comparison with the reference method, as well
as by proficiency test programmes.

The organizers of this Seminar emphasized that I was invited
to participate in order that the disciplines of clinical
pathology and clinical biochemistry would be represented.
Therefore, I feel obliged to direct attention to the omission

of clinical pathologists and clinical biochemists from Dr Nelson's extensive tabulation of disciplines. Occupational physicians, industrial hygienists, and analytical chemists need the specialized expertise of clinically trained laboratory scientists in the collection analysis and interpretation of measurements of xenobiotics, and metabolites in body fluids, excreta and tissues.

Finally, I draw attention to the recent applications of saliva analysis of xenobiotics for biological monitoring. Collection of saliva from Stensen's duct by suction capsule is non-invasive, and it does not encounter the employee resistance to urine collection - it is also less susceptible to contamination.

R. HART An agreed upon and uniform training programme for a GLP inspector has little to do with a lack of trust between individuals, institutes or governments but rather it is a method to ensure fair and equitable evaluation and treatment of those inspected. Such an agreed upon training programme enhances the communication and evaluation of data and thus lessens debate as to the validity of such data. Extension of such a programme to the international level could have similar benefits, but may be difficult to achieve.

A. BERLIN The question of international training of GLP inspectors is interesting and important but outside the scope of this discussion. Considering the area of applicability of GMP in the concept of ambient and biological monitoring at the workplace, I feel that the need for international training of GMP inspectors is not compelling.

A. M. THIESS Education of the worker in the FRG is recognized as very important and has been offered for many years through:

1.   Factories

Management took the initiative and developed a special
Safety-Education programme agreed to by the Union representatives (training on the job; advice through psychologists;
special training for the guest workers, foreign workers,
immigrants) - special training in their own languages; analysis after accident or intoxication.

2.   Berufsgenossenschaft (Professional society or
      association)

Insurances of Liability Association have run for many years
special courses with excellent results.

3.   Institutions - Courses

We started this education training in the FRG because the
best prevention of any accident or intoxication is good
information and education of workers.

R. L. ZIELHUIS I would like to add two groups to Dr Nelson's
list.

1.   Worker's family, particularly wife
2.   Journalists; press; TV.

J.D.G. HAMMER Training of workpeople in health and safety is
a legal obligation of every employer in Great Britain. The
quality of training obviously varies. Tripartite Industrial
Training Boards have developed vocational training modules
and the Inspectorate has been concerned to ensure that health
and safety is treated as an integral part of job training.
In the training of statutorily appointed safety representatives trade unions have insisted on controlling the content
of such courses. Clearly however such courses have to be

supplemented by technical training and major companies at least have done this systematically. We have also urged, with some success, the better training of junior and middle managers.

N. NELSON Several suggestions were made for the inclusion of additional persons in the list of potential participants in optimizing good health. Dr Sunderman recommends the inclusion of clinical pathologists or clinical biochemists, and Zielhuis recommends the inclusion of a family member or a representative of the media. These useful suggestions should be added.

Two other suggestions can be linked.

Barnard from the UK pointed out the many ways in which the nurse can be helpful in informing the worker. This is very much the case; the nurse has a close and continuing relationship with the worker. In addition the worker has a high degree of confidence in the nurse. Thus the nurse can play a critical role in instructing the worker in correcting some of the difficulties in the collection of biological samplers as described by Dr Kazantzis.

R. E. YODAIKEN Endorsing Barnard's plea to use nurses more frequently, I would like to turn that around and suggest that where possible nurses use their initiative to participate in occupational health activities. It has frequently been demonstrated that nurses are not only competent, but they frequently exhibit greater competence than physicians because they are able to engender confidence in patients/ workers.

In the United States we have long been concerned with education of both professionals and public. Under the 1977 Clean Air Act a Task Force was set up to examine environmental

causes of cancer, heart and lung disease. One project group
of this Task Force has addressed the education of professionals and the public. Professionals are often outside the
workplace. There are not enough trained professionals in
industry, and workers (and management) often rely on professionals in the surrounding area who are not adequately
trained - in fact many professionals are unaware that occupational disease is an entity. The project group has attempted
to come to grips with this problem - ways and means of educating these professionals and has sent recommendations to
Congress suggesting ways and means this can be achieved.

NIOSH has also tackled this problem and has set up 12 Educational Resource Centers around the country which have the
responsibility for training all disciplines of occupational
health - physicians, nurses, industrial hygienists, engineers, etc. One major fact of their training programmes are
outreach programmes designed to provide professionals who do
not have the benefit of any other educational background in
occupational medicine.

As Nelson indicated we have an aggressive press in the United
States and our problem is not so much to provide the press
with information, as to provide them with accurate information. We are entertaining the idea of setting up a clearing
house which will not only be a focal point for environmental
news but also offer an interpretation service so that the
press will have a point of reference - a professional organization that can interpret or explain.

B. GOLDSTEIN I am concerned about who will be subject to GLP
codification. Although Hart used the terms scientific
research and toxicological research, I am sure that he does
not mean that research into mechanisms of toxicity be subject
to the standardization. Further, I would urge that those who
will be responsible for codification of GLP make this point
concerning non-applicability to basic toxicological research.

Otherwise one may find the legal process discarding perfectly valid scientific information which may be pertinent to understanding and regulating workplace hazards.

A second point concerns the education of workers in the United States about health hazards. I envy what I have heard from our European colleagues. Obviously the easiest way to approach the worker is through the large institutions of unions and industry. However, in the United States well over 50% of the work force is both non-unionized and employed by small companies. The difficulty in educating these workers is a major problem in the United States.

C. FALLING   Danish journalists have themselves called for further training in work environment studies. Training is difficult in small firms. In Denmark the problem is being tackled with the aid of an "information bus" which visits some of these firms.

Motivation is very important. Management must also be motivated. They have an interest in acquiring knowledge in this field if only to avoid falling behind the level acquired by the workers and shop stewards.

A further important objective is the integration of work environment studies into the basic training of nursing staff. This will also make it easier to improve the training of personnel in factory health services.

L. MIKSCHE   Information to workers on possible risks or dangers at the workplace is provided usually twice a year in the workshop and this has some legal background.

Concerning Good Monitoring Practice, the importance of sample collection has to be taken into account. Sampling technique can be crucial to the importance of AM (E. King: Techniques

for the measurement of cadmium in air. In: Occupational
Exposure to cadmium: Seminar, London 20 March 80 Cadmium
Association, London 1980) and BM. In BM the time of sampling
is of great importance for the validity of the results.
Preshift samples will give results different from postshift
samples. Xenobiotics excreted or metabolized within a short
time need different sampling time schedules to slowly excreted substances. These are only some of the arguments that
point out the importance of the use of standardized or at
least comparable sampling techniques and sampling strategies
in AM and BM.

J. V. HOMEWOOD With reference to the education and training
of the occupational team, to avoid the professional isolation
of the health professional, it might be useful when training
profiles are developed, to base the total programme on the
philosophy of a team approach to problem solving.

In pursuance of this philosophy each training module should
offer the opportunity to develop interpersonal skills as an
aid to team building, and where appropriate modules should be
developed which are open to several disciplines.

D. C. LOGAN Education and training of criteria is an
important priority to which we all must be committed. The
difficulty of reaching workers, particularly workers in small
operations where there are no unions is a problem not only
for government agencies but for the private sector as well.
In a recent medical investigation where there were fatalities
and serious illness in workers exposed to pentachlorophenol,
the problem was found to be primarily due to the inappropriate use of a product sold to the small employer, despite
transmission of safety-data information by the primary manufacturer to all users. The large manufacturer was clearly
concerned about the mis-use of their product but felt power-
less to adequately educate all downstream users. Joint

cooperation between OSHA and the primary manufacturers will hopefully lead to creative approaches in dealing with this particular problem.

OSHA is clearly committed to worker education and training and a substantial financial commitment is given to this end. "New Directions" grants and video-tape series "Spectrum", the OSHA consultation programme, worker pamphlets, Health Hazards, Alerts, joint OSHA-NIOSH Current Intelligence Bulletins and a large publications office are a few of the ways OSHA attempts to accomplish this objective.

OSHA also has an occupational physician elective programme where physicians can spend from 1-3 months at OSHA to gain first hand field experience in occupational medicine. We also give lectures and talks to physician groups, and unions on occupational health topics, in a further effort to extend our education and training.

OSHA sponsored a Seminar in September of 1979 for the news media to inform them of important issues in occupational medicine.

R. HART   Three points should be clarified to this morning's discussion.

1.   Relative to Goldstein's comments: in the area of toxicity testing and toxicology research, many aspects of laboratory operations fall under the general concept of GLP principles but are currently excluded because of their association with basic research, methods development, validation and toxicokinetics.

2.   Relative to Gompertz's comments: duality assurance and GLP do not speak to the value of one procedure over another but rather how the procedure is carried out.

3. Cooperative training is suggested only as a means to enhance communication and evaluation of data and events thus lessening debate as to the validity of data and consequence of events.

A. M. THIESS Concerning the statement: "In the USA the mass media is very aggressive"

We should ask ourselves what could be the reasons: these could be
-   accidents in the past
-   sometimes restrictive behaviour in discussing these accidents
-   increased worldwide consciousness of the environment and workplace areas
-   improved analysis techniques (we measure ppm and ppb and only experts know what that means)
-   loss of confidence in experts' statements in past years

We should try to get this confidence back worldwide: one way would be: not only the workers need education and real information but also the reporters, because what they report will be read by thousands of people.

J. T. WILSON With respect to teamwork among occupational health professionals, we have observed a deficiency of this in the US. However, in recent years joint training of physicians, nurses and industrial hygienists all being prepared for occupational health professions, has occurred. Also, field experience is jointly arranged through health hazard evaluations, all of which may improve cooperative practice later.

Reference laboratory methods are highly desirable especially as related to analysis of complex substances, e.g. volcanic ash which contains silicates as well as free silica.

J. P. STEINER It was indicated that a paper presented at an earlier meeting on Cd underlined the importance of air sample collection.

Experience suggests that such factors as sampling time, location, position and type are of different degrees of criticality if one deals with gases, mists and fumes dispersing uniformly or heavy dusts sedimenting rapidly.

A. J. LEBRUN A couple of factors that have not been discussed so far are the enforcement of the safety measures and the liability of the employers and the employees.

Every time I visit a plant I see employees not wearing hearing protective devices provided by the company or respirators hanging around necks rather than on noses; yet the workers were properly informed. Are the unions going to help enforce protection of health?

What is the liability of the company which has done what it was supposed to do to protect its employees health? Is it not time to introduce the concept of shared responsibility and liability?

D. M. RADWANSKI We cannot devise what nurses in other countries should do without asking them what they are prepared to be trained to do.

During one term of their courses, joint teaching of physicians and nurses being prepared for occupational health practice has gone on for the last 10 years.

S. CRISP I wish to refer to three areas that impinge on my paper:

Standardization of methods

I would make the following comments based on Gompertz's statement:

Multiple choice of analytical methods will always be available. This is after all what analytical chemistry is about and probably one of the main reasons for standardization. I do not understand how Gompertz knows he has no bias without reference samples - even different methods producing the same or similar, results does not logically mean no bias. The approach of Gompertz seems to amount to a cooperative study and is an acceptable one. Often precision sufficient for decision is all that is required of an analytical method. But a cooperative study will always be less certain than a collaborative study. Let us remember there are other areas in occupational hygiene besides clinical analysis.

International Inspection

There may be a need for internationally agreed principles but I feel inspection should be done nationally.

Standardization of sample strategy

There is an ad hoc group of ISO TC 146 on the standardization of sampling strategy in the workplace.

D. DALY There is a need when talking of education of workers to do so in simple layman's terms. This would also apply to Middle Management who can do most to implement a good Health and Safety programme.

With regard to Personal Protection it should be suitable and should not cause discomfort.

It is worrying that laboratories do not have harmonized methods. It is like the saying "Doctors differ and patients die".

C. COURTOUX   To what extent should one go into detail and
what emphasis should be placed on form? The most simple
language is not necessarily the most appropriate.

L. DE BOER Occupational Health should only be practised by
fully qualified occupational health doctors if the purpose is
proper prevention which is more than just diagnosis of occupational diseases. It is indeed important to build safety
and health education in to every course not just in separate
special courses.

A. J. LEBRUN In response to my colleague. I chose those two
examples because they are readily verifiable at any time of
the day. Although I am ready to accept that wearing a respirator for a full day may be inconvenient or even somewhat
stressful for some individuals, I hardly see that wearing
proper hearing protection may be so. Be it as it may, there
are other safety precautions that are regularly violated
despite their importance, such as smoking or eating in the
workplace, not washing hands before eating, showering or
changing dirty clothes before going home, etc... I do not
think those safety precautions would be that stressful.
Although properly informed the employee is still not heeding
advice designed for his protection. Clearly some incentive
for acting and some sanction for not acting should be considered. Safety is indeed a two way street.

GENERAL DISCUSSION

C.   COURTOUX   I should like to say the group has emphasized
protection of the worker but this Seminar has lost time
discussing terminology. The first activity is ambient monitoring and every work person knows its importance. Chemists,
and engineers and doctors - a number of different disciplines
contribute to it.   The point of this seminar has been to
bring together issue groups with different opinions particularly those from the U.S. and from Europe. They are able to
see the difference in the importance that's attached to
biological monitoring. In Europe our tendency is to consider
biological monitoring as an important element in the health
of the worker and the health protection of the worker.
Whether carried out once or repeatedly it is important to
look at the practical implications.   The third important
element in the promotion of the health of the worker is the
organization of adequate medical surveillance. The importance of medical surveillance is different in industrialized
countries, so you have ambient monitoring, biological monitoring and health surveillance, three complementary activities which contribute to protect the health of the worker. I
think that the presence of Trade Unions has been a great
benefit.   In Europe if the prevention and protection of the
worker is to be improved, we must start to find a course. The
people who have participated to this Seminar are people who
are really experts in their fields and have defined their
points of view with intelligence. But dogmatic positions go
against not only understanding our different disciplines but
also against finding a solution. I think we are in the first
stages.   What we have done has been enriching but it has to
be followed up by a second phase. Personally I find that the
term "clinical scientist" is not appropriate but we can find
other words, other terms.   We have a confusing problem of
terminology, we have to consider all international labour and
we have several points of view. Many different activities
are complementary in achieving the health protection of the

worker.   Another   point   is   the   difference between various
agencies   according   to   the   country and tradition.   For the
health   of   the   worker   we need the contribution of a lot of
complementary disciplines.

W. J. HUNTER Definitions are not meant to be a requirement
but to state what is done within a certain context and who is
to   do   it.   I think that one has to react to references made
to terms such as "clinical scientists" "screening" and so on.
One   has to remember that these words came out of discussions
between   scientists   on   two sides of the Atlantic so that at
the   worst   a sort of agreement was reached as the best words
to use in a particular context.

But   of   course   it   is   possible   to   change them.   There is
another point that I would like to make.   Irreversible health
effects rarely fit into biological monitoring but relate more
to health surveillance.

From a personal point of view I have tried to act as a reporter   and so reflect the views that have been expressed during
this meeting.   I think one of the things that may be a disappointment   on   a personal basis is that there have been a lot
of   criticisms   made   of   biological monitoring.   The fact is
that   it   has   just been of limited use now but in the future
biological   monitoring   will   probably   be   one   of   the most
important developments to come.   I think these things haven't
come   out very clearly from the discussions and I regret this
because   I   think   the   interaction between these two concepts
has   to   be   strengthened.   As a reporter I recorded what the
meeting   said and then produced my own report on what I would
like to see.

One   problem   that   has   not been resolved concerns the place
within   the definitions of certain tests such as ZPP and ALAD
that previously were called "biological monitoring".

The place of irreversible health effects within the definition of health surveillance needs further discussion since
there is a general conclusion that such effects should not be
included in biological monitoring.

A. BERLIN   The following matrix defining the training profile
requirements could be considered:

Object	Ambient Monitoring					Biological Monitoring				
	Design	Sampling	Analysis	Eval	Action	Design	Sampl	Analy	Eval	Action
Compliance with standards	Indus Hyg	Indus Hyg	Chem/ Ind Hyg	Ind Hyg	Ind Hyg Eng	Med Nurs	Nurs	Chem	Nurs Med	Med/ Ind Hyg
Epidemiology	Epid/ Ind Hyg	Indus Hyg	Chem	Stats Epid		Epid/ Med	Nurs	Chem	Epid/ Med	
Eval Control Technologies	Ind Hyg Eng	Indus Hyg	Ind Hyg	Ind Hyg Econ	Eng					

F. H. MEPPELDER   In the matrix presented by Berlin the training requirements for the various disciplines in connection with ambient and biological monitoring have been systemised, monitoring being the central theme of the present seminar.

In setting up training programmes and in devising procedures for the cooperative activities of the multidisciplinary hygiene teams, it should however not be overlooked that monitoring is only one part of occupational hygiene care and in chronological order not the first. Assurance of good working conditions as regards agents should start at the laboratory where chemical processes are now being developed. We still see that solvents like benzene and carbon tetrachloride for instance are used where safety alternatives exist and that in devising the chemical route, little attention is paid to noxious intermediates.

Another important phase where hygiene disciplines should be involved to assure clean technology is in devising installations where chemical and/or physical processes are performed and where toxic agents can be generated and emitted.

Further the spatial planning of installations in connection with minimising numbers and levels of exposures, requires the involvement of certain hygiene disciplines. Another obvious subject is the development of good procedures and working practices for the operation, inspection, maintenance, etc. of the installations.

I think we should stress the importance of the contribution of the hygiene team in this respect and tune the training profiles to these needs. Protection of the health workers should start with the best technological prevention.

I suggest that the Commission considers the possibility of organising a seminar which focuses on the questions of technological prevention and good operating practices.

I am disappointed because by 1980 in no European country has the work of the occupational physician been more limited than by the definition of biological monitoring. The physician uses methods which help to pin point or identify harmful substances. He also tries to highlight effects which without being defined, are indicators of reaction in the human body.

I find myself close to the definition of biological monitoring as presented by Zielhuis. The physician has an important role because of his knowledge, in the multidisciplinary team even when building or developing industrial plans. Their profiles drawn, plans actually take you back into the past. They break up competences in a very rigid manner. From experience biological monitoring choices which have been implemented are based on all the components of the worker environment. We should give up assessing environmental or ambient monitoring results provided only by specialists instead of multidisciplinary teams in which physicians have acquired a role.

R. L. ZIELHUIS I am not happy with what I understood Dr Hunter to say although there are some good points. The term "screening" has a different meaning and should be deleted.

Second "clinical scientists" may be confusing I should consider associated with hospital work. I suggest "medical scientists" or better "occupational physicians".

Another remark: you say somewhere that where biological monitoring refers to effect parameters it should not be discussed under the heading of biological monitoring. This creates confusion again. Now, a remark which is more directed to CEC as police doctors. I wonder if official policy of CEC biological monitoring would be changed by the meeting the effect parameter. I refer to ambient monitoring and to biological monitoring and the lead directive to point out the consequences of this definition of biological monitoring. I have one remark for Berlin and his very beautiful brief representation. I think that it's an important point to design health care for the man who has been exposed often.

P. B. MEYER Though ambient air monitoring might sometimes correlate poorly with "internal exposure", biological monitoring on the other hand might give no correlation with the exposure which takes place at the workplace. This drawback of biological monitoring should be added to Dr Hunter's summary.

A definition of a hygienist which I propose is: the hygienist is the manager of the environment of the workplace as far as this environment can be described by physical or chemical parameters. To keep this environment within accepted limits is his responsibility. His responsibility is the collective protection of persons who are exposed. Protection of the individual worker by biological monitoring periodic health examinations is the responsibility of the physician.

A. J. LEBRUN Not having the written text in front of me I apologise if I have misunderstood any of the speakers I refer to.

One remark for which we have a text is access to medical and monitoring records. I think that this should be precise and that the employees should have access to their own medical records.

My second remark concerns the dose in biological monitoring and that dose should be related to health effects. I think that this is a very broad statement because there is not necessarily a dose relationship with health effects. I am thinking particularly of pesticides where there is no relationship between dose of exposure and clinical effect or even with physiological effects.

A third remark is about standardization of techniques. I recognise that this is an ideal goal but by my own personal experience it's a very difficult one to reach. The local hospital which serves a small plant is not going to have a standardized technique because it has not the equipment so I would like to suggest that we also consider something perhaps more easily done viz. a standardization of the units in which results are reported. We have been told also that most of the workforce is covered by physicians practising in small communities who have no particular training in Occupational Medicine. We have the same problem as in the United States and maybe this Seminar should recommend that more attention be given in the curriculum at the universities in the train- ing of physicians.

A remark was made about the fact that Government should make a decision on cost benefit. I think that there should be an addition here to correct that by saying that the cost benefit is not measured only in money but in other units too.

As far as the decision of how to deal with information resulting from biological monitoring I have some difficulties there. I do not see how it's possible not to say that such an employee has to be removed from work because he has such a raised level. The manager would understand that this parti- cular employee has a level above a particular figure. We tell the manager so and so has a broken leg or a torn liga- ment. I do not see basically why it would be unethical to say he has so many mc/g of this in his blood.

In summary

- access to medical records should be restricted to access to his/her own medical records by the employee only

- dose is not always related to health effects of even physiological effects

- the ordinary practitioner needs better background in occupational medicine and medical schools should improve their curriculum

- cost/benefit analysis should not be measured in money <u>alone</u> but also in human terms

- it is difficult not to divulge directly or indirectly the result of biological monitoring when requesting that an employee be removed from work since the active levels set in regulations will by themselves give away at least the levels above which the employee is.

B. GOLDSTEIN   I would just emphasize a point that has been made very well by others that the distinction between biological monitoring, health surveillance and health effects is arbitrary. A last point is to express disappointment that the multidisciplinary approach did not include the laboratory scientist. We have said biological monitoring detects agents which produce reversible effects before they become irreversible effects. We cannot do without biological monitoring and it is really the laboratory scientists who detect such reversible effects.

I would feel very unhappy if the reported negative impressions from the USA would have negative "spill over" on disciplines in Europe.

I would therefore recommend a check on the negative statements relating to the situation in the USA, and action upon the positive recommendations.

L. DE BOER   Just a short general remark. The time we have had here with representatives from the States and Europe has been very useful. Of course there are differences because of different experiences, especially negative experiences. I

appreciate that but I would regret it if these spill over on
the images of certain disciplines. These negative experiences are less common in Europe perhaps than in the United
States so my request to the secretary is to look carefully
into the statements made. After all it is not the statements which are important but the recommendations.

N. J. ROBERTS We must face the reality that when we examine
a worker we cannot artificially look only at evidence of
exposure, calling it biological monitoring, and not continue
to look for health effects, whether adverse or not, which it
is proposed that we call health surveillance. We must coin or
invent a new term which couples biological monitoring and the
surveillance of the health of workers to detect the many
effects of exposure to work hazards.

J. R. FROINES I want to take this opportunity to thank the
CEC for the excellent conference. This has been an important
attempt to bring together the views of the United States and
Europe. I am pleased with the unanimity in the conclusions
expressed here today. I did not expect the agreement we find
here when the conference began earlier this week. While
there is significant agreement there remain unsolved issues
which I believe would be appropriately discussed at a following meeting perhaps a year from now. Once again, thank you
for your hospitality and best wishes.

LIST OF PARTICIPANTS

BELGIUM

BEST F.W.   Everslaan 45
                                   3078 EVERBERG

BUNGE G.   Directeur Général CEFIC
                                   Avenue Marie-Louise 250
                                   1000 BRUXELLES

COLLIGNON R.   Directeur du Service Médical
                                   General Motors Continental N.V.
                                   Noorderlaan 75
                                   Postbus 9
                                   2030 ANTWERPEN

DE GREVE J.   Ministère de l'Emploi et du Travail
                                   Rue Belliard 53
                                   1040 BRUXELLES

DE PLAEN P.   Docteur en médecine (MD)
                                   Institut d'Hygiène et
                                   d'Epidemiologie (IHE)
                                   14 rue Juliette Wytsmans
                                   1050 BRUXELLES

DEURINCK L.   Ecological and Technical Department
                                   Federate der Chemische Nijverheid
                                   van Belgie
                                   Maria Louiza Square 49
                                   1040 BRUXELLES

GROSJEAN R.   Administration de l'Hygiène
                                   Ministère de l'Emploi et du Travail
                                   Rue Belliard 53
                                   1040 BRUXELLES

HEUSE A.   Université Libre de Bruxelles
                                   Laboratoire de Médecine de Travail
                                   et d'Hygiène du Milieu
                                   campus Erasme
                                   808 route de Lennik
                                   1070 BRUXELLES

JOURDAN L.   Délégué a l'Environnement
                                   CEFIC
                                   250 avenue Louise (bte 71)
                                   1050 BRUXELLES

LAUWERYS R.   Unité de Toxicologie Médicale et
                                  Industrielle
                                  Université Catholique de Louvain
                                  20 avenue Chappelle-aux-Champs
                                  1200 BRUXELLES

MATTSON J.   Labor attache
                                  U.S. Mission to the EC
                                  Bd. du Regent 40
                                  1000 BRUXELLES

MUNN A.   Director
                                  Medicine & Environmental Health
                                  Monsanto Europe S.A.
                                  Avenue de Tervuren 270-272
                                  1150 BRUXELLES

RONDIA D.   Laboratoire de Toxicologie
                                  Université de Liège
                                  151 Boulevard de la Constitution
                                  4000 LIEGE

SILON P.   Verantwoordelijke Dienst
                                  "Onderbeming"
                                  van het algemeen Christelijk
                                  Vakverbond
                                  Wetstraat 121
                                  1040 BRUXELLES

TASSIGNON J. P.   Solvay et Cie
                                  33 rue du prince Albert
                                  1050 BRUXELLES

VANDEBORNE E.   Médicin à l'Administration de
                                  l'Hygiène et Médecine de Travail
                                  Ministère de l'Emploi et du Travail
                                  Rue Belliard 53
                                  1040 BRUXELLES

DENMARK

ANDERSEN I.   National Institute of Occupational
                                  Hygiene
                                  73 Baunegardsvej
                                  2900 HELLERUP

ELIKOFER J.   Landsorganisationen i Danmark
                                  Rosenørnsalle 14
                                  1970 KØBENHAVN

FALLENTIN B.

Director
National Institute of Occupational
Hygiene
73 Baunegardsvej
2900 HELLERUP

FALLING C.

Arbejdsmiljøfondet
Vesterbrogade 69
1620 KØBENHAVN V

GRANDJEAN P.

National Institute of Occupational
Hygiene
73 Baunegardsvej
2900 HELLERUP

GYNTELBERG F.

Arbedjdsmedicinsk Klinik
Rigshospitalet
KØBENHAVN

JAROSZEWSKI M.

Direktoratet for Arbejdstilsynet
Rosenvaengets Alle 16-18
2100 KØBENHAVN

SCHNEIDER T.

National Institute of Occupational
Hygiene
73 Baunegardsvej
2900 HELLERUP

SVANE O.

Direktoratet for Arbejdstilsynet
Rosenvaengets Allé 16-18
2100 KØBENHAVN

FEDERAL REPUBLIC OF GERMANY

BROCKHAUS

Med. Institut fur Lufthygiene
Universitat Dusseldorf 28-30
Gurlittstrasse 63
4 DUSSELDORF

COENEN W.

Berufsgenossenschaftliches
Institut für Arbeitssicherheit
53 BONN

HENSCHLER D.

Institut für Toxikologie und
Pharmakologie der Universitat
Würzburg
Versbacher Landstrasse
8700 WURZBURG

KLIESCH G.

Bundesministerium für Arbeit und
Sozialordnung
Postfach 140280
5300 BONN 1

LEHMANN M.

Bundesanstalt fur Arbeitsschutz
und Unfallforschung
Postfach 170202
4600 DORTMUND 17

LEHNERT G.

Zentralinstitut für Arbeitsmedizin
Adolph-Schönfelderstr. 5
HAMBURG 76

LEWALTER J.

Arzliche Abteilung Bayer A.G.
5090 LEVERKUSEN-BAYERWERK

MIKSCHE L.

Artzliche Abteilung
Bayerwerk
5090 LEVERKUSEN

PARTIKEL H.

Abteilung Arbeitsschutz
Vorstand IG Metall
Wilheim-Leuschner-Strasse 79-85
6000 FRANKFURT/MAIN

ROBOCK K.

Asbest-Institut für Arbeits-und-
Umweltschutz
Görlitzer Strasse 1
404 NEUSS

SCHAFER K.

Hoechst AG
Abt. Sicherheitsüberwachung
Postfach 800320
6230 FRANKFURT/MAIN 80

SCHALLER K. H.

Universität Erlangen/Nürnberg
Schillerstrasse, 25-29
8520 ERLANGEN

SCHUETZ A.

Staubforschunginstitut
Postfach 150140
5300 BONN 1

SEGEWITZ

Berufsgenossenschaft der chemischen
Industrie
Postfach 10 14 80
6900 HEIDELBERG 1

STEINHOFF D.

Bayer ag
Institut fuer Toxikologie
Friedrich-ebert Str. 217
5600 WUPPERTAL 1

THIESS A. M.

BASF AG
6700 LUDWIGSHAFEN/RHEIN

VALENTIN H.

Institut für Arbeits-und
Sozial-Medizin
Universität Erlangen-Nürnberg
Schillerstrasse 25/29
8520 ERLANGEN

WAGNER R.

Ministerialrat
Bundesministerium fur Arbeit und
Sozialordnung
5300 BONN

FINLAND

PEKARI K.

Institute of Occupational Health
Biochemistry Laboratory/KP/EF
Arinatie 3
SF - 00370 HELSINKI 37

FRANCE

CAILLARD L.

Chef du Département Toxicologie
Rhône Poulenc
B.P. 753
75360 PARIS cedex 08

CAVELIER

I.N.R.S.
Centre de Recherche de Nancy
Avenue de Bourgogne
54500 VANDOEUVRE

DE CEAURRIZ

I.N.R.S.
Centre de Recherche de Nancy
Avenue de Bourgogne
54500 VANDOEUVRE

COURTOUX C.

Ministère du Travail
Inspection Médicale
1 Place de Fontenoy
75007 PARIS

FISCHOFF R.

IBM's Europe
8-10 Cité du Retiro
75008 PARIS

FOURNIER E.

Hôpital F. Widal
200 rue du Faubourg St. Denis
75010 PARIS

JEAMMAUD A.

Les Genêts
Chemin du Plat
69360 TERNAY

LAFOREST J. C.

I.N.R.S.
30 rue Olivier Noyer
75680 PARIS Cedex 14

LARDEUX P.

I.N.R.S.
30 rue Olivier Noyer
75680 PARIS Cedex 14

LEVY J.

191 rue d'Alésia
75014 PARIS

MORIN B.

Inspection Médicale du Travail
17 rue Cdt l'Herminier
38000 GRENOBLE

PRAT C.

MICHELIN (service GV
Place des Carmes)
6300 CLERMONT FD

REBIERE A.

Ministère du Travail et de la
Participation
Direction des Relations du Travail
1 Place de Fontenoy
75007 PARIS

TAIB A.

Ministère de la Santé et de la
Securité Sociale
8 Avenue de Segur
75700 PARIS

GREECE

GEORGOPOULOU H.

Centre Health and Safety
Directorate
Ministry of Labour
Fhrakis 8 Trahones. Ano Kalamaki
ATHENS

PELORIADIS G.

Centre of Occupational Safety
and Health
Ministry of Labour
40 Piraeus str.
ATHENS

SIGONI D.

Ministère de cooordination
Direction Générale des Relations
de la Grèce avec les Communautés
Européennes
Direction de Politique Sociale
Place de la Constitution
ATHENS

IRELAND

CLARKE R. G.

Personnel Director
Brooks Thomas Limited
Bluebell
Naas Road
DUBLIN 12

DALY D.

Irish Transport & General
Workers' Union
10 Palmerston Park
DUBLIN 6

O'CALLAGHAN M.

Department of Labour
Mespil Road
DUBLIN 4

ITALY

ALESSIO L.

University of Milan
Clinica del Lavoro
Via S. Barnaba 8
20122 MILANO

ARMELI G.

MONTEDISON
Via Appiani 12
20121 MILANO

BIOCCA M.

Istituto Superiore di Sanità
Viale Regina Elena 299
ROMA

CECCHETTI G.

Instituto de Medicina del Lavoro
dell Università Cattolica del
Sacro Cuore
Via della Pineta Sacchetti 644
00168 ROME

FOA V.

Clinica del Lavoro
Via S. Barnaba 8
20122 MILANO

GUERRIERI M.

Ministero del Lavoro
Previdenza Sociale
Via Flavia 12
00187 ROMA

MATTIUSSI R.

Responsable di Medicina
e Igiene del Lavoro
MONTEDISON
Via Appiani 12
20121 MILANO

PERUZZO G. F.

Clinica del Lavoro
Via S. Barnaba 8
20122 MILANO

POCCHIARI F.

Istituto Superiore di Sanità
Viale Regina Elena 299
00161 ROME

ROSSI L.

Instituto Superiore de Sanità
Viale Regina Elena 299
00161 ROME

SORDELLI D.

MONTEDISON
Viale Montegrappa 3
20121 MILANO

LUXEMBOURG

DAUBENFELD J.P.   Goodyear
                             Colmar - Berg
                             LUXEMBOURG

SCHUSTER A.   Inspection du Travail et des
                             Mines
                             2 Rue des Girondins
                             LUXEMBOURG

THE NETHERLANDS

DE BOER L.   Lange Kerkdam 84
                             WASSENAAR

DEL CASTILHO P.   Wetenschaps Winkel
                             University of Amsterdam
                             Sarphatiestraat 133
                             AMSTERDAM

MEPPELDER F. H.   Directorat-Generaal van de arbeid
                             Ministerie van Sociale Zaken
                             Postbus 69
                             2270 VOORBURG

MEYER P. B.   Instituut voor milieuhygiene en
                             Gezondheidstechniek
                             Postbus 214
                             2600 AE DELFT

de MIK G.   Medish Biologish Laboratorium TNO
                             Lange Kleiweg 139
                             Postbus 45
                             2200 AA RYSWYK

TWISK J. J.   Ministerie van Sociale Zaken
                             Directorat Generaal van de arbeid
                             Medische afdeling
                             Balen van Andelplein 2
                             VOORBURG

ZIELHUIS Rainier L.   Universiteit van Amsterdam
                             le Constantijn Huygensstraat 20
                             AMSTERDAM

ZWENNIS W. C. M.   Medish Biologish Laboratorium TNO
                             Lange Kleiweg 139
                             Postbus 45
                             2200 AA RYSWYK

SWEDEN

MALKER H.   National Board of Occupational
                                   Safety & Health
                                   171 84 SOLNA

OSTERBERG Carl-Johan   The Swedish Work Environment Fund
                                   Box 1122
                                   111 81 STOCKHOLM

SWITZERLAND

DROZ   Responsable du Secteur d'Hygiène
                                   Industrielle
                                   Institut Universitaire de Médecine
                                   du Travail et d'Hygiène
                                   Route de la Clochatte
                                   1052 LE MONT-SUR-LAUSANNE

UNITED KINGDOM

BARNARD J.   Occupational Health Service
                                   Manor Farm
                                   The Granary
                                   Sherborne St. John
                                   BASINGSTOKE RC24 9HX

BAXTER R.   CISHEC
                                   Occupational Hygiene Committee
                                   LONDON

BURGESS C. D.   Health & Safety Executive
                                   25 Chapel Street
                                   LONDON NW1

CRISP S.   Laboratory of the Government Chemist
                                   Cornwall House
                                   Stamford Street
                                   LONDON SE1 9NQ

DUNSTER H. J.   Deputy Director General &
                                   Director of Nuclear Safety
                                   Health & Safety Executive
                                   25 Chapel Street
                                   LONDON NW1 5DT

GOMPERTZ D.

Occupational Medicine Laboratory
405 Edgware Road
LONDON NW2 6LN

HALL J. G.

Chief Employment Medical Adviser
Department of Manpower Services (NI)
Netherleigh House
Massey Avenue
BELFAST BT4 2JP

HAMMER J. G. D.

Chief Inspector of Factories
Health & Safety Executive
25 Chapel Street
LONDON NW1

HENMAN B. A.

Royal Society of Chemistry
30 Russell Square
LONDON WC1B 5DT

HIGGINS R.I.

Chloride Group Ltd.
Wynne Avenue
Swinton
MANCHESTER M 27248

HOMEWOOD J. V.

ICI Central Medical Group
Harefield House
PO Box 3, Fulshaw Hall
Wilmslow
CHESHIRE SK9 1QB

HUGHES E.G.

Johnson Matthey
100 High Street
South Gate
LONDON N14

JOHNSTON R.

Shell International Petroleum Co.
Shell Centre
LONDON SE1

KAZANTZIS G.

The Centenary Institute of
Occupational Health
London School of Hygiene
LONDON WC1

LAWTHER P. J.

Medical Research Council
Air Pollution Unit
St. Bartholomew's Hospital
Medical College
Charterhouse Square
LONDON EC1 6BQ

RADWANSKI D. M.

Chief Employment Nursing Adviser
Health & Safety Executive
25 Chapel Street
LONDON NW1 5DT

SORRIE G.

Health and Safety Executive
25 Chapel Street
LONDON NW1

STAFFORD J.

DSO-14
ICI Plastics Division
Bessemer Road
Welwyn Garden City
HERTFORDSHIRE AL7 1HD

STEINER

BNF
Denchworth Road
Wantage
OXFORDSHIRE OX12 9BG

SWANN Peter G.

Director of Medical Services
Esso Europe Incorporated
50 Stratton Street
LONDON W1X 6AU

THOMPSON R. H.

Chief Inspector of Factories
Department of Manpower Services (NI)
Netherleigh House
Massey Avenue
BELFAST BT4 2JP

USA

BARAM M. S.

Bracken & Baram
33 Mount Vernon Street
Boston
MASSACHUSETTS 02108

BELL R. H.

US Department of Labor
Occupational Safety & Health
Administration
Room N 3651
200 Constitution Avenue NW
WASHINGTON DC 20210

BETTINGER G. E.

Manager
Technical Services Division
Haskell Laboratory for Toxicology
& Industrial Medicine
DUPONT
WILMINGTON, DELAWARE 19898

CORN M.

Division of Environmental Health
& Engineering
Johns Hopkins School of Hygiene &
Public Health
BALTIMORE, MARYLAND 21205

EPSTEIN S.

Professor of Occupational &
Environmental Medicine
Room 416
19/9 West Taylor Street
University of Illinois Medical
Center
CHICAGO, ILLINOIS 60680

EVANS J.

Coal Conversion Energy
9822 Ridge Road
BETHESDA, MARYLAND 20034

FISHBEIN L.

National Center for Toxicological
Research
JEFFERSON, ARKANSAS 72079

FROINES J. R.

National Institute for
Occupational Safety & Health
Room 805
5600 Fishers Lane
ROCKVILLE, MARYLAND 20857

GOLDSTEIN B.

Department of Environmental &
Community Medicine
College of Medicine & Dentistry
Rutgers Medical School
University Heights
PISCATAWAY, NEW JERSEY 08854

HART R.

National Center for Toxicological
Research
JEFFERSON, ARKANSAS 72079

HOCHSTRASSER John M.

Tenneco Chemicals Incorporated
Park 80
Plaza West - 1
SADDLE BROOK, NEW JERSEY 07662

HRICKO Andrea M.

American Labor Education Center
1808 Belmont Road N.W.
WASHINGTON DC 20009

HUGHES James P.

Kaiser Aluminium & Chemical Company
300 Lakeside Dune
OAKLAND, CALIFORNIA 94643

LANDRIGAN P.

National Institute for Occupational
Safety & Health
4676 Columbia Parkway
CINCINNATI, OHIO 45226

LAVE L.

Brookings Institute
1775 Massachusetts Avenue NW
WASHINGTON DC 20036

LEBRUN Andre J.

2000 Market Street
PHILADELPHIA, Pa. 19103

LOGAN David C.

United States Department of Labor
Occupational Safety & Health
Administration
Room No. 3656
200 Constitution Avenue NW
WASHINGTON DC 20120
(present affiliation Mobil
Corporation)

MATANOSKI G.

Johns Hopkins School of Hygiene
& Public Health
615 North Wolfe Street
BALTIMORE, MARYLAND 21205

NELSON N.

Institute of Environmental
Medicine
New York University
550 First Avenue
NEW YORK, NEW YORK 10016

PERRY M.

Washington University
School of Medicine
660 S. Euclid
Box 8048
ST. LOUIS, MISSOURI 63118

RADFORD Edward P.

School of Public Health
University of Pittsburgh
PITTSBURGH, PENNSYLVANIA 15261

RAHJES Mary E.

Colorado Department of Health
4210 East 11th Avenue
DENVER, COLORADO 80220

RHONE David H.

United States Department of Labor
OSHA
Gateway Building, Suite 2100
3535 Market Street
PHILADELPHIA, PENNSYLVANIA 19144

ROBERTS Norbert J.

Exxon Company
1251 Avenue of the Americas
NEW YORK, NEW YORK 10020

SMITH C.

Dupont Co.
F + F Dept.
Concord Plaza
WILMINGTON, Del.

SUNDERMAN William F.

University of Connecticut
School of Medicine
PO Box G
FARMINGTON, CONN. 06032

WEINER P.

California Departments of
Industrial Relations
525 Goldengate Avenue
Room 614
SAN FRANCISCO, CALIF. 94102

WOLKONSKY P.

Medical & Environmental
Health Service
Standard Oil of Indiana
PO Box 5910'A
200 East Randolph Dune
CHICAGO, ILLINOIS 60680

WILSON J. T. M. D.

Professor & Chairman
Department of Environmental Health
School Public Health &
Community Medicine
University of Washington
SEATTLE (WASHINGTON) 98195

YODAIKEN R. E.

Director of Occupational Medicine
OSHA
200 Constitution Avenue NW
WASHINGTON DC 20120

YODER John D.

Director
Environmental Health
I.T.T.
320 Park Avenue
NEW YORK, NEW YORK 10022

COMMISSION OF THE EUROPEAN COMMUNITIES

BERLIN A.	Health and Safety Directorate LUXEMBOURG
BONINI A.	Health and Safety Directorate LUXEMBOURG
DEGIMBE J.	Director General Employment and Social Affairs BRUSSELS
HUNTER W.	Health and Safety Directorate LUXEMBOURG
LANGEVIN M.	Health and Safety Directorate LUXEMBOURG
LEMOINE P.	Health and Safety Directorate LUXEMBOURG
RECHT P.	Health and Safety Directorate LUXEMBOURG
ROI R.	Joint Research Centre ISPRA
VAN BOCKSTAEL G.	Health and Safety Directorate LUXEMBOURG

INDEX OF CONTRIBUTORS TO DISCUSSION SESSIONS

Typed on word processor for

Directorate General 5
Employment, Social Affairs & Education

of

The Commission of the European Communities

by

Freelance Services
(Joan Wilkins Associates Limited)
37 Maida Vale
London W9 1TP
01-286 0115